Disguising Disease in Italian Political and Visual Culture

Although considered an isolated event, the Italian government's initial resistant response to COVID-19 has deep historical roots. This is the first interdisciplinary book to critically examine the ongoing phenomenon of disguising contagious disease in Italy from Unification to the present.

The book explores how governments, public opinion, social entities and cultural production have avoided or sublimated contagion during cholera, typhoid, syphilis, malaria, HIV and COVID-19 to impose narratives of the nation's healthy body in Italy and its colonies. Examples range from a tuberculosis sanatorium in Capri that masked as a luxury hotel and hideaway for queer couples to an obscure but talented professor who found a new cure for syphilis; from denial of disease in governmental actions to sublimated representations in Italian art, literature and films such as Luchino Visconti's cinematic adaptation of Thomas Mann's *Death in Venice* to a sociological study of the need to include fragile figures based on the lessons of COVID-19.

Intended for scholars, students and general readers interested in the history of medicine, political and cultural history, and Italian studies, this volume shows how contagious diseases clash with the official narrative of emerging modernized urban settings and challenge the desire for political and economic stability.

Sharon Hecker is an art historian and curator specializing in Modern and Contemporary Italian art. She is the author of *A Moment's Monument: Medardo Rosso and the International Origins of Modern Sculpture* and co-editor of *Curating Fascism: Exhibitions and Memory from the Fall of Mussolini to Today*.

Arianna Arisi Rota is Professor of Contemporary History at the University of Pavia. She specializes in the history of politics and diplomacy in the nineteenth century, with special attention to generations, and memory-building. Her publications include *I piccoli cospiratori*, *Risorgimento*, *Il cappello dell'imperatore* and *Profughi*.

Routledge Studies in the Modern History of Italy

Edited by Carlotta Ferrara degli Uberti (*University College London*), Marco Mondini (*University of Padua and Italian German Historical Institute-FBK Trent*), Silvana Patriarca (*Fordham University*) and Guri Schwarz (*University of Genoa*)

The history of modern Italy from the late 18th to the 21st centuries offers a wealth of dramatic changes amidst important continuities. From occupying a semi-peripheral location in the European Mediterranean to becoming one of the major economies of the continent, the Peninsula has experienced major transformations while also facing continuing structural challenges. Social and regional conflicts, revolts and revolutions, regime changes, world wars and military defeats have defined its turbulent political history, while changing identities and social movements have intersected with the weight of family and other structures in new international environments.

The series focuses on the publication of original research monographs, from both established academics and junior researchers. It is intended as an instrument to promote fresh perspectives and as bridge, connecting scholarly traditions within and outside Italy. Occasionally, it may also publish edited volumes. The sole criteria for selection will be intellectual rigour and the innovative character of the books.

It will cover a broad range of themes and methods – ranging from political to cultural to socio-economic history – with the aim of becoming a reference point for groundbreaking scholarship covering Italian history from the Napoleonic era to the present.

Racism and Antisemitism in Fascist Italy
The Politics, Ideology, and Imagery of *La Difesa della razza*
Francesco Cassata, translated by Stuart Oglethorpe

Italian Fascism in Rhodes and the Dodecanese Islands, 1922–44
Edited by Valerie McGuire and Aron Rodrigue

Disguising Disease in Italian Political and Visual Culture
From Post-Unification to COVID-19
Edited by Sharon Hecker and Arianna Arisi Rota

For more information about this series, please visit: www.routledge.com/Routledge-Studies-in-the-Modern-History-of-Italy/book-series/ITALIANHISTORY

Disguising Disease in Italian Political and Visual Culture

From Post-Unification to COVID-19

**Edited by Sharon Hecker
and Arianna Arisi Rota**

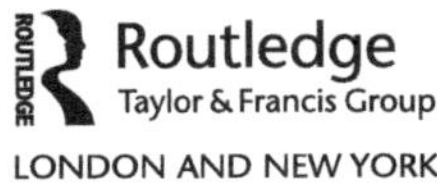

LONDON AND NEW YORK

First published 2025
by Routledge
4 Park Square, Milton Park, Abingdon, Oxon OX14 4RN

and by Routledge
605 Third Avenue, New York, NY 10158

Routledge is an imprint of the Taylor & Francis Group, an informa business

British Library Cataloguing-in-Publication Data
A catalogue record for this book is available from the British Library

Library of Congress Cataloging-in-Publication Data
Names: Hecker, Sharon, editor. | Arisi Rota, Arianna, 1964– editor.
Title: Disguising disease in Italian political and visual culture :
    from post-unification to COVID-19 / edited by Sharon Hecker and
    Arianna Arisi Rota.
Description: Abingdon, Oxon ; New York, NY : Routledge, [2025] |
    Series: Routledge studies in the modern history of Italy | Includes
    bibliographical references and index.
Identifiers: LCCN 2024015430 (print) | LCCN 2024015431 (ebook) |
    ISBN 9781032466798 (hardback) | ISBN 9781032466804 (paperback) |
    ISBN 9781003382805 (ebook) | ISBN 9781040121856 (adobe pdf) |
    ISBN 9781040121863 (epub)
Subjects: LCSH: Communicable diseases–Italy–History. |
    Communication in public health–Italy–History. | Communicable
    diseases in literature. | Communicable diseases in art.
Classification: LCC RA643.7.I8 D57 2025 (print) | LCC RA643.7.I8
    (ebook) | DDC 362.196900945–dc23/eng/20240521
LC record available at https://lccn.loc.gov/2024015430
LC ebook record available at https://lccn.loc.gov/2024015431

ISBN: 978-1-032-46679-8 (hbk)
ISBN: 978-1-032-46680-4 (pbk)
ISBN: 978-1-003-38280-5 (ebk)

DOI: 10.4324/9781003382805

Typeset in Sabon LT Pro
by Apex CoVantage, LLC

To all those who suffered during the COVID-19 pandemic
Sharon Hecker

To the memory of my beloved parents
Arianna Arisi Rota

Contents

Figures

Tables

Contributors

Arianna Arisi Rota, PhD, is Professor of Contemporary History in the Department of Political and Social Sciences at the University of Pavia. She specializes in the history of political mobilization and diplomacy in the nineteenth century, with special attention to generations, and memory-building. Her publications include *I piccoli cospiratori. Politica ed emozioni nei primi mazziniani* (2010); *1869: il Risorgimento alla deriva* (2015); *Risorgimento. Un viaggio politico e sentimentale* (2019, Spanish edition 2021); *Il cappello dell'imperatore. Storia, memoria e mito di Napoleone Bonaparte attraverso due secoli di culto dei suoi oggetti* (2021); and *Profughi* (2023).

Gabriele Bassi holds a PhD in contemporary history. He has focused on colonial history, with a particular emphasis on the significance of cultural studies as a tool for understanding society and overseas policies. His areas of expertise include the history of Italian public security forces in the liberal and fascist eras, as well as the phenomenon of military internment during World War II. He has published *Sudditi di Libia* (2018); *Il diritto come strumento di politica coloniale nella Libia italiana (1911–1943)* (2018); and *Una straziante incertezza: internati militari italiani fra guerra, morte e riconoscimenti da parte della Repubblica* (2022).

Sharon Hecker (PhD UC Berkeley) is an independent art historian and curator specializing in modern and contemporary Italian art. Her publications include *Curating Fascism: Exhibitions and Memory from the Fall of Mussolini to Today* (with Raffaele Bedarida, 2022); *Female Cultural Production in Modern Italy: Literature, Art and Intellectual History* (with Catherine Ramsey-Portolano 2023); *A Moment's Monument: Medardo Rosso and the International Origins of Modern Sculpture* (2017, CAA Milliard Meiss Prize, translated into Italian); *Posthumous Art, The Market and Art Law* (with Peter J. Karol, 2022); *Postwar Italian Art History Today. Untying "the Knot"* (with Marin Sullivan, 2018). Her research awards include Fulbright, Mellon, Getty and Gladys Krieble Delmas Foundations.

Brendan Hennessey is Associate Professor of Italian in the Department of Romance Languages and Literatures at Binghamton University. His specializations include Italian cinema and photography, the interrelationships between film and the other arts, and the technology of Italian moviemaking. Hennessey is the author of *Luchino Visconti and the Alchemy of Adaptation* (SUNY Press, 2021) and has published articles in journals such as *The Italianist, Italian Culture, Modern Language Notes* and *Italian American Review.* He is co-editor of book reviews at the *Journal for Italian Cinema & Media Studies.*

Ewa Kawamura is Professor in the Department of Tourism Design at the Atomi University of Tokyo, Japan. She specializes in the history of architecture, tourism and landscape paintings in the nineteenth and twentieth centuries, with special attention to hotel buildings and iconographical art. Her publications in Italian include *Alberghi storici dell'isola di Capri: una storia dell'ospitalità tra Ottocento e Novecento* (2005), *Il Quisisana. Biografia del Grand Hotel di Capri* (2011, English edition 2011) and *Storia degli alberghi napoletani dal Grand Tour alla Belle Époque nell'ospitalità della Napoli "gentile"* (2017).

Louise Marshall is Honorary Senior Lecturer in the Department of Art History at the University of Sydney, where she taught medieval and Renaissance art for many years. Her primary field of research, on which she has published extensively, is the intersection of art and bubonic plague in Renaissance Italy. Her recent publications include studies on epidemics and religion, St. Roch and the angel and the role of emotions in plague images. Her research has been supported by the Gladys Krieble Delmas Foundation, the Renaissance Society of America and the ARC Centre for the History of Emotions.

Federica Massia holds a PhD in modern philology from the University of Pavia (2020). As a research fellow, she pursued her academic interests in Italian literature between the nineteenth and twentieth centuries and in literary translation. Noteworthy among her scientific publications is the monograph *Il* Fogliame *americano. Whitman in Italia e la nascita del verso libero* (2021), which was awarded the 2023 Marino Moretti Finalist Prize for philology, history and criticism in the field of Italian literature.

Paolo Mazzarello is Professor of History of Medicine in the Department of Brain and Behavioral Sciences and President of the Museum System of the University of Pavia. He wrote the biography of Camillo Golgi (*Il Nobel dimenticato,* 2006; 2019), translated into English by Oxford University Press (2010). His other publications include *Il genio e l'alienista. La strana visita di Lombroso a Tolstoj* (2005), *E si salvò anche la madre* (2015), *L'intrigo Spallanzani* (2021) and *Storia avventurosa della* *medicina* (2023). He also edited (with Marco Beretta and Maria Conforti) the book *Savants Relics. Brains and Remains of Scientists* (2016).

Catherine Ramsey-Portolano (PhD, U of Chicago) is Director and Associate Professor of Italian Studies at The American University of Rome. Her research interests are gender studies, nineteenth- and twentieth-century Italian women writers and Italian film. Her publications include *Female Cultural Production in Modern Italy: Literature, Art and Intellectual History* (edited with Sharon Hecker, 2023); *Nineteenth-Century Italian Women Writers and the Woman Question* (2020); *Performing Bodies: Female Illness in Italian Literature and Cinema* (2018); *The Future of Italian Teaching: Media, New Technologies and Multi-Disciplinary Perspectives* (2015); and *Rethinking Neera* (supplement to *The Italianist*, edited with Katharine Mitchell, 2010).

Marco Rovinello is Assistant Professor of Contemporary History at the University of Calabria. His research has been devoted to migrations, national identity, conscription and the military in nineteenth-century Italy. His published works include *Cittadini senza Nazione. Migranti francesi a Napoli (1793–1860)* (2009), *Fra servitù e servizio. Storia della leva in Italia dall'Unità alla Grande Guerra* (2020 – *Acqui Storia* award 2021), and *Drafting Italy. Conscription and the Military from 1814 to 1914* (2023). Currently, he is working on the history of HIV/AIDS in Italy as Deputy Principal Investigator of the National Research Project (PRIN2022) *Historicizing AIDS. Policies, rights, discourses and memories in the Italian case.*

Marco Terraneo, PhD, is Professor of Sociology in the Department of Sociology and Social Research at the University of Milano-Bicocca, where he teaches courses in the Sociology of Health. He is Director of the Professional Master's Program in Deviance, Justice System and Social Services. He is involved in numerous national and international research projects. His main research interests include social and health inequalities, healthcare systems, material deprivation and dimensions of social stratification. Some of his recent publications include *La salute negata: Le sfide dell'equità in prospettiva sociologica* (2018) and *Studiare la salute: La prospettiva della sociologia* (2023).

Acknowledgments

The authors express appreciation to the Schoff Fund at the University Seminars at Columbia University for their help in publication. Material in this work was first presented to the University Seminar: Studies in Modern Italy, and the ideas in this volume have benefited from discussions at the Seminar. We also would like to thank Rebecca Bauman, former Chair, for inviting us to present the joint paper that launched the idea for this volume, and Molly Tambor, current Chair, for her continued support. Nick Geller did a meticulous copy-editing job, and Jane Friedman carefully indexed the volume.

We are grateful to the publishing team at Routledge Taylor & Francis, especially Robert Langham, Editor, for shepherding this volume to publication.

Our deep gratitude goes to all the contributing authors who have devoted countless hours to their individual contributions. Responding to our endless queries was a true labor of love.

A particular thanks goes to Vivien Greene, Kara Kirk and Michele Rostan, as well as Silvana Patriarca for their suggestions as well as for connecting us to authors and editors who contributed to the volume and for suggesting Routledge as a possible publisher. Sharon Hecker would like to thank Claudio and Barbara Calabi, Giovanna Ginex, Maria Flora Giubilei, Anna Mazzanti, Ughetta Orlando, Judith Hecker, Melissa Larner and Elisabetta Staudacher. Arianna Arisi Rota wishes to thank Geoffrey R. Berridge for the exchange of views on the rise of sanitary diplomacy and all those who gave inspiration to the volume.

We express thanks to all the rightsholders and institutions who graciously allowed us to reproduce the images in this volume.

Finally, we thank our families for their love and support.

1 Denying Disease

An Introduction

Sharon Hecker and Arianna Arisi Rota

Authors' note: We have chosen to present this opening chapter together while maintaining our separate voices by adopting a dialogic approach. This method underlies not only our opening chapter but also the way in which we have chosen to work on editing the volume. It has the advantage of allowing us to challenge, expand and nuance our own and each other's views from different disciplines. We have followed the same dialogic format in our discussions with authors whose chapters are presented in this book.

Sharon Hecker (SH): In January 2020, the COVID-19 pandemic began spreading aggressively around the globe with lightning speed, forcing the world into intermittent periods of lockdown. Over the following three years, the pandemic wrought havoc on every aspect of life, from healthcare systems to social, economic, political, educational and cultural institutions. The strength of the virus and a lack of understanding of how to cure it caused nearly seven million reported deaths, a truly staggering number.

Three years later, vaccinations became readily available. People developed greater immunity to COVID-19, either due to having been infected or thanks to inoculations. By May of 2023, the pandemic was declared to be over. The world desperately wished to return to normal. Facial masks were abandoned; people went back to their daily lives, work and free circulation. Social distancing was abandoned as a form of human interaction, and we returned to meeting in person, shaking hands, hugging and kissing.

So hungry were people to return to their normal pre-pandemic lives that the disease's dramatic daily unfolding of the past three years seemed to fade. Newspaper headlines, which had been updated online by the minute on the pandemic's surge, were now rapidly superseded by more immediate world concerns, such as wars in Ukraine and the Middle East. The pandemic seemed essentially over and done. But this was not necessarily a positive step. In the

DOI: 10.4324/9781003382805-1

case of the United States, on May 11, 2023, the *New York Times*' "Opinion" section ran an article by the editorial board and staff writer Jeneen Interlandi, who writes about issues of public health, titled "America Is Forgetting the Lessons of the Covid Health Emergency." Interlandi became concerned and critical about this cultural amnesia, remarking, "It's a good time for the country to absorb the many lessons of the crisis. Instead, we seem to be actively forgetting them."[1]

The rapidity of an epidemic disease's appearance and its equally swift attempt at historical forgetting, which is largely aspirational – for can we ever truly forget what the pandemic was like? – turn out not to be unique to the COVID-19 evolution, for willful disregard is a recurring feature of human reactions to pandemics. From the beginning of a disease's emergence and after the wave has passed, many different forms of downplaying, disguise and outright denial recur. These features can have dire consequences for how we come to understand past contagious diseases and react to future ones.

Academic scholarship is able to take a wider and longer viewpoint. It can allow for an ongoing and reflective space to process, study and critically question the history of diseases. The volume that follows is the first interdisciplinary study to analyze the ongoing phenomenon of disguising contagious disease in modern Italy through underinvestigated cases in sociology, political and cultural history, history of medicine, art history, literature and film studies. The book examines how governments, public opinion, social entities and cultural production have avoided or sublimated contagion during cholera, typhoid, syphilis, malaria, HIV and COVID-19 to impose narratives of the nation's healthy body in Italy and its colonies.

Arianna Arisi Rota (AAR): The specific focus of this volume is contagious disease in Italy from the country's unification in the nineteenth century to the present. In the broadest sense, this book is intended as a historical record, a way not to forget what we have just lived through and at the same time to better understand some of the less-discussed aspects of pandemics in Italy over a longer historical range. While the volume has its origins in the life cycle of COVID-19, it seeks to tease out commonalities in ways in which humans have negated or minimized the numerous pandemics that have afflicted Italy over the past two centuries.

The idea to write this book developed during the first lockdown of 2020, after the journal *Modern Italy* asked me to contribute to the August 2020 issue by recounting my experience of the COVID-19 emergency in Italy. My dual sensibility as a citizen and historian was challenged. My personal account of daily life in Milan, the so-called *Milano da bere* ("Swinging Milan") according to a popular advertisement from the early 1980s, with its inhabitants' new fears and concerns, became interlaced with an awareness of the fact that I was living a historical experience. I realized that the many private and collective memories of the Before and After needed to be recorded for future generations. From an academic point of view, I felt that the Italian government's initial resistant response to the COVID-19 crisis has a history in post-unification Italy that is worth examining: the denial of social risk during cholera, typhoid, syphilis and malaria outbreaks. These occurred repeatedly because the notion of disease clashed with the official narrative of an emerging modernized urban setting, challenging a myth of political stability and vigor.

The so-called Spanish Flu epidemic of 1918–20 has urged scholars to engage with broader historical tools and disciplinary approaches: oral history, history of mentalities and of political practices. This subject has long been monopolized by the history of medicine and has been well researched by this field, but not from other scholarly approaches and perspectives. When I shared my published reflections with the art historian and my long-time friend Sharon Hecker, also based in Milan, she commented that such a participatory observation could produce further brainstorming if we joined together our experiences during the emergency in a form of cultural mediation. Borrowing a term from sociologists and anthropologists, such participatory observation involves prolonged participation of the researcher in the life of the social group under observation. We were both at once living the experience and reflecting on it at the same time. Our ongoing conversations during lockdown led us to compare and interlace our respective fields of expertise – in political and cultural history and art history – to investigate questions of absence and denial, minimization and forgetting of diseases in post-unification Italy, from both the perspective of governmental crisis management and the representation of disease in the arts.

SH: While still under lockdown, Arianna and I shared our initial findings in an online seminar in September of 2020 at the Seminars of Columbia University's Studies in Modern Italy. We examined links between the political realm and the visual arts in the case of Italy. In her part of our seminar, Arianna found numerous historical examples in Italy related to diseases that had been denied and disguised in the nineteenth century. This opening led us to wish to consider more deeply other diseases of the past century and how they, too, were denied and disguised with dire consequences.

In my part of the seminar, I noted a relative lack of an artistic language in modern and contemporary Italian visual arts. I felt that the isolated case studies of artworks that I was able to unearth did not lay the groundwork for a robust modern artistic language for representing contagious diseases in

Italian art in ways that would develop in other countries in the twentieth and twenty-first centuries. By contrast, I immediately thought of Swiss painter Arnold Böcklin's dramatic *Plague* (1898), Austrian painter Egon Schiele's *Gustav Klimt on His Death Bed*, *The Family* and *Portrait of the Dying Edith Schiele*, a tragic representation of his ill pregnant wife, all of 1918. Schiele himself died a few days later of the same influenza epidemic. Another example is Norwegian painter Edvard Munch's *Self-Portrait with the Spanish Flu* and *Self-Portrait after the Spanish Flu* (both 1919) when he recovered. These might be exceptional cases, but they have gained a place in the canon of representing contagious disease in art. They further resonate with the methodological stance of participatory observation that seems to be a key component of such an experience.

Thinking further about art on other epidemics in other countries, I wondered why Italy did not participate in this group of representations or in representations of the AIDS epidemic of the 1980s, which produced an outpouring of international artistic response, again participatory: Keith Haring's protest posters *Ignorance=Fear* (1989) before he died of AIDS; the work of General Idea in the 1980s; Helen Chadwick's government-commissioned *Viral Landscapes* (1989); Felix Gonzàles-Torres's *Untitled (Portrait of Ross in LA)* (1991), a candy pile offered to viewers to touch, take away and eat, so that the weight of the candy diminishes, as did his lover dying of AIDS (the artist died of AIDS, as well); Zoe Leonard's *Strange Fruits* (1992–97), empty fruit skins sutured together honoring the tragic loss of her friends from AIDS, metaphors of life's fragility as decomposition unfolds before our eyes. These and other powerful images showed me that art had a fundamental participatory role to play in providing coping mechanisms for processing and coming to terms with disease's overwhelming power. I pondered whether this absence in Italy suggested a recurring reluctance to show the fragile, sick body in art, and how this could be related, for example, to national needs to appear strong during periods of exaltation of the healthy body – for example, in the fascist *Ventennio* and the postwar recovery period. Our audience of scholars who participated in the Columbia webinar suggested that Italian literature and film had something to offer to the discussion here.

AAR: During our seminar, we played with flashbacks and flashforwards, examining cases from late nineteenth- and early twentieth-century Italian history, as well as from recent narratives of the current pandemic that were shaped in the Italian environment. We emphasized the perspective from the north – the most severely hit area of the country, the one we both witnessed. We also considered the physical anthropomorphized representations of the state/nation. After the seminar, we began to enlarge our field of inquiry to consider Southern Italian experiences of past pandemics and how contagious disease was represented in the colonies.

SH: One of our flashforwards during the seminar was to the COVID-19 outbreak. On February 27, 2020, in the early days of the epidemic, the video/hashtag #milanononsiferma (#milandoesnotstop) appeared online. The video/hashtag immediately went viral, its sponsors hoping to combat the fear of potential lockdown. We can see here the return of the nineteenth-century Italian disguising of disease but in a new form. This time, it was not the government that issued the image but rather a private group of restaurateurs concerned about losing clientele. The video's makers were not artists but rather a hip Italian advertising company called Brainpull.[2] The imagery was a rapid succession of photos and slogans suggesting a fast-paced metropolis: no pandemic would stop Milan. The music was not national but rather global, a clip from an Israeli singer who was inspired by blues musicians of Mississippi in the United States.[3]

AAR: Milan's mayor, Beppe Sala, quickly reposted the video/hashtag. In doing so, he contributed to a narrative that I would call more arrogant than consoling. A month later, Sala admitted the mistake and apologized, saying that nobody at the end of February had understood the seriousness of the situation.[4] As a historian, I think that humility is the most appropriate form of communication in the face of a new invisible enemy. Therefore, in addition to not denying or mystifying the existence of danger and emergency – medical or otherwise – those who govern have the responsibility to inform and call for caution, without letting themselves be overwhelmed by easy optimism or be conditioned by pressures of individual lobbyists and commercial stakeholders.

SH: What happened next in Italy was unexpected. Press criticism of the Berlusconi-style video images of denial admitted that Italy is sick, and Milan should stop.[5] A new, more realistic hashtag, #iorestoacasa (#istayathome), emerged. On March 10, during lockdown, a second image hit Facebook: a drawing of a masked female doctor with angel's wings cradling a wounded and sick Italian peninsula wrapped in the Italian flag. The drawing's author, Veneto artist Franco Rivolli, depicted the country as fragile, ill and small. He explained the image's genesis: "In these days of emergency . . . I've been thinking a lot about someone I know who works in pulmonology. And everyone who, like her, devotes their energy to taking care of the weakest. This drawing is meant as a heartfelt thanks to them."[6] Newspapers as far as Sardinia commented:

> For the first time, after many, many years, thanks to Rivolli's illustration, the image of a country united and proud of those three colors of its flag re-emerges, not for the victory at a World Cup, but for the silent sacrifice of doctors, nurses and the whole civil society. Even those at home. All "brothers of Italy," like our national anthem, returns, today more than ever, to teach us.[7]

AAR: Today, just as at the origins of a united Italy, the courage to visually represent the country as sick is rare, often an expression of opposition groups far from the prevailing government narrative.[8] In contrast to historian Suzanne Stewart-Steinberg's characterization of Italy as an immature, eternal adolescent, the courage to show reality can be seen as a maturation, a taking of responsibility that, despite initial errors, has made the subsequent Italian management of the COVID-19 emergency a model for other countries, not least the US.[9]

SH: This has been a lockdown project through and through. Given social distancing, our discussion developed via ideas exchanged on WhatsApp, email, Skype and Zoom. In keeping with the way this work originated, our approach in this volume is dialogic. We intend the volume to shed light on our lived experience of the current pandemic, as well as to make connections between past and present, noting similarities and differences in the ways in which disguising disease occurred both then and now. We wish to do something more through this volume, for as we can see in the essays by our authors, the lessons from the past suggest that the temptation to conceal vulnerability ultimately does not pay.

AAR: In contrast to the general tendency to deny and disguise, during the COVID-19 crisis we witnessed the opposite approach in academic circles. Scholarship on the theme expanded significantly during the period of the pandemic. Being forced to stay home allowed colleagues more time to brainstorm, discuss and compare experiences and to study past models of how epidemics had been handled. Between 2021 and 2022, during the height of COVID-19, a plethora of conferences, seminars, calls for papers and special issues of academic journals arose, offering evidence of how the COVID-19 pandemic had urged historians to look back and revisit historical experiences of contagion with new eyes and sensibilities.

In fact, for the first time, the entire world was equally affected by the same invisible threat at the same historical moment. The sense of history itself was at stake, in the sense that the never previously experienced planetary emergency needed visions and forecasting based on lessons from the past, while the feeling of being part of and living through a turning point was shared by the intellectual community. There were, however, some exceptions. On April 7, 2020, still in the early phases, Richard Haass, president of the Council of Foreign Relations, went against the mainstream when he titled his article published in *Foreign Affairs* "The Pandemic Will Accelerate History Rather Than Reshape It: Not Every Crisis Is a Turning Point."[10] Historians felt obligated to participate, as if in a call to arms. This was because, besides the larger issue of life and death, such a global challenge was deeply affecting the memory-building processes of different generations.

The revival of interest in contagious disease is evident in many realms. For one, publishers hastened to reprint classic volumes to feed an eager and disoriented general audience. This was the case, for example, with the multiple reprints of historian Alfred W. Crosby's *America's Forgotten Pandemic*, first published in 1989, reprinted in 2003 during the SARS virus explosion and again rediscovered during COVID-19.[11] Additionally, around the globe, scholars of different generations and disciplines engaged in online brainstorming sessions about contagion and its communication and representation. In some cases, the autobiographical experience of the COVID-19 lockdown became mixed with professional knowledge and gave life to timely journal articles, such as the one I published in the August 2020 issue of *Modern Italy*.[12] Books and short essays appeared, like the one written in late 2020 by French historian Xavier Tabet, who effectively wrote about denial, social control, politics and biopolitics according to the lesson of philosopher and sociologist Michel Foucault.[13] Among historians, collective efforts contributed to revisiting the history of single epidemics. This was the case, for example, of the volume edited in 2020 by historian Guy Beiner, pointedly titled *Pandemic Re-Awakenings: The Forgotten and the Un-Forgotten "Spanish" Flu of 1918*, which was based on testimonial stories of the post–World War I so-called Spanish flu, paving the way to a renewed approach to the phenomenon of social forgetting and to memory dynamics. The same phenomenon of social forgetting and memory building is enmeshed in the fabric of our current edited volume.[14]

Historians of the early modern age found it easy to turn back to the territory of the plague experience as a seminal laboratory: to give one of the many examples, the recent issue of the Italian academic journal *Studi storici* is devoted to public health policies, practices, agents and rules in the Mediterranean area from the sixteenth to the nineteenth centuries.[15] The British historian Fiona Johnstone's 2023 volume, *AIDS and Representation*, offers an example of the shift in the scientific interest in the past produced by the recent emergency (in this case, the 1980s and 1990s AIDS crises in the United States). Her work urges us to focus on narratives, perceptions and self-perceptions of the disease as portrayed by artists, following the fruitful path opened up by the pioneering, now overquoted essay by feminist US author, philosopher and historian Susan Sontag, "Illness as Metaphor," first published in 1978.[16]

The search for an unconventional perspective on epidemics that includes the dimension of the visual arts produced outcomes before the COVID-19 era. An example is an edited volume published in late 2019 titled *A Visual History of HIV/AIDS: Exploring The Face of AIDS Film Archive*, which documented how a multidisciplinary approach can help to record and preserve experiences of an initially deadly, socially stigmatized disease, which has now become a living condition for many. Reinforcing such an expanded, interdisciplinary approach to the cultural history of epidemics is part of the aim of our volume, as well, in order to cast light on uninvestigated or under-investigated perspectives that rely on different fields of scholarly expertise and genealogies.

With specific reference to Italy, since Italy was one of the European countries affected most severely by the first wave of the COVID-19 pandemic, the Italian scholarly community reacted with a wide range of initiatives where senior historians of medicine were often joined by younger historians who had recently become committed to researching how politics and society had dealt with the invisible enemies raging across the peninsula from the modern to the contemporary age. Shocked by the initial COVID-19 experience, where the historically less fortunate southern part of the country was safe and free, while the prosperous industrial north was struggling against the virus, junior and senior researchers launched a wide range of initiatives, such as online workshops made possible by newly improved Zoom connections online. Academic journals could easily promote and host forums and individual research, urged on by the current emergency, as was the case of the beautiful review article by Emmanuel Betta, "Pandemia come metafora?" (Pandemic as metaphor?) published in the historical journal *Contemporanea* in 2020.[17] This was also the case abroad, where Italy-focused academic journals began to invest in the issue of contagion, approached from a broad perspective of cultural history. One such initiative was launched by the University of California at Berkeley's *California Italian Studies*, which issued a call for papers for a special issue devoted to "Italy and the Epistemes of Contagion: Touch, Contact, Distance" in 2021, published in 2022.[18] A similar experience was produced by the Italian academic historians' journal *Genesis*, which focuses on gender studies, with its special issue simply titled *Contagi* published in 2022.[19] In late 2022, historian of medicine Gilberto Corbellini's monograph *Storia della malaria in Italia* (History of malaria in Italy) appeared, the first outline of how science, ecology and society were entangled in the battle against malaria. This subject had already been examined by historian of medicine Frank Snowden's pioneering monograph *The Conquest of Malaria: Italy, 1900–1962*, published in 2006 and translated into Italian two years later.[20] The historian of medicine Eugenia Tognotti, who had been investigating the so-called Spanish flu, cholera, syphilis, phthisis and malaria in the Italian context for many years, became a subject of renewed interest in the topic of contagion, as documented by the inspiring interview published on the website of the journal *Ricerche di storia politica*.[21]

After nearly four years since the tragic events that began in February 2020, contagious diseases are still popular in the Italian academic setting and collective projects have been funded to favor scholarly cooperation. One example is the PRIN 2022 (Research Project of National Interest) funded by the Italian Ministry for Universities and for Research, currently devoted to *Historicizing AIDS: Policies, Rights, Discourses, and Memories in the Italian Case*. The fruits of recent research have become evident in new monographs and articles that attest to an enduring commitment to historicizing the impact, narrative and collective memory of contagious diseases in contemporary Italy.[22] The case of cholera in the experience of Naples is also under the spotlight thanks to very recent initiatives, such as the conference *Prima e dopo il colera del 1973: Le epidemie nella storia di Napoli*, on October 25–26, 2023.[23]

Almost no attention has been given to studies of this theme in Italian visual arts. One rare example is the special bilingual issue of the online journal of Sapienza University of Rome, *Novecento transnazionale: Letterature, arti e culture*, which was edited during the pandemic by Sharon Hecker and Carla Subrizi, titled "Sull'orlo di un cambiamento: L'arte immagina il mondo dopo la pandemia/On the Brink of Change: Art Imagines the World after the Pandemic."[24]

Notwithstanding this enormous academic output, the attitude of minimizing, concealing and disguising evidence of contagion waves in the long arc of Italian history has been conspicuously absent in this revival of interest in the subject of pandemics. The way the central government, single communities, as well as medical experts, hotel managers and artists dealt with the issue of contagious disease seems to be a promising perspective for unveiling the long-lasting hypocrisy and contradictions that we all were confronted with during the first wave of the COVID-19 pandemic. The chapters in this volume discuss case studies and aim at offering some answers to the many questions still open, both for our time and for future generations.

> *SH and AAR:* What follows is a roadmap of the rest of the chapters in this volume and a rationale for their inclusion. We begin by widening the historical lens of disease with a view into the past. In Chapter 2, art historian Louise Marshall shows a different approach to how diseases were pictured in early modern times as compared to the nineteenth, twentieth and twenty-first centuries. She examines a variety of strategies adopted to represent bodies and those dying from epidemics during the second global bubonic plague beginning with the Black Death of 1348 and up to the early eighteenth century. Marshall highlights disjunctions between textual and visual descriptions of plague victims: while writers detailed symptoms, images showed no physical signs of buboes until the later fifteenth century, when these images began to appear. Marshall considers how visual representations ultimately came to shape cultural attitudes and responses to the epidemic experience.

Moving into the nineteenth century in Italy, we find various forms of disguising and denial of pandemics. In Chapter 3, historian Arianna Arisi Rota analyzes the clash between the protection of public health and the defense of commerce, two opposing values that are elicited recurrently by pandemics. She focuses on the underexamined case of post-Napoleonic Europe during the cholera, typhus and yellow fever outbreaks. Her chapter shows how in the Italian case the health-commerce dilemma continued to puzzle policy-makers and renowned experts of public health from the 1830s and up to Italy's jubilee in 1911, on the eve of the military campaign to conquer Libya.

The link between the challenges brought on by pandemics and political, social and economic changes is the focus of Chapter 4 by historian Gabriele Bassi. The author hones in on the Italian war for the conquest of Libya, during which cholera ended up being inadvertently exported from Italy to its colonies because it had not been made public. The country's desire for military prestige as well as strategic political choices led the government not to report the cholera epidemic back home and to partially neglect measures to contain it in the colonial spaces.

From the perspective of the history of medicine, Paolo Mazzarello analyzes the case of syphilis in Italy in the 1860s in Chapter 5. Mazzarello focuses on the efforts of Angelo Scarenzio, a little-remembered professor of dermatology at the University of Pavia in the last decades of the nineteenth century, to work on a new treatment of the disease. Despite its positive results, the treatment was initially opposed and marginalized by the international scientific community. Mazzarello suggests that the disappearance of therapy from medical practice at the beginning of the twentieth century is the reason why Scarenzio is not considered a pioneer scientist today.

Cultural production in the nineteenth and twentieth centuries supports Mazzarello's assessment of Scarenzio's difficulties in having his cures legitimized. As literary historian Federica Massia suggests in Chapter 6, doctors and medicine in Italian literature were viewed with the same skepticism as medical science, which accompanied the disillusionment citizens felt toward the Risorgimento's ideals and positivist thought. Writings of the time on contagious diseases range from negative depictions of doctors in novels by Giovanni Verga and Luigi Capuana to Southern Italian narratives about the Sicilian cholera epidemic, which was accompanied by a mistrust in local and national authorities. Doctors and priests were believed to be spreading the disease intentionally. Northern Lombard Scapigliati writers, some themselves dying of tuberculosis, considered medicine and science as lacking sensitivity for understanding human nature, as did Crepuscolari poets, who condemned medicine, instead fading into melancholic resignation.

In contrast to the literary production, nineteenth-century images of disease in visual arts were rare. In Chapter 7, art historian Sharon Hecker contends that the few images produced elicited revulsion, expressions of sadness, or a pivoting away from the unappealing subject toward aesthetic discussions of artistic form and style. Most of these works did not find buyers in Italy: they either languished in the artist's studio, were painted over or were shipped abroad, leading to these images' invisibility today. Hecker unearths a few examples that involved the personal, public and scientific spheres, all of which address the horror and fear of epidemics, invisible lethal enemies for which no cure had been found. They provoked anxieties ranging from the private to the social, cultural and political.

Cinema took yet another approach to denying or disguising disease. Literary historian Catherine Ramsey-Portolano's Chapter 8 focuses on how tuberculosis was described in the 1875 novel *Tigre reale* (*The Royal Tiger*) by Verga and then masked in its 1916 film adaptation by Giovanni Pastrone. The female protagonist's illness is rephrased as an excess of passion, in accordance with cultural stereotypes about women. The protagonist's death by tuberculosis in the novel is reconfigured in the film to showcase the character portrayed by a cinematic diva and creates for her a regenerative role in the movie.

A similar masking of disease is evident later in twentieth-century cinema as well, as shown by historian of cinema Brendan Hennessey, who devotes Chapter 9 to the denial of cholera in Luchino Visconti's *Death in Venice* (1971). In Thomas Mann's 1912 novel, upon which the film is based, the protagonist dies of cholera, but in the film, he is said to have died of a heart attack. Hennessey contends that this is not simply a creative liberty or adaptation by the director. Visconti uses cholera to focus on the casualty of old people in post-unification Italy, by referring to Prime Minister Giovanni Giolitti's personal silencing of the outbreak in 1911, thereby placing the most vulnerable citizens at risk. This relates to Visconti's concern late in life with questions of aging, mental and physical decline, as well as intergenerational misunderstanding, equating old age with disease to highlight the elderly as victims of Italy's ambitions for modern statehood.

Historian Ewa Kawamura's Chapter 10 turns to tuberculosis at the Grand Hotel Quisisana of Capri, founded in the nineteenth century by a doctor for travelers and invalids recovering from consumption due to Capri's salutary climate. The hotel later developed into a luxury hotel, transforming patients into clients, as well as a hideaway for queer couples. Literary works celebrated the hotel and guaranteed its continued fame. In the early twentieth century, the name "Quisisana" became widespread for hotels, pensions and villas around the world, no longer associated with disease and erasing the name's unpleasant origins in contagious infection.

Turning to pandemics that have afflicted the twentieth century in Chapter 11, historian Marco Rovinello focuses on the HIV/AIDS epidemic of the 1980s and 1990s. Rovinello analyzes the coverage of news on the epidemic by the Italian mass media. He utilizes quantitative and qualitative analysis of newspaper titles to show the terms in which HIV/AIDS was framed, reported and illustrated and to ascertain whether and why HIV/AIDS was simply forgotten or intentionally disguised when it became a chronic disease. He compares the coverage to that in other countries to determine whether Italy was unique or not in its reporting. His chapter discusses how an Italian narrative of otherization in space and time functions as a form of miscommunication with respect to the disease.

A quantitative analysis from the perspective of the social sciences seemed important to the theme of the volume. We therefore decided to end the volume with a chapter dedicated to a view of today and a lesson for the future. In Chapter 12, sociologist Marco Terraneo examines how the Italian National Health Service responded to the COVID-19 pandemic, especially with respect to the most vulnerable population in Italy. His work dovetails with other chapters in the volume that focus attention on fragile people. Using qualitative and quantitative analysis and working from a sociological perspective, Terraneo examines how marginalized groups are often forgotten by the public health system due to structural factors, as well as institutional and organizational characteristics. Terraneo suggests new avenues for the reform of Italian healthcare, toward a more inclusive system based on a social and community perspective.

Ultimately, this book derives from personal urgencies linked to an *ego-histoire* dimension. It aims to offer to the scholarly community and to general audiences further interdisciplinary tools for understanding long-term processes. Such tools can help broaden the current scholarly interest by paying attention to the issue of denial of contagious disease in the history of Italy. The book is only a start. Future generations should keep in mind the need to include fragility and marginalization within our broader social horizon.

Notes

1 Jeneen Interlandi, "America Is Forgetting the Lessons of the Covid Health Emergency," *Opinion, New York Times*, May 11, 2023, www.nytimes.com/2023/05/11/opinion/covid-pandemic-emergency-lessons.html.
2 Brainpull, "Milano NON si ferma," *YouTube video*, February 27, 2020, www.youtube.com/watch?v=Gr0Nsrz7W3s. Brainpull did not accept our request to be interviewed for this essay.
3 The musician is Tomer Katz ("D Fine Us"). The song is "Howling at the Moon."
4 The TV talk show was *Che tempo che fa* ("Giuseppe Sala," *YouTube Video*, March 22, 2020, www.youtube.com/watch?v=oT7f_ea-SLA).
5 See, for example, Alessandro Rovellini, " 'Milano non si ferma' è un video orrendo: E non dobbiamo nascondere di avere paura," *Milano Today*, March 3, 2020, www.milanotoday.it/attualita/coronavirus/milano-non-si-ferma-commento.html.
6 L'Unione sarda/v.l., "L'Italia ferita e malata: La suggestiva immagine che sta facendo il giro del web," *L'Unione sarda*, March 13, 2020, www.unionesarda.it/articolo/cultura/2020/03/13/l-italia-ferita-e-malata-la-suggestiva-immagine-che-sta-facendo-i-8-997097.html.
7 Ibid.
8 A rare example is a caricature by the satirical cartoonist Casimiro Deja, published on January 26, 1857, in the illustrated magazine *Il Fischietto*. It shows a dying woman representing Italy lying in her bed while a doctor – the satirical magazine itself – checks her pulse and takes care of her. The image is reproduced in Sandro Morachioli, "Il volto del giornale: Usi e funzioni della personificazione nella stampa satirica risorgimentale," *Mélanges de l'École française de Rome: Italie et*

méditerranée modernes et contemporaines 130, no. 1 (2018): 30, https://journals. openedition.org/mefrim/3667?lang=en.

 9 Suzanne Stewart Steinberg, *The Pinocchio Effect: On Making Italians, 1860–1920* (Chicago, IL: University of Chicago Press, 2008), 6. For Italy as a model for the United States, see, among others, Paul Krugman, "Why Can't Trump's America Be Like Italy?," *Opinion, New York Times*, July 23, 2020, www.nytimes. com/2020/07/23/opinion/us-italy-coronavirus.html; Jason Horowitz, "How Italy Turned Around Its Coronavirus Calamity," *New York Times*, July 31, 2020, www.nytimes.com/2020/07/31/world/europe/italy-coronavirus-reopening.html; and Roger Cohen, "The Unlikely Triumph of Italian Nationhood: Italy Coheres as American Breaks Apart," *Opinion, New York Times*, August 14, 2020, www. nytimes.com/2020/08/14/opinion/italy-coronavirus.html.

10 Richard Haass, "The Pandemic Will Accelerate History Rather Than Reshape It: Not Every Crisis Is a Turning Point," *Foreign Affairs*, April 7, 2020, www. foreignaffairs.com/articles/united-states/2020-04-07/pandemic-will-accelerate-history-rather-reshape-it.

11 Alfred W. Crosby, *America's Forgotten Pandemic: The Influenza of 1918*, 2nd ed. (Cambridge: Cambridge University Press, 2003).

12 Arianna Arisi Rota, "The Invisible Enemy: A Historian's Short Tale of Covid-19 in Italy," *Modern Italy* 25, no. 3 (2020): 237–41, www.cambridge. org/core/journals/modern-italy/article/invisible-enemy-a-historians-short-tale-of-covid19-in-italy/1FD8A38E45F6F72A1D3913FC7941D4AC.

13 Xavier Tabet, *Lockdown: Diritto alla vita e biopolitica* (Dueville, Vicenza: Ronzani, 2021).

14 Guy Benier, ed., *Pandemic Re-Awakenings: The Forgotten and the Un-Forgotten "Spanish" Flu of 1918* (Oxford: Oxford University Press, 2022).

15 Giulia Delogu, "Politiche della sanità: Pratiche, agenti, norme in area mediterranea (secoli XVI–XIX)," Special Issue, *Studi storici* 64, no. 3 (2023): 521–27.

16 Susan Sontag, *Illness as Metaphor* (New York: Farrar, Straus & Giroux, 1978).

17 Emmanuel Betta, "Pandemia come metafora?" *Contemporanea* 4 (October–December 2020): 681–97, www.rivisteweb.it/doi/10.1409/99941.

18 Cristiana Giordano and Rhiannon Noel Welch, eds., "Epistemes of Contagion," Special Issue, *California Italian Studies* 11, no. 1 (2022), https://escholarship.org/uc/ismrg_cisj/11/1.

19 Francesca Arena and Giulia Calvi, eds., "Contagi," Special Issue, *Genesis* 21, no. 1 (2022), www.viella.it/rivista/9791254691021.

20 Frank M. Snowden, *The Conquest of Malaria: Italy, 1900–1962* (New Haven, CT and London: Yale University Press, 2006); and Snowden, *La conquista della malaria: Una modernizzazione italiana, 1900–1962*, trans. Valentina Besi and Cinzia Di Barbara (Turin: Einaudi, 2008).

21 Eugenia Tognotti, "Pandemia e governo dell'emergenza sanitaria," interview by Salvatore Botta, *Ricerche di storia politica*, July 30, 2020, www.arsp. it/2020/07/30/pandemie-e-governo-dellemergenza-sanitaria/. Botta is a historian of natural disasters and emergencies.

22 See, for instance, Fiammetta Balestracci, Fabio Guidali and Enrico Landoni, eds., *L'Aids in Italia (1982–1996): Istituzioni, società, media* (Pisa: Pacini, 2022); and Silvia Inaudi, "La tubercolosi nell'Italia del secondo dopoguerra: L'azione dell'UNRRA," *Italia contemporanea* 301 (2023): 16–42. The issue is dedicated to the health system in Republican Italy during the postwar decades.

23 *Convegno: Prima e dopo il colera del 1973, le epidemie nella storia di Napoli*, October 25–26, 2023. The conference program is available online at www.scienzepolitiche.unina.it/?p=3313.

24 Sharon Hecker and Carla Subrizi, eds., "Sull'orlo di un cambiamento: L'arte immagina il mondo dopo la pandemia/On the Brink of Change: Art Imagines the World After the Pandemic," Special Issue, *Novecento transnazionale: Letterature, arti e culture* 5, no. 1 (March 2021), https://doi.org/10.13133/2532-1994/17457.

References

Arena, Francesca, and Giulia Calvi, eds. "Contagi." Special Issue, *Genesis* 21, no. 1 (2022). www.viella.it/rivista/9791254691021.

Arisi Rota, Arianna. "The Invisible Enemy: A Historian's Short Tale of Covid-19 in Italy." *Modern Italy* 25, no. 3 (2020): 237–41. www.cambridge.org/core/journals/modern-italy/article/invisible-enemy-a-historians-short-tale-of-covid19-in-italy/1FD8A38E45F6F72A1D3913FC7941D4AC.

Balestracci, Fiammetta, Fabio Guidali, and Enrico Landoni, eds. *L'AIDS in Italia (1982–1996): Istituzioni, società, media.* Pisa: Pacini, 2022.

Benier, Guy, ed. *Pandemic Re-Awakenings: The Forgotten and the Un-Forgotten 'Spanish' Flu of 1918.* Oxford: Oxford University Press, 2022.

Betta, Emmanuel. "Pandemia come metafora?" *Contemporanea* 4 (October–December 2020): 681–97. www.rivisteweb.it/doi/10.1409/99941.

Brainpull. "Milano NON si ferma." *YouTube Video*, February 27, 2020. www.youtube.com/watch?v=Gr0Nsrz7W3s.

Cohen, Roger. "The Unlikely Triumph of Italian Nationhood: Italy Coheres as American Breaks Apart." *Opinion, New York Times*, August 14, 2020. www.nytimes.com/2020/08/14/opinion/italy-coronavirus.html.

Convegno: Prima e dopo il colera del 1973, le epidemie nella storia di Napoli. October 25–26, 2023. www.scienzepolitiche.unina.it/?p=3313.

Crosby, Alfred W. *America's Forgotten Pandemic: The Influenza of 1918.* 2nd ed. Cambridge: Cambridge University Press, 2003.

Delogu, Giulia, ed. "Politiche della sanità: Pratiche, agenti, norme in area Mediterranean (secoli XVI–XIX)." Special Issue, *Studi storici* 64, no. 3 (2023): 521–94.

Giordano, Cristiana, and Rhiannon Noel Welch, eds. "Italy and the Epistemes of Contagion: Touch, Contact, Distance." Special Issue, *California Italian Studies* 11, no. 1 (2022). https://escholarship.org/uc/ismrg_cisj/11/1.

Giuseppe Sala. "Che tempo che fa" *YouTube Video*, March 22, 2020. www.youtube.com/watch?v=oT7f_ea-SLA.

Haass, Richard. "The Pandemic Will Accelerate History Rather Than Reshape It: Not Every Crisis Is a Turning Point." *Foreign Affairs*, April 7, 2020. www.foreignaffairs.com/articles/united-states/2020-04-07/pandemic-will-accelerate-history-rather-reshape-it.

Hecker, Sharon, and Carla Subrizi, eds. "Sull'orlo di un cambiamento: L'arte immagina il mondo dopo la pandemia/On the Brink of Change: Art Imagines the World after the Pandemic." Special Issue, *Novecento transnazionale: Letterature, arti e culture* 5, no. 1 (2021). https://doi.org/10.13133/2532-1994/17457.

Horowitz, Jason. "How Italy Turned Around Its Coronavirus Calamity," *New York Times*, July 31, 2020. www.nytimes.com/2020/07/31/world/europe/italy-coronavirus-reopening.html.

Inaudi, Silvia. "La tubercolosi nell'Italia del secondo dopoguerra: L'azione dell'UNRRA." *Italia contemporanea* 301 (2023): 16–42.

Interlandi, Jeneen. "America Is Forgetting the Lessons of the Covid Health Emergency." Opinion. *New York Times*, May 11, 2023. www.nytimes.com/2023/05/11/opinion/covid-pandemic-emergency-lessons.html.

Krugman, Paul. "Why Can't Trump's America Be Like Italy?" *Opinion, New York Times*, July 23, 2020. www.nytimes.com/2020/07/23/opinion/us-italy-coronavirus.html.

L'Unione sarda/v.l. "L'Italia ferita e malata: La suggestiva immagine che sta facendo il giro del web." *L'Unione sarda*, March 13, 2020. www.unionesarda.it/articolo/cultura/2020/03/13/l-italia-ferita-e-malata-la-suggestiva-immagine-che-sta-facendo-i-8–997097.html.

Morachioli, Sandro. "Il volto del giornale: Usi e funzioni della personificazione nella stampa satirica risorgimentale." *Mélanges de l'École française de Rome: Italie et méditerranée modernes et contemporaines* 130, no. 1 (2018): 30. https://journals.openedition.org/mefrim/3667?lang=en.

Rovellini, Alessandro. " 'Milano non si ferma' è un video orrendo: E non dobbiamo nascondere di avere paura." *Milano Today*, March 3, 2020. www.milanotoday.it/attualita/coronavirus/milano-non-si-ferma-commento.html.

Snowden, Frank M. *The Conquest of Malaria: Italy, 1900–1962*. New Haven, CT: Yale University Press, 2006.

______. *La conquista della malaria: Una modernizzazione italiana, 1900–1962*. Translated by Valentina Besi and Cinzia Di Barbara. Turin: Einaudi, 2008.

Sontag, Susan. *Illness as Metaphor*. New York: Farrar, Straus & Giroux, 1978.

Stewart-Steinberg, Suzanne. *The Pinocchio Effect: On Making Italians, 1860–1920*. Chicago, IL: University of Chicago Press, 2008.

Tabet, Xavier. *Lockdown: Diritto alla vita e biopolitica*. Dueville; Vicenza: Ronzani, 2021.

Tognotti, Eugenia. "Pandemia e governo dell'emergenza sanitaria." Interview by Salvatore Botta. *Ricerche di storia politica*, July 30, 2020. www.arsp.it/2020/07/30/pandemie-e-governo-dellemergenza-sanitaria/.

2 Diseased Bodies in Early Modern Europe

Picturing Plague Victims

Louise Marshall

The power of the image to compel attention and rouse emotions was starkly evident in drone footage published in *The New York Times* and other news outlets in April 2020, at the height of the coronavirus epidemic, showing hazmat-clad workers burying stacks of coffins in a newly dug trench on Hart Island, New York (Figure 2.1).[1] Visual affect works through conjoined absence and presence, the bodies of the dead invisible to the eye yet still vividly present via the mute witness of their coffins, their numbers and anonymity equally eloquent in evoking the horrendous mortality then overwhelming the city.[2] Historical resonances with mass burials during earlier epidemics were inevitable. In his famous account of Florence during the Black Death of 1348, Giovanni Boccaccio describes how,

> when all the graves were full, huge trenches were excavated in the churchyards, into which new arrivals were placed in their hundreds, stowed tier upon tier like ships' cargo, each layer of corpses being covered over with a thin layer of soil till the trench was filled to the top.[3]

Writing a few decades later, when bubonic plague had become a recurrent scourge, another Florentine chronicler described bodies buried in deep pits, piled in layers and covered with earth "like garnishing lasagne with cheese."[4]

Imagined Bodies: Coffins and Shrouds

Visual echoes were also not far to seek, including what is probably the earliest representation of the Black Death in Western Europe, a much-reproduced if little-analyzed miniature from the fourth chronicle (*Tractatus quartus*) of Tournai abbot Gilles Li Muisis (Figure 2.2).[5] The text was composed in 1349–53, immediately after the Black Death, and survives in the original mid-fourteenth-century manuscript. This collection of Li Muisis's writings was probably prepared by the author himself, preserving his works for posterity in a manuscript copied, illuminated and bound by his monastery's book restorer Pierart dou Tielt.[6] As in the modern photograph, the miniature's impact relies on a combination of the seen and the unseen. With the

DOI: 10.4324/9781003382805-2

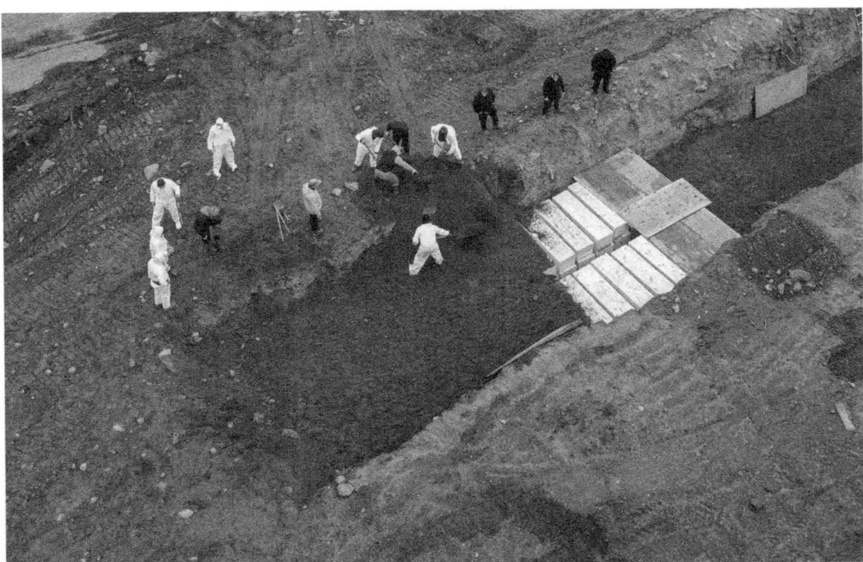

Figure 2.1 Drone pictures show bodies being buried on New York's Hart Island, where the Department of Corrections is dealing with more burials overall, amid the coronavirus disease (COVID-19) outbreak in New York City, U.S., April 9, 2020.

Source: Photo: REUTERS/Lucas Jackson.

exception of a shrouded corpse being lowered into a grave, the plague's victims are both here and not here, sensed but for the most part not visible, haunting the viewer's imagination by their very absence. Pars pro toto, the anonymous body about to be buried provides the emotional and literal center of the composition, even as it is about to disappear from view.

In both images, multiplied coffins are shocking indices of the catastrophic numbers of dead. In the Tournai painting, a group of six coffins form a cresting wave at left, drawing the eye inward to the burial at the center through a series of assertive rising diagonals, the foremost aligned with the exposed body in a purposeful visual rhyming. Yet the connection of corpse and casket is one of potential, a grimly predictive futurity, since by the way they are so easily hefted over shoulders, these coffins must be empty. A later plague picture, discussed below, represents a gravedigger carrying an empty casket in similar fashion as he arrives to collect a body (see Figure 2.3). In Northern Europe, wooden caskets were normally used only to transport bodies from locus of death to church and cemetery; timber was too valuable to be buried and would only hinder the process of decomposition which might facilitate subsequent reuse of the same ground.[7] However, during plague epidemics, authorities – including those in Tournai, as Li Muisis reports in his

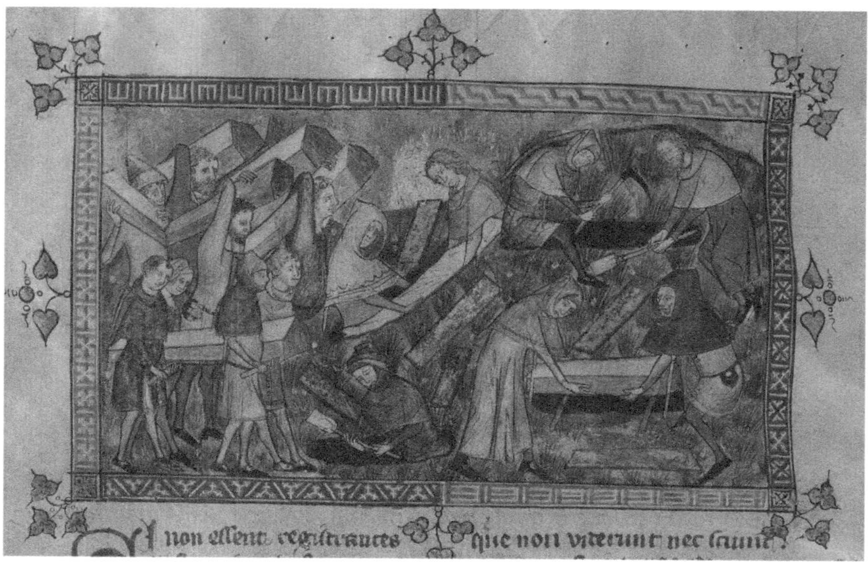

Figure 2.2 Pierart dou Tielt, *Burial of Plague Victims in Tournai in 1349*, c. 1353. Miniature in Gilles Li Muisis, *Tractatus quartus*. Brussels, KBR, ms 13076–13077, fol. 24v.

Source: Photo: KBR.

chronicle – often mandated coffin burials to prevent infection.[8] Hence the need for ever-more coffins, requisitioned from elsewhere or, as seems more likely, newly made to meet escalating demand and brought to the cemetery by the carpenters.

Unlike these empty caskets, the coffin in the foreground is carried horizontally, its corpse-filled weight requiring the concerted action of four men. Their bowed heads and sober mien contrast with the more casual attitudes of the workers above, acknowledging the presence of the dead they carry. Still being excavated by a gravedigger standing waist-deep in the hole, an open grave in front of the arriving coffin is its likely destination. The next stage in the process is already in train to the right, where two workers balance a laden coffin on its makeshift bier above a finished grave, about to slide the casket into the ground. The discarded planks from these biers litter the graveyard, their numbers yet another telling register of the multitude of burials already completed.

Both past and present images share a focus on the mechanics of mass burial, registering the epidemic's effects through the intense concentration of cemetery workers in burying the dead as efficiently and expeditiously as possible. In the miniature, sharply observed details create a veristic effect. Not surprising in view of the likely close collaboration between illuminator and author, many correspond with the civic decrees reported by Li Muisis. In the

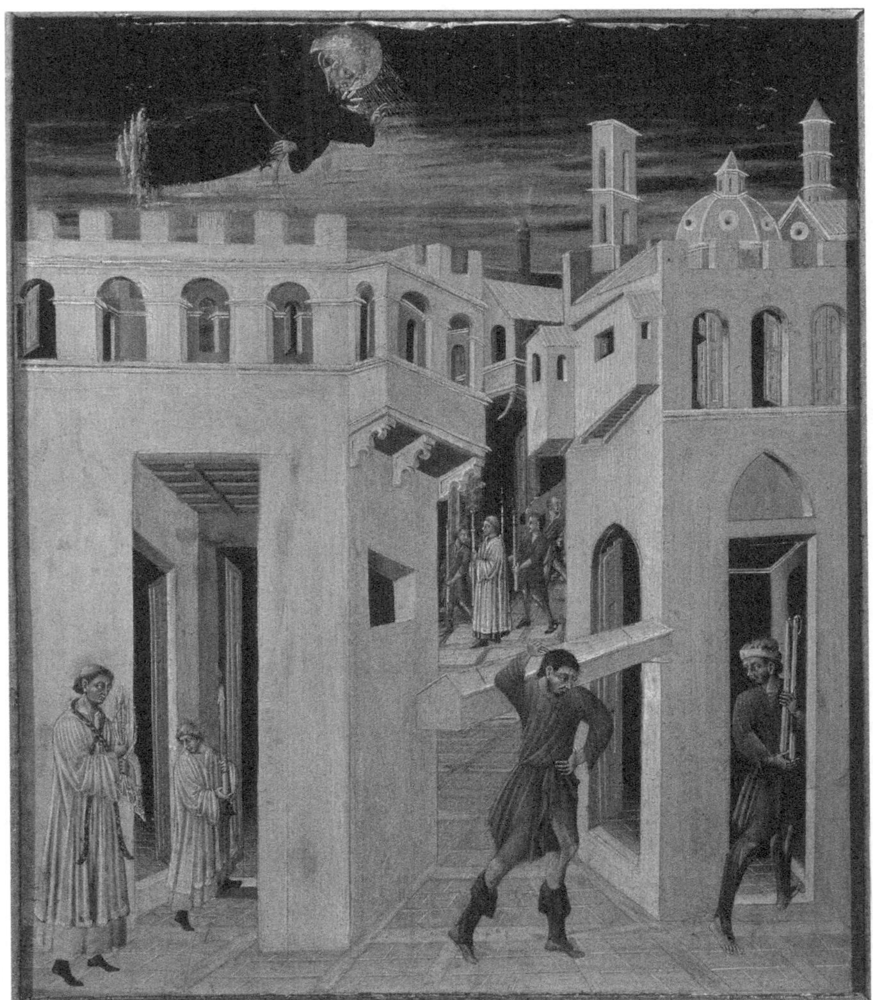

Figure 2.3 Giovanni di Paolo, *St. Nicholas of Tolentino Saving a City from Plague*, 1457. Panel from the altarpiece of St. Nicholas of Tolentino in S. Agostino, Montepulciano. Wien, Gemäldegalerie der Akademie der bildenden Künste/Vienna, Academy of Fine Arts, Paintings Gallery.

Source: Photo: Akademie der bildenden Künste.

foreground, the alignment of arriving casket and partially excavated grave is one of cause and effect. According to Tournai regulations, a grave should be dug as soon as a plague death was reported, irrespective of the victim's status and "at whatever hour of the day or the night."[9] Notably, too, unlike the situation seen in New York and reported by Boccaccio and other chroniclers for Florence, following Tournai resolutions, these burials are individual rather than collective. The human effort required to dig down to the six feet mandated by the Flemish city is demonstrated by the depiction of no less than three excavators. In addition to the gravedigger in the foreground, two more are at an earlier point in the process, one standing with his foot in a shallow depression to break ground with a pick, while another shovels away the earth. Even the number and varying stages of readiness of the four visible graves seem to invoke, if only to exceed, the magistrates' provision that "in each parish there should always be three graves ready prepared."[10]

The combination of shroud and coffin burial within the one scene has thus far escaped attention. Differing practices might be depicted to signal the haste and urgency of the ever-mounting number of victims requiring immediate burial. Yet the abundance of coffins suggests otherwise. Instead, the exposed body should be recognized as a function of artistic rather than reportorial aims, deployed to provide a compelling focus of spectatorial engagement and affect. Singularity only enhances emotional impact. Fear and grief, horror and repulsion are stimulated by the pathetic spectacle of the shrouded body, its corporeality both revealed and concealed, the viewer in turn tantalized and frustrated in the desire for closer inspection. Impersonal and anonymous, with neither social nor gender identity, the body is unknown and unknowable, an every-person for the pandemic's extraordinary virulence and universal reach.

This chapter focuses precisely on what is absent or only partially glimpsed in modern footage and fourteenth-century miniature – that is, the bodies of those dying from epidemic disease. Analysis of the variety of strategies adopted to depict the victims of the second global pandemic of bubonic plague, which opened in the West with the infamous Black Death of 1348 and lasted until the early eighteenth century, provides instructive parallels and divergences with the visual regimes of later periods. In particular, I focus on the hitherto little-noticed disjunction between text and image in descriptions of those suffering and dying from plague. While contemporary chroniclers in Italy and elsewhere itemized symptoms in detail, for a century or more after the Black Death, Renaissance depictions of plague dead showed no such physical signs. Exploring the motives and impact of a range of artistic strategies in representing plague victims, my investigation sheds light on the role of visual representations in articulating and shaping cultural attitudes and responses to the experience of epidemic disease.

The conflicting dynamic of revelation and concealment that I have identified as key to the Tournai miniature is rarely found in Italian representations of plague victims, where coffins almost never appear, despite the provisions enacted by city governments for casket burials during epidemics.[11] The sole instance known to me is a 1457 panel by the Sienese artist Giovanni di Paolo, representing Augustinian St. Nicholas of Tolentino intervening to save a plague-stricken city (Figure 2.3). This was part of a dismembered altarpiece of the saint, made for the Order's church in Montepulciano.[12] Even more stringently than in the Flemish miniature, visual access to the bodies of the dead is withheld. Occupying the center of the picture, coffins are key protagonists, fraught pictorial surrogates for the invisible but no less vividly imagined dead. Empty and laden caskets define a similar trajectory of absence and occupation that dramatizes the epidemic's ubiquity and appalling body count. In the right foreground, gravediggers with an empty coffin and unlit candles arrive to collect a corpse for burial, while the coffin of another victim, draped with a pall, is carried in procession by their colleagues in the street behind. A priest bringing the viaticum to the dying in the house at the left further enhances the sense of ever-present death, the better to celebrate the epidemic's rout at the hands of the saint, who emerges from the clouds above with blessing at the ready.

Blocking, deflecting, limiting or masking the vision of plague victims relies on the viewer to complete the prospect, as if the full charnel horrors of death by bubonic plague could be evoked more vividly in the imagination than in any figuration. However, this is only one pictorial strategy, and not the most common in Italian art, where representations of the bodies of victims begin to appear from the 1370s. This coincides with the disease's return in the 1360s and 1370s, demonstrating that the Black Death of 1348 was not the singular disaster that contemporaries assumed, but only the first of many – a realization in some senses even more shocking than the first onset. As I have argued, visual images were a crucial coping strategy for early modern populations confronting the ever-present threat of plague.[13] Belief in divine causation of plague as punishment for sin was universal, but an offended God could nonetheless be persuaded to change his mind by the efforts of his mother and his friends the saints. Activated through prayer and penitential procession, plague pictures offered worshippers consolation and hope by articulating contemporary understandings of the disease's origins and enlisting the aid of a range of heavenly protectors.

In this salvific economy, representation of plague victims served a variety of affective and hortatory purposes. Clinical accuracy was never the aim, nor can such depictions be neatly corralled into a teleological history of increasingly secular public health narratives.[14] For more than a century after the first appearance of bubonic plague in Italy, the bodies of its victims were represented following two distinct visual conventions, showing the dead either intact and unmarked or pierced with arrows. Although it would be easy to characterize these two representational strategies in oppositional terms, as naturalistic or symbolic, this would be a misrepresentation. Both modes were created at the same time and coexisted, sometimes within the context of a single work, throughout the fourteenth and fifteenth centuries.[15] Neither are completely veristic, but both would be read as true and convincing by their makers and viewers. The existence of these two representational modes underlines the artifice at work in plague images, undercutting presumptions of unmodified documentary reportage, as is still too often assumed. As I will argue, both choices articulate the same worldview of disease causation and necessary remedial action; what differs is the ways in which the visual is shaped to communicate with and affect the viewer.

The Reality Effect: Dead Bodies in the City

Just as in the later picture by Giovanni di Paolo so an earlier representation of city and countryside devastated by plague by Florentine Giovanni del Biondo hammers home the message of saintly deliverance by confronting viewers with plague's horrifying effects, made plain to see by the plethora of corpses spilling down the hillside (Figure 2.4). The subject is a celebrated epidemic in seventh-century Pavia, halted by St. Sebastian.[16] Thanks to his intervention, an angel (due to paint loss, now visible only through the surrounding incised rays of heavenly light) drives off the demon responsible for the epidemic.[17] The episode closes a cycle of the saint's life and miracles on an altarpiece for Florence Cathedral, probably commissioned soon after the city's third

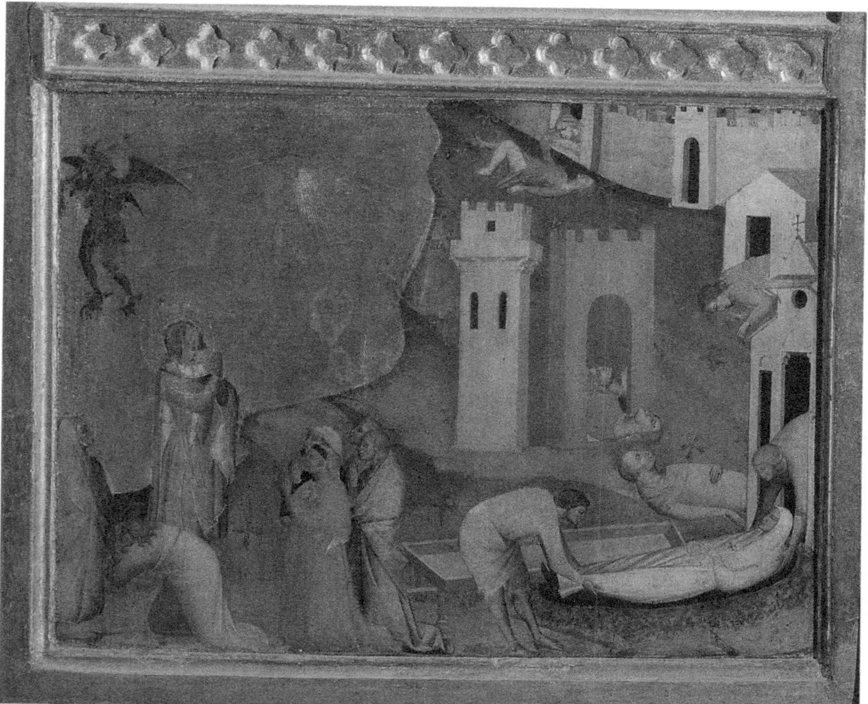

Figure 2.4 Giovanni del Biondo, *St. Sebastian Saving Pavia from Plague*, c. 1374. Panel from the altarpiece of St. Sebastian in Florence Cathedral. Florence, Museo dell'Opera del Duomo.

Source: Photo: Courtesy of the Opera di S. Maria del Fiore.

outbreak of plague in 1374.[18] Carefully observed details of costume, architecture, objects and funerary practice recast seventh-century Pavia as a contemporary town. Viewed through the prism of recent experience, the past is made shockingly present and immediate. Sprawled over gates and doors, piled in houses, lying on the ground or lowered by two gravediggers into a newly dug grave, the superabundance of corpses presents a hyperbolic vision of horror and dread, deliberately rousing and manipulating the viewer's emotions for hortatory and hagiographic effect.

Plague is shown to be remorseless and all-consuming: city walls are no defense, whole households perish and efforts to escape divine judgment by flight are useless. Thrice repeated, the dead bodies lying across thresholds emblematize the disease's overwhelming assault, breaching all boundaries. Town and houses alike are broken open and gutted by the virulence of plague's attack. The catastrophic cascade of bodies begins at the top with the corpse of a young man picked out in eye-catching red. Collapsed across the open city gate, as if struck down in the very act of attempting to flee, he reaches toward a woman lying on her back, her naked legs shamefully exposed.[19] The pairing suggests they may be lovers, justly punished for their sinful lust. However, other victims appear blameless, like the woman lying face up across the door of the castellated residence further down the hill. By their domestic location and more decorous poses, she and the man lying behind her seem to offer a corrective mirror of licit conjugality to the pair above. Yet if so, they have nonetheless perished in their turn, a reminder that God's thirst for vengeance might strike innocent and sinful alike.

This harsh lesson was encoded in the Old Testament, when God punished David's sin of taking a census by inflicting plague on the entire nation of Israel. This biblical precedent of mass mortality was retold in the special mass against plague created by the administration of Pope Clement VI during the Black Death, which became the standard liturgical response to pestilence.[20] The enormity of the mortality exacted upon humanity then and in later epidemics was widely understood as an indictment of the extraordinary extent of human sin, that would require such a severe and blanket punishment that took no heed of collateral damage. Writing soon after 1348, Piacenza notary Gabriele de Mussi envisaged God unleashing the plague with fearsome commands for the wholesale destruction of a world sinful beyond measure: "Let no one be spared, either for their sex or their age; let the innocent perish with the guilty and no one escape."[21] Balance was restored by the divergent fates of souls in the exacting accountancy of the afterlife, where the good, bad and middling received their just deserts by allocation to heaven, hell or purgatory. But such discriminations are not visible in Giovanni's picture. Hence the ambiguity of these bodies, their spiritual status undetermined, rousing guilt and grief, condemnation and compassion, as the viewer might decide.

Lying where no bodies should, the exposure and isolation of these corpses play on beholders' worst fears of the social and spiritual deprivations wrought by plague. Oft-repeated stories by Boccaccio and others, of victims abandoned by family and friends, dying alone without the services of doctor, notary or priest and buried without mourners or funeral rites, are brought vividly to life.[22] Although historians have demonstrated that such tales are more fanciful than accurate, this does not lessen their efficacy as visual shock tactics. Although widespread negative stereotypes of callous and avaricious gravediggers are contradicted by the workers' careful handling of the body of a professed religious or confraternity member, the absence of any priest, despite the churchyard setting, is telling. In every respect, these victims represent the polar opposite of what Roger Wieck has aptly dubbed "the death desired."[23] Left alone to die by those who should care for them, shunned by the professionals who would normally support them in their final hours, potentially dying with their sins unconfessed and buried without religious or social ceremony, the altarpiece's representation of plague victims offered audiences a negative mirror, stirring repentance and urging recourse to Sebastian as the only remedy.

Giovanni del Biondo's panel works on the viewer by its perceived naturalism, its compelling reality effect. Yet plausible evocation of contemporary experience extended only so far. Although the social horrors of death by plague are evoked in detail, it is noteworthy that the bodies of the victims are unmarked by any physical signs of the disease. Such absences cannot be attributed to disinterest or lack of familiarity with plague's clinical features, since virtually every account of the Black Death in Italy and elsewhere in Europe included a detailed exposition of symptoms. Amidst universal recognition that plague was a new disease, authors were at pains to itemize its characteristics in detail, creating scrupulous checklists for future reference.[24] Subsequent recurrences would only make the symptoms more familiar.

The absence of clinical signs on these plague bodies is another reminder, if one were needed, of the artifice at work in Italian Renaissance plague pictures. Lived experience is drawn upon but is also purposefully shaped for affective impact. In Giovanni del Biondo's panel, as in later fifteenth-century depictions of this same miracle, representations of the dead emphasized not the disease symptoms of individual sufferers, but the catastrophic disorder which such bodies showed forth. Plague signaled the world as out of joint, a disastrous upset of normal relations between heaven and earth. Yet the aim of the evocation of plague's horrors in both literature and art was to reverse them – behind the gruesome details and dramatic vignettes was an intense desire for restoration and wholeness, for reconciliation between heaven and earth. Like preachers including vivid anecdotes of contemporary life to drive home the moral message of their sermon, these abandoned bodies roused emotions for therapeutic aims. Horror, fear, guilt and remorse were deliberately manufactured to stir the soul and set in motion the necessary repentance and renewal.

Wounded by God: Death by Arrows

Alternatively, from the fourteenth to the early sixteenth century, plague victims in Italian Renaissance art were often represented pierced with arrows (Figure 2.5). Swift, silent and deadly, a killing blow loosed from the heavens to strike unsuspecting victims, the arrow is an apposite means by which to conceptualize the sudden onset of unexpected afflictions, disease and death. From the Old Testament, Renaissance worshippers were familiar with many instances of God punishing sinners in this way, and from 1300 if not earlier, bow and arrow often figured as the weapon of choice of personified Death. Such habits of thought shaped responses to the plague in literature and art. Chroniclers described plague's advent as arrows of death sent down by an angry God. In Gabriele de Mussi's account of the Black Death, the "darts of death" are launched by a furious deity proclaiming, "No one will be given rest, poisoned arrows will strike everyone, fevers will throw down the proud, and incurable disease will strike like lightning."[25] Italian plague pictures portray a variety of heavenly agents – God the Father, Christ the Son, as well as angels and demons, working as divine subcontractors in the task of punishing humanity – unleashing the plague on humanity by hurling or shooting arrows.[26]

In a miniature from the illustrated chronicle of Lucchese notary Giovanni Sercambi (Figure 2.5) – one of seven marking the sequence of plague

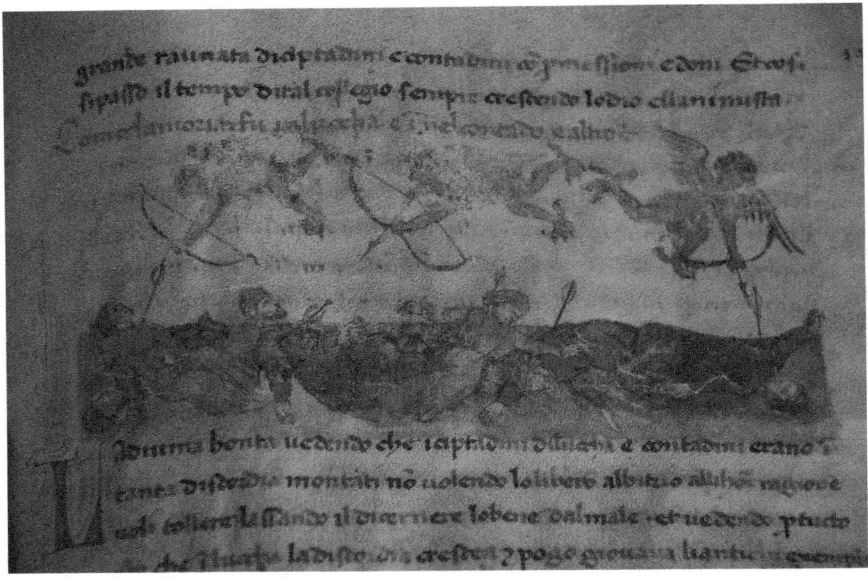

Figure 2.5 Lucchese illuminator, *1390 Plague Epidemic in Lucca*, c. 1400. Miniature in Giovanni Sercambi, *Croniche*. Lucca, Archivio di Stato, ms. 107, fol. 120r.

Source: Photo: author, courtesy of the Archivio di Stato di Lucca. Reproduction prohibited.

epidemics in Lucca over the 50-year period from 1348 to 1400 – the bodies of five men and one woman lie scattered on the ground.[27] Their tumbled disarray of ungainly, sprawling poses, arms flung wide, flat on their backs or face down, dramatizes the suddenness with which they were felled in the midst of ordinary life. The only exception to this pattern of expansively gesticulating corpses is the sole woman, lying second from the left, her arms folded protectively in front of her crotch in a doubled version of the classical modesty gesture, as if guarding her chastity amongst this otherwise all-male company. These victims' adversaries were evidently crack shots, since each has been killed by a single large arrow protruding from the back or chest. Taloned demons swoop low over the corpses with arrows notched to the string of their bows, patrolling to make certain all their prey is dead. In this stark rendition, variations of which accompany each accounting of plague in the chronicle, the world is time and again reduced to corpses, with no survivors.

In the gestural language of Italian Renaissance art, the outflung arms of the male bodies could be read as voicing protest or astonishment, anguish or appeal. Like Giovanni del Biondo's panel, their spiritual status is left for the viewer to decide, although the dead woman's decorous pose might suggest virtue rather than vice. Other Renaissance paintings, however, explicitly identify arrow-pierced victims as sinners by virtue of their location outside the charmed circle of the Virgin Mary's protective mantle.[28] Pietro Alemanno's 1485 altarpiece for the collegiate church of San Ginesio (Figure 2.6) shows hordes of grinning demons emerging from storm clouds to reenact the biblical sixth plague of the Egyptians, shooting arrows from their bows and vomiting, blowing, and throwing giant hailstones.[29] Secure within the textile womb of the universal mother of all Christians, most of the populace of San Ginesio escape the deadly rain unscathed.

The contrast between their upright, intact selves and the prostrate, pierced bodies beyond demonstrates the selectivity of Marian favor and protection. Issuing an invitation to the viewer to approach her ("Come to me, all ye that desire me"), an offer seconded by town patron St. Ginesius ("Children, hasten to her that you will find grace") and Dominican plague protector St. Vincent Ferrer ("Trust in her, all ye people"), Mary is nonetheless implacable in the fealty she demands of her devotees. Scrolls above the heads of the sheltering townspeople spell out the criteria for admission to her sanctum, professing their devotion and fidelity in the words of well-known Marian prayers.[30] The grim fate of those insufficiently devoted or faithful, as they themselves confess ("Justly we suffer this, because we did not love you"; "Alas for us, that we did not trust in you") is represented with dreadful clarity in the battered and wounded bodies on display (Figure 2.7). By their own admission, these sinners deserve their fate, spurning the recommendations of the saints and Mary's own loving invitation. Hence the serenity of the holy figures amidst the carnage and the resolute fixity of the saved, turning their backs and even

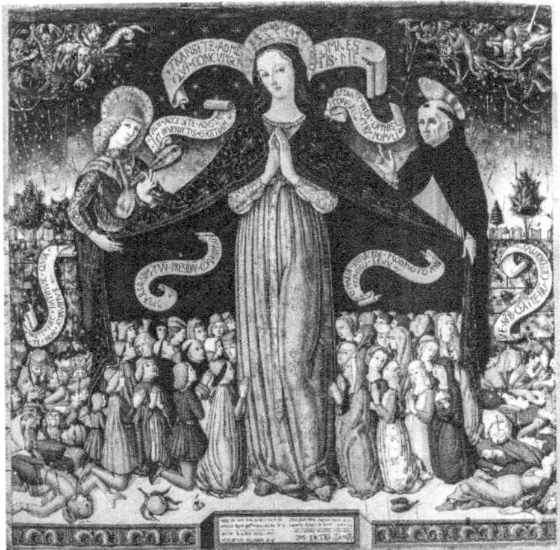

Figure 2.6 Pietro Alemanno, *Plague Virgin of Mercy with Sts Ginesius and Vincent Ferrer*, 1485. San Ginesio, Collegiata.

Source: Photo: courtesy of Ministero della Cultura-Soprintendenza Archeologia, Belle Arti e Paesaggio per le Province di Ancona e Pesaro e Urbino.

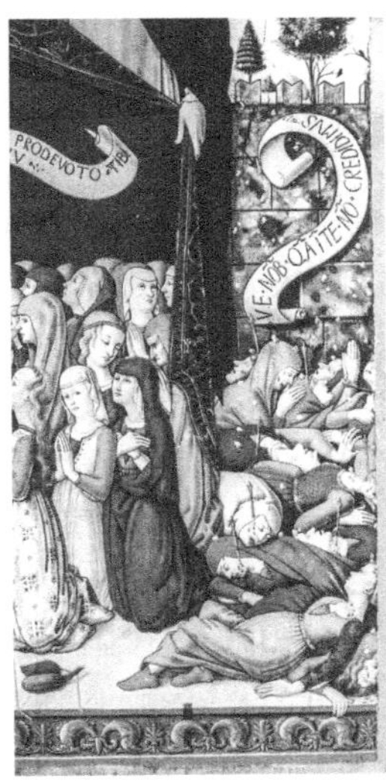

Figure 2.7 Pietro Alemanno, *Plague Virgin of Mercy with Sts Ginesius and Vincent* Ferrer, detail: *Plague Dead*, 1485. San Ginesio, Collegiata.

Source: Photo: courtesy of Ministero della Cultura-Soprintendenza Archeologia, Belle Arti e Paesaggio per le Province di Ancona e Pesaro e Urbino.

kneeling on top of an outstretched dead arm. Yet the beholder does not have the same luxury but is forced to see and understand their deaths.

These victims' suffering is terrible to witness, for many are still alive and struggling vainly against their fate. Open mouths invite us to hear their cries of pain and confession of guilt; heads are bowed in resignation or despair. Some seem to protest or beg for mercy, while others show last-minute signs of repentance that might save their souls if not their bodies, like the two women praying in the uppermost row, alongside a third who gazes upward and beats her breast with a fist in a common gesture of grief and penance. Dying before our eyes, these plague victims present a confronting mirror that urges penitence and right behavior by the force of their example. The psychic shock of these deaths is almost physical in its assault on viewers. In the right foreground, a young woman bleeding from her wounds and pinned to the ground by the press of corpses grasps one-handed at the edge of the marble parapet, as if to pull herself into the actual space occupied by the beholder. Spattering onto the marble floor, her blood, along with the blood spooling out from under the head of the young man dying so flamboyantly at left, is about to drip into our space.

Death by arrows creates a more physically visceral representation of plague's onset in Italian Renaissance representations of victims. The violence of this imagery is chilling and confronting. Against armed supernatural beings, whether divine, angelic or demonic, mere mortals cannot defend themselves. Heaven-sent arrows penetrate deeply; victims can bleed profusely. Body speaks to body in a process of empathetic seeing that cannot be unseen. As the arrows find their targets, challenged viewers are made to feel the sickening impact of the sharp points against their own vulnerable flesh. Identification with the fallen rouses conflicting emotions of compassion and condemnation to spur reform of life. One might wonder whether there is any significance in the location of the missiles. In some instances, arrows seem to pierce victims' bodies at sites where inflamed lymph nodes, or buboes, commonly appear: in the groin, armpits or neck. Yet the correspondences are not consistent; just as often, even in the same work, arrows are embedded in places where buboes do not form, including chests and backs, heads, faces, cheeks and foreheads. Rather than a literal mapping of plague buboes, the key issue is disfigurement, the shocking breach of the body's boundaries, a mortal rupturing of corporeal integrity that defines human frailty in the face of divine omnipotence. In any contest between God and humanity, the outcome is foreordained. For those marked for death, there is no escape.

The longevity of the visual formula of victims pierced with arrows in Renaissance art, from the 1370s through to the early sixteenth century, is due to its combination of explanatory clarity and emotional ferocity. Bodies shot with arrows visualized both plague's heavenly origins and its horrendous, usually mortal, assault on its victims. Naturalistically rendered weapons of mass destruction embedded in realistically wounded, suffering and dying bodies rendered the invisible workings of the divinely ordained universe visible and tangible. Such pictures revealed the truth behind the appearances, showing what everyone knew to be true. As ever in Italian Renaissance art, naturalism was deployed in the service of the convincingly realistic presentation of the supernatural.

Suffering and Cure: St. Roch and the Appearance of Plague Buboes

During the fifteenth century, schematized plague buboes begin to appear in a handful of medical illustrations plotting wound or bloodletting sites (Figure 2.8).[31] These diagrams are not without emotional affect in the way they visualize a beleaguered male body standing upright on the page, the buboes appearing as discolored circular masses superimposed on naked flesh. Significantly, too, these imagined victims are in their own fashion still alive, offering reassurance for practitioners and patients alike. In this, one might see them as expressive of the same desires and hopes that brought into being the cult of the French pilgrim St. Roch, whose meteoric rise as new plague saint in the latter fifteenth century in Italy and throughout Europe brought recognizable depictions of plague buboes into wide circulation. Recently unmasked as

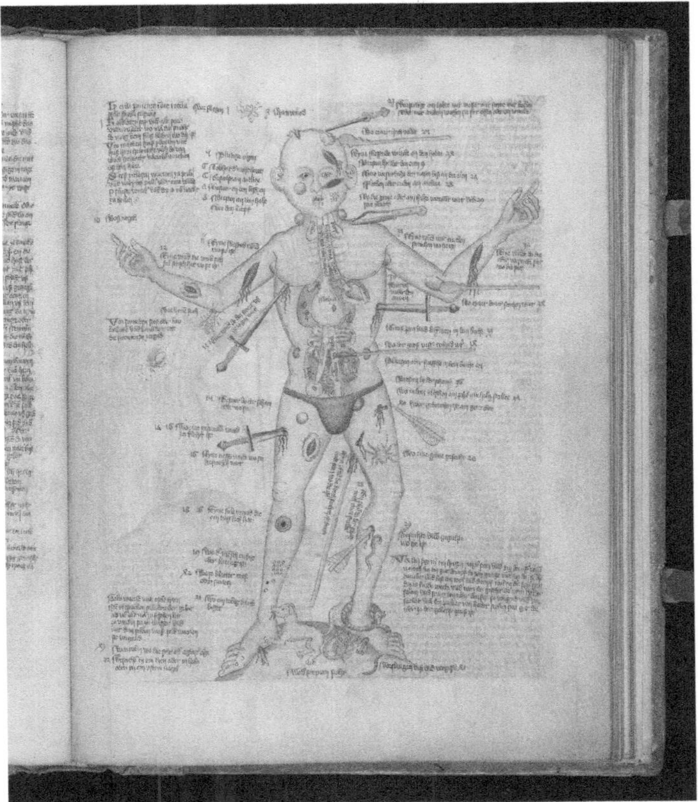

Figure 2.8 South German artist, *Wound Man*, c. 1420–30. One of a set of anatomical drawings in the pictorial encyclopedia known as the Wellcome Apocalypse. London, Wellcome Library, ms. 49, fol. 35r.

Source: Photo: Wellcome Collection. Public Domain Mark.

fictional, Roch owed his appeal to his dual status as both healer and victim of the plague.[32] According to his confected biography, he was a French pilgrim who cured plague victims before himself contracting the disease. Healed by divine fiat, he was imprisoned as a spy and died in prison after being assured by God that his sufferings had merited the reward of intercessory power over the plague. His veneration was thus intensely somatic, defined by and approached through the body of the saint – the actions it performed and the afflictions it endured.

In Italian Renaissance art, Roch's characteristic gesture is the ritualistic presentation of his plague bubo to audiences earthly and heavenly.[33] For worshippers, this must have been an emotionally charged vision of hoped-for protection and cure. On a 1462 pier fresco in the parish church of Volpedo (Figure 2.9), Roch opens his cloak to display his bubo in a calculated act of

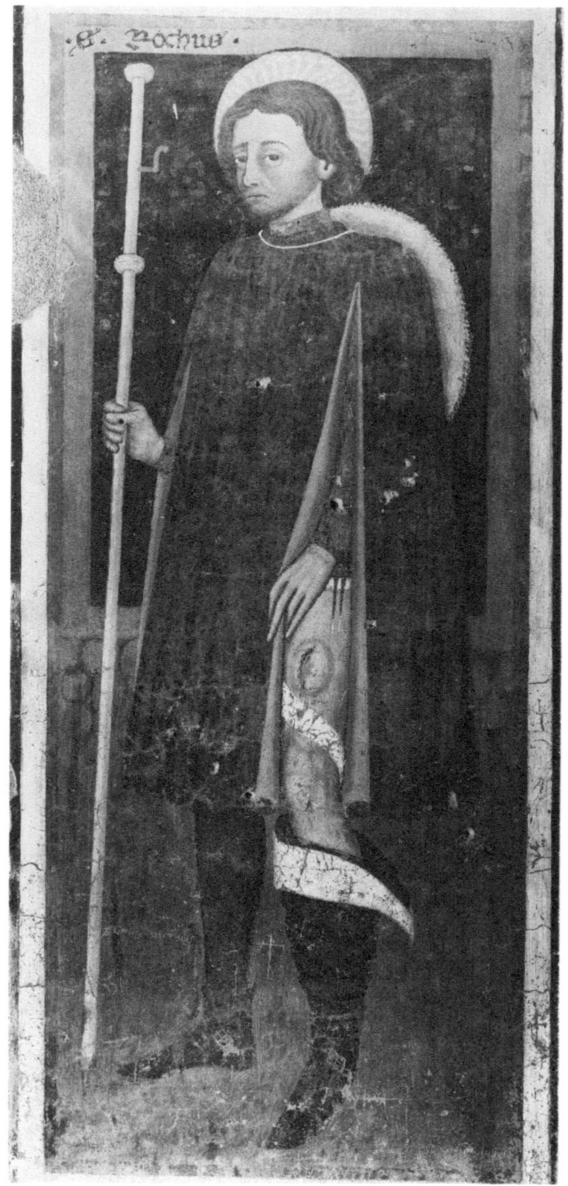

Figure 2.9 Magister Antonio, *St. Roch*, 1462. Pier fresco, S. Pietro, Volpedo.
Source: Photo: Sansoni, Courtesy of the Frick Art Reference Library, New York.

self-revelation. His tunic and a cloth wrapped about his leg frame the bubo like a relic in a reliquary or the host in a monstrance. Bearing the death mark of the plague yet manifestly alive and healthy, the saint triumphs in his own flesh over the very disease threatening his worshippers. Here was tangible proof that one could survive its onslaught. The bubo's poisonous presence draws the eye and stirs the emotions, binding together the similarly marked bodies of the saint and supplicants.

Scenes of Roch's cures, which proliferated throughout Northern and Central Italy from the 1480s on, resonate with a differing dynamic, since they took place before the saint was afflicted with plague (Figure 2.10).[34] Instead, healthy and diseased bodies are inversely mirrored, the saint bringing

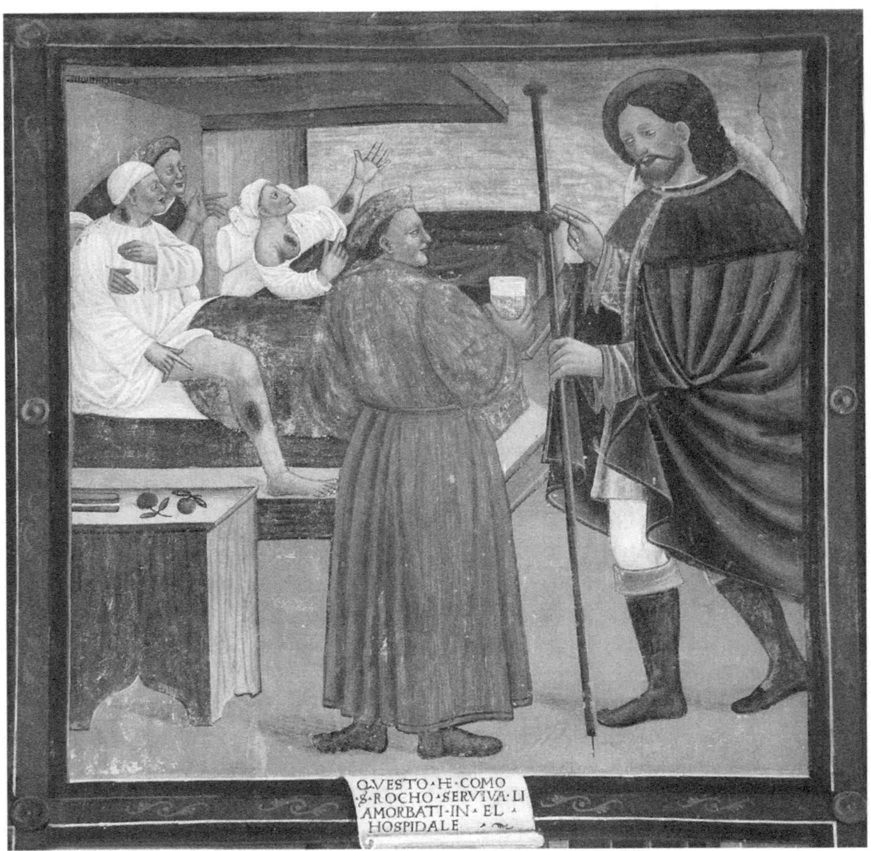

Figure 2.10 Battista da Legnano, *St. Roch Healing Plague Victims*, 1534. Crana, Oratorio di S. Rocco.

Source: Photo by author.

miraculous healing to infected victims whose sufferings predict his own. Contemporaneity of setting – a hospice ward with beds lined neatly against the wall, patients in nightshirts and caps cared for by nurses and supervised by the hospital guardian – confers plausibility for worshippers seeking the same miracle for themselves. Naturalism climaxes in the demonstrative display of patients' buboes. Although not clinically accurate, these are immediately recognizable, magnetizing the gaze as dreaded signs of death imprinted on the bodies of otherwise healthy men, women and children. The pathos of their bared and disfigured flesh calls upon the saint for cure and plays on contemporary familiarity with the disease to celebrate Roch's healing powers.

Yet here, too, representational strategies follow the logic of religious purpose. Thus, Renaissance depictions of plague's most characteristic physical sign both connect and differentiate the bodies of victims and the saint (see Figures 2.9, 2.10). While patients' buboes may be multiple, his is singular; whereas theirs may occur on legs, arms, neck and breasts, his is always on the thigh, gesturing toward but decorously quarantined from groin and genitals. Most notably, while victims' buboes may be painfully swollen or red and inflamed, as in the 1534 fresco by Battista da Legnano, Roch's is most often shown broken open, red and bloody or copiously bleeding. Naturalism combines with a hyperrealism of bodily excess. At Volpedo, the painter carefully detailed the jagged edges of the gaping flesh.

A certain degree of verism is at work, since buboes may spontaneously rupture and discharge a bloody pus. But such messy and distasteful reality is only distantly evoked. Roch's bubo bleeds cleanly, not a stinking sore but an honorable wound. Just like the victims we have seen pictured, Roch was wounded by a deadly heaven-sent arrow (or in one case a sword), as his biographers described.[35] Ardently welcoming the atrocious pain as a means of imitating the sufferings of Christ, he was venerated as a martyr.[36] By its bloodiness, Roch's bubo testifies to his heroic endurance of extraordinary suffering in imitation of Christ, so extreme as to be rewarded with the power to turn aside that suffering from others. Hence the salvific charge of the saint's bubo, displayed before God to sway him from anger to mercy, and shown to viewers as promise of salvation from that selfsame disease. By contrast, victims' buboes are signs of pathos, mortal wounds that will kill them without the saint's curative intervention.

This chapter has analyzed a range of strategies for representing victims of epidemic disease in Italian Renaissance art during the first two centuries after bubonic plague's appearance, from invisibility and displacement to corpses abandoned in doorways and shockingly convincing depictions of supernatural attacks. Renaissance art used the bodies of the dead to represent plague's civic and social desolation. Empathetic seeing endowed the vision of stricken and dying victims with extraordinary psychological and moral force. Specific disease signs were for a century or more after the Black Death not so much disguised as irrelevant to prophylactic purpose. The cult of St. Roch brought recognizable buboes into widespread circulation, but victim and saintly bodies were nonetheless differently configured. Above all, representations of epidemic disease were culturally specific; bodies are variously deployed for affect and impact.

Notes

1 Corey Kilgannon, "As Morgues Fill, N.Y.C. to Bury Some Virus Victims in Potter's Field," *New York Times Online*, April 10, 2020, www.nytimes.com/2020/04/10/nyregion/coronavirus-deaths-hart-island-burial.html.
2 For the history of Hart Island, where more than a million unidentified, unclaimed or otherwise marginalized dead have been buried by prison labor since 1869, see Sally Raudon, "Huddled Masses: The Shock of Hart Island, New York," *Human Remains and Violence: An Interdisciplinary Journal* 8, no. 1 (2022): 84–101; and Diane O'Donoghue, "Last Place: Burying the Dead in Times of Pandemic," *Human Remains and Violence: An Interdisciplinary Journal* 8, no. 2 (2022): 74–93.
3 Excerpted in Rosemary Horrox, trans. and ed., *The Black Death*, Manchester Medieval Sources (Manchester: Manchester University Press, 1994), 33.
4 Jonathan Usher, trans., "Florentine Chronicle of Marchionne di Coppo di Stefano Buonaiuti (1327–1385)," *Decameron Web*, Brown University, accessed February 18, 2010, www.brown.edu/Departments/Italian_Studies/dweb/plague/perspectives/marchionne.php.
5 Brussels, KBR, ms. 13076–77, f. 24v; digital facsimile, https://uurl.kbr.be/2028135. See Pieter-Jan De Grieck, "Li Muisis, Giles," in *Encyclopedia of the Medieval Chronicle Online*, ed. Graeme Dunphy and Cristian Bratu (Leiden: Brill, 2021), http://dx.doi.org/10.1163/2213-2139_emc_SIM_01137. See also Li Muisis's account of the Black Death in Tournai translated in Horrox, *Black Death*, 47–54.
6 Albert D'Haenens, "Pierart dou Tielt, enlumineur des oeuvres de Gilles Li Muisis: Note sur son activité à Tournai vers 1350," *Scriptorium* 23, no. 1 (1969): 88–93.
7 Roger S. Wieck, "The Death Desired: Books of Hours and the Medieval Funeral," in *Death and Dying in the Middle Ages*, ed. Edelgard E. DuBruck and Barbara I. Gusick (New York: Peter Lang, 1999), 437, 439–40.
8 Horrox, *Black Death*, 52.
9 Ibid.
10 Ibid.
11 See the 1348 Pistoia regulations translated in ibid., 194–203.
12 Louise Marshall, "Plague in the City: Identifying the Subject of Giovanni di Paolo's Vienna *Miracle of Saint Nicholas of Tolentino*," *Renaissance Studies* 27, no. 5 (November 2013): 654–80.
13 Louise Marshall, "Manipulating the Sacred: Image and Plague in Renaissance Italy," *Renaissance Quarterly* 47, no. 3 (Autumn 1994): 485–532.
14 For the opposing approach, cf. Sheila Barker, "Picturing the Plague, 1250–1630," in *Plague Image and Imagination from Medieval to Modern Times*, ed. Christopher Lynteris (Cham: Palgrave Macmillan, 2021), 37–67.
15 Both are found in Sercambi's chronicle, discussed below.
16 For Sebastian's cult, see Marshall, "Manipulating the Sacred," 488–500; and Marshall, "Reading the Body of a Plague Saint: Narrative Altarpieces and Devotional Images of St. Sebastian in Renaissance Art," in *Reading Texts and Images: Essays on Medieval and Renaissance Art and Patronage in Honour of Margaret M. Manion*, ed. Bernard J. Muir (Exeter: Exeter University Press, 2002): 237–72.
17 This significantly revises the original miracle, where angel and devil worked together to spread the plague. See Louise Marshall, "The Collaboration from

Hell: A Plague Strike Force in S. Pietro in Vincoli, Rome," in *Religion, the Supernatural and Visual Culture in Early Modern Europe: An Album Amicorum for Charles Zika*, ed. Jennifer Spinks and Dagmar Eichberger (Leiden: Brill, 2015), 19–45. Barker, "Picturing the Plague," 44, misidentifies the demon's weapon as arrows being thrown at the city. However, the long shaft carried over the devil's right shoulder indicates either the hunting spear or mallet described in texts, with which the demon struck house doors at angelic direction to kill those inside.

18 See Louise Marshall, "Coping with the Black Death: Giovanni del Biondo's St Sebastian Altarpiece for Florence Cathedral," in *Trecento Studies: Andrew Ladis Memorial Conference*, ed. Trinita Kennedy and Theresa Flannigan (Turnhout: Brepols, forthcoming).

19 Barker, "Picturing the Plague," 45, misreads this pair as a woman pushing a body out of a house window. Other errors include a nonexistent road down the hill, used to identify the body of the man in pink as a traveler cut down en route. However, since no path is visible and he lies next to the church, his elbow almost grazing the just vacated bier, it might be more plausible to see this corpse as next in line for burial in the churchyard by the gravediggers.

20 Horrox, *Black Death*, 122–24; and Christopher Macklin, "Stability and Change in the Composition of a 'Plague Mass' in the Wake of the Black Death," *Plainsong & Medieval Music* 25, no. 2 (October 2016): 167–89.

21 Horrox, *Black Death*, 16.

22 Ibid., pt. 1, "Narrative Accounts."

23 Wieck, "The Death Desired."

24 Horrox, *Black Death*, 3–8, with many examples. For the relative paucity of such descriptions in medical tracts, see Lori Jones "'Apostumes, Carbuncles, and Botches': Visualizing the Plague in Late Medieval and Early Modern Medical Treatises," in *Disease and Disability in Medieval and Early Modern Art and Literature*, ed. Rinaldo F. Canalis and Massimo Ciavolella (Turnhout: Brepols, 2021), 173–200.

25 Horrox, *Black Death*, 16, 19.

26 Marshall, "Manipulating the Sacred," 515–29; Marshall, "Collaboration from Hell"; and Marshall, "God's Executioners: Angels, Devils and the Plague in Giovanni Sercambi's Illustrated Chronicle," in *Disaster, Death and the Emotions in the Shadow of the Apocalypse, 1400–1700*, ed. Jennifer Spinks and Charles Zika (London: Palgrave Macmillan, 2016): 177–99.

27 For these, see Marshall, "God's Executioners."

28 For the Plague Virgin of Mercy, see Marshall, "Manipulating the Sacred," 506–15; and Marshall, "Affected Bodies and Bodily Affect: Visualising Emotion in Renaissance Plague Images," in *Performing Emotions in Early Europe*, ed. Philippa Maddern, Joanne McEwan, and Anne M. Scott (Turnhout: Brepols, 2018), 90–94.

29 Marshall, "Manipulating the Sacred," 512–16; Stefano Papetti and Sandra Di Provvido, ed., *Pietro Alamanno: Un pittore austriaco nella Marca* (Milan: Motta, 2005), 134–37; and Marshall, "Affected Bodies," 94–95.

30 Marshall, "Affected Bodies," 93n39, 94n40.

31 Jack Hartnell, "Wording the Wound Man," *British Art Studies* 6 (2017), https://doi.org/10.17658/issn.2058-5462/issue-06/jhartnell; and Lori Jones, "Bubo Men? Repurposing Medieval Anatomic Illustrations for Plague Therapy in the Fifteenth and Sixteenth Centuries," in *Death and Disease in the Medieval and Early Modern World: Perspectives from Across the Mediterranean and Beyond*, ed. Jones and Nükhet Varlık (Woodbridge: Boydell & Brewer, 2022), 221–46.

32 Pierre Bolle, "Archival Documents, Early Printed Books, and Manuscripts: The Backwards Text-Tradition of St. Roch 'of Montpellier,'" in *The Saint Between*

Manuscript and Print: Italy, 1400–1600, ed. Alison K. Frazier (Toronto: Centre for Reformation and Renaissance Studies, 2015), 143–82, with earlier bibliography.
33 For Roch's imagery, see Marshall, "Manipulating the Sacred," 500–06; Marshall, "Affected Bodies," 94–98; and Marshall, "St. Roch and the Angel in Renaissance Art," *Studies in Iconography* 41 (2020): 165–211.
34 Louise Marshall, "A New Plague Saint for Renaissance Italy: Suffering and Sanctity in Narrative Cycles of Saint Roch," in *Crossing Cultures: Conflict, Migration, Convergence: Acts of the 32nd Congress of the International Committee of the History of Art*, ed. Jaynie Anderson (Melbourne: Melbourne University Publishing, 2009), 543–49.
35 See critical editions of the fifteenth-century *vite* on the website of the Italian Association of St. Roch of Montpellier (Associazione Italiana San Rocco di Montpellier, "Agiografie," accessed December 1, 2021, www.sanroccodimontpellier.it/2022/12/01/agiografie/).
36 For Roch as martyr, see Marshall, "Manipulating the Sacred," 505.

References

Associazione Italiana San Rocco di Montpellier. "Agiografie." Accessed December 1, 2021. www.sanroccodimontpellier.it/2022/12/01/agiografie/.

Barker, Sheila. "Painting the Plague, 1250–1630." In *Plague Image and Imagination from Medieval to Modern Times*, edited by Christos Lynteris, 37–67. Cham: Palgrave Macmillan, 2021.

Bolle, Pierre. "Archival Documents, Early Printed Books, and Manuscripts: The Backwards Text-Tradition of St. Roch 'of Montpellier.'" In *The Saint Between Manuscript and Print: Italy, 1400–1600*, edited by Alison K. Frazier, 143–82. Toronto: Centre for Reformation and Renaissance Studies, 2015.

De Grieck, Pieter-Jan. "Li Muisis, Giles." In *Encyclopedia of the Medieval Chronicle Online*, edited by Graeme Dunphy and Cristian Bratu. Leiden: Brill, 2021. http://dx.doi.org/10.1163/2213-2139_emc_SIM_01137.

D'Haenens, Albert. "Pierart dou Tielt, enlumineur des oeuvres de Gilles Li Muisis: Note sur son activité à Tournai vers 1350." *Scriptorium* 23, no. 1 (1969): 88–93.

Hartnell, Jack. "Wording the Wound Man." *British Art Studies* 6 (2017). https://doi.org/10.17658/issn.2058-5462/issue-06/jhartnell.

Horrox, Rosemary, trans. and ed. *The Black Death*. Manchester: Manchester University Press; Manchester Medieval Sources, 1994.

Jones, Lori. "'Apostumes, Carbuncles, and Botches': Visualizing the Plague in Late Medieval and Early Modern Medical Treatises." In *Disease and Disability in Medieval and Early Modern Art and Literature*, edited by Rinaldo F. Canalis and Massimo Ciavolella, 173–200. Turnhout: Brepols, 2021.

———. "Bubo Men? Repurposing Medieval Anatomic Illustrations for Plague Therapy in the Fifteenth and Sixteenth Centuries." In *Death and Disease in the Medieval and Early Modern World: Perspectives from Across the Mediterranean and Beyond*, edited by Jones and Nükhet Varlık, 221–46. Woodbridge: Boydell & Brewer, 2022.

Kilgannon, Corey. "As Morgues Fill, N.Y.C. to Bury Some Virus Victims in Potter's Field." *New York Times Online*, April 10, 2020. www.nytimes.com/2020/04/10/nyregion/coronavirus-deaths-hart-island-burial.html.

Macklin, Christopher. "Stability and Change in the Composition of a 'Plague Mass' in the Wake of the Black Death." *Plainsong & Medieval Music* 25, no. 2 (October 2016): 167–89.

Marshall, Louise. "Manipulating the Sacred: Image and Plague in Renaissance Italy." *Renaissance Quarterly* 47, no. 3 (Autumn 1994): 485–532.

———. "Reading the Body of a Plague Saint: Narrative Altarpieces and Devotional Images of St. Sebastian in Renaissance Art." In *Reading Texts and Images: Essays on Medieval and Renaissance Art and Patronage in Honour of Margaret M. Manion*, edited by Bernard J. Muir, 237–72. Exeter: Exeter University Press, 2002.

———. "A New Plague Saint for Renaissance Italy: Suffering and Sanctity in Narrative Cycles of Saint Roch." In *Crossing Cultures: Conflict, Migration, Convergence; Acts of the 32nd Congress of the International Committee of the History of Art*, edited by Jaynie Anderson, 543–49. Melbourne: Melbourne University Publishing, 2009.

———. "Plague in the City: Identifying the Subject of Giovanni di Paolo's Vienna *Miracle of Saint Nicholas of Tolentino*." *Renaissance Studies* 27, no. 5 (November 2013): 654–80.

———. "The Collaboration from Hell: A Plague Strike Force in S. Pietro in Vincoli, Rome." In *Religion, the Supernatural and Visual Culture in Early Modern Europe: An Album Amicorum for Charles Zika*, edited by Jennifer Spinks and Dagmar Eichberger, 19–45. Leiden: Brill, 2015.

———. "God's Executioners: Angels, Devils and the Plague in Giovanni Sercambi's Illustrated *Chronicle*." In *Disaster, Death and the Emotions in the Shadow of the Apocalypse, 1400–1700*, edited by Jennifer Spinks and Charles Zika, 177–99. London: Palgrave Macmillan, 2016.

———. "Affected Bodies and Bodily Affect: Visualising Emotion in Renaissance Plague Images." In *Performing Emotions in Early Europe*, edited by Philippa Maddern, Joanne McEwan and Anne M. Scott, 73–106. Turnhout: Brepols, 2018.

———. "St. Roch and the Angel in Renaissance Art." *Studies in Iconography* 41 (2020): 165–211.

———. "Coping with the Black Death: Giovanni del Biondo's St Sebastian Altarpiece for Florence Cathedral." In *Trecento Studies: Andrew Ladis Memorial Conference*, edited by Trinita Kennedy and Theresa Flannigan. Turnhout: Brepols, forthcoming.

O'Donoghue, Diane. "Last Place: Burying the Dead in Times of Pandemic." *Human Remains and Violence: An Interdisciplinary Journal* 8, no. 2 (2022): 74–93.

Papetti, Stefano, and Sandra Di Provvido, eds. *Pietro Alamanno: Un pittore austriaco nella Marca*. Milan: Motta, 2005.

Raudon, Sally. "Huddled Masses: The Shock of Hart Island, New York." *Human Remains and Violence: An Interdisciplinary Journal* 8, no. 1 (2022): 84–101.

Usher, Jonathan, trans. "Florentine Chronicle of Marchionne di Coppo di Stefano Buonaiuti (1327–1385)." *Decameron Web, Brown University*. Accessed February 18, 2010. www.brown.edu/Departments/Italian_Studies/dweb/plague/perspectives/marchionne.php.

Wieck, Roger S. "The Death Desired: Books of Hours and the Medieval Funeral." In *Death and Dying in the Middle Ages*, edited by Edelgard E. DuBruck and Barbara I. Gusick, 431–76. New York: Peter Lang, 1999.

3 Experiencing Transnational Health Challenges

The Safety/Commerce Dilemma in Italy's Long Nineteenth Century

Arianna Arisi Rota

> He took no precautions against the pestilence; he caught it, and died, like Metastasio's hero, complaining of the stars.
> – Alessandro Manzoni, *The Betrothed*, chapter 36

Like the seventeenth-century Milan of Alessandro Manzoni's masterpiece *The Betrothed*, in which Don Ferrante stubbornly denied the existence of the plague to the point of death, the long nineteenth century also had its advocates for the nonexistence of contagion. Flagellated by several waves of cholera, the Mediterranean region proved particularly fragile in the face of a disease whose biological origin and geographical directions were still being studied.[1] Contemporaneously, in a Europe shocked by the French Revolution and Napoleon, its most disruptive product, the metaphor of contagion was being applied to the spread of liberalism by conservatives and reactionaries alike.[2] Against this political plague of transnational scope, government authorities, legitimists and policemen called for the adoption of ideological and institutional sanitary cordons. In those same decades, sanitary cordons as public health measures ended up at the center of a heated debate in the embryonic community of experts.

Because of its geographical location in the center of the Mediterranean and the strategic nature of its ports, the Italian peninsula suffered every nineteenth-century wave of cholera epidemics. This led the country to preserve memories of the plague of the modern age and to deal with the persistence of popular beliefs and superstitions that medical science could not erase.[3] Individual states of Italy's fragmented political checkerboard participated in the first attempts at international coordination on public health and the fight against epidemics. Doctors and consuls discussed preventive measures in an emergent culture of containing health crises originating from outside, divided between the defense of public health and the reasons of commerce that required protection in turn. From the 1830s until the first international health conference in Paris in 1851 and the subsequent multilateral meetings on public health, the scientific community made progress that often did not find adequate responses in the politics and society of a by now unified

DOI: 10.4324/9781003382805-3

Italy. This took place perhaps only after the epidemic wave of 1867 showed a greater awareness of Europe's interdependence in coping with health crises, as evidenced, for example, by parliamentary debates.[4] However, this did not prevent the fact that when facing the test of yet another epidemic in 1910–11, Italy could not resist the temptation to conceal the alarming extent and numbers of the contagion amidst its half-century celebrations of national independence and preparations for launching its longed-for colonial conquest of Libya.[5]

In the following pages, I will analyze the dilemma between the demands for public safety, on the one hand, and those for ensuring the success of economy and commerce, on the other, as they developed in the long term. I will contend that this dilemma was the main reason why local and central governments tended to minimize or even deny the existence of epidemic outbreaks. I will give voice to the isolated critics who on various occasions spoke out against the contradictions and hypocrisy of politicians, arguing that priority should always and without exception be given to safeguarding public health.

Contagionists versus Localists

Europe's cholera wave of 1830 – which arrived from the Southern coast of the Caspian Sea and rose northward, reaching Poland and central Europe via Moscow – struck France with particular ferocity between 1831 and 1832. In Paris alone, 44,119 victims were recorded out of a population of 785,862, causing hysteria and massive flights from the capital. In Italy, cholera peaked in 1835.[6,7] Between July and August, it reached Genoa by sea from Marseilles and overland by smugglers from Provence to Piedmont. From there, the contagion penetrated the Kingdom of Lombardy-Venetia and moved on to Central Italy, also through the ports of Leghorn and Ancona, and thence to Puglia, Naples and Sicily, causing almost 150,000 deaths in the three-year period from 1835 to 1837, of which 5,000 were in Rome alone.[8] This first experience of a contagion domino effect left a deep trace in the minds of Italy's healthcare personnel, who in the following years made themselves heard in the debate on the disease and on containment and prevention measures. At the same time, scientific research made significant though undervalued progress thanks to the pioneering microscope observations of Filippo Pacini, an Italian pathologist from Pistoia, who succeeded in identifying the vibrio pathogen of Asian cholera, which was isolated in Calcutta decades later, bringing fame to the German microbiologist Robert Koch.

The late recognition of Pacini's discovery was only one of the outcomes of the persistent uncertainty of the Italian and European scientific environment. This community was divided between the so-called contagionists, who were convinced that the disease was transmitted from person to person, and the localists, whose orientation, which emerged in the 1850s, attributed the infectious agent to the structural conditions of individual cholera-ridden localities, fertile for its development. While the contagionists pressed for the adoption of sanitary cordons, quarantines, inspections on land and by sea of ships, lazarets, disinfection centers and more, the localists left "commerce free" and sought "first of all to make the large localities resistant to cholera, as they are the main points of commerce."[9] The two theories resulted in a conflict between the lockdown measures supported by the contagionists and intervention at the source of the problem advocated by the localists, among whom the German physiologist and hygienist Max von Pettenkofer became a leading exponent. According to him, "in Europe since 1830 billions have been sacrificed to this contagionist theory, without achieving anything."[10] For their part, the contagionists defended themselves by arguing that governments should not implement what were deemed the outmoded measures of completely blocking the movement of people and things, but rather targeted measures, such as "isolating the sick, limiting the outbreaks of infection, impeding the useless and excessive agglomerations of people, and adopting a series of hygienic practices."[11]

This debate, which went on for decades inside and outside of Italy, was fueled by the political problem of reconciling the protection of public safety with the freedom of universal commerce. This is what Agostino Cappello, the Papal State's delegate to the first international health conference held in Paris from July 1851 to January 1852, wrote in one of his pamphlets. For Cappello, adviser emeritus of the Supreme Roman Magistrate of Health, the experience of 1836 had been illuminating. To prevent the spread of cholera from Lombardy-Venetia and Trieste, the traditional Senigallia fair was forbidden in the Papal States, but "since this measure undermined commerce," the fair of Ancona was instead authorized. "I opposed this measure," the councilor recalled, adding that while in that instance trade had prospered, so did cholera.[12] The awareness of doctors like Cappello was shared by experts from other Italian states, such as the Grand Duchy of Tuscany and the Kingdom of the Two Sicilies, while the Kingdom of Sardinia aligned itself with the British position, opposed to the system of quarantines and blockade of goods in its ports: "This disease is not contagious at all," Anthony Perrier, consul in Brest and British delegate to the second health conference in Paris, could still maintain in 1859, adding that "the development of European railway networks in the meantime today renders illusory any system of quarantine against arrivals by sea from cholera-infected places."[13]

The surgeon Pietro Betti, the Tuscan delegate in Paris, was Perrier's opponent and therefore Cappello's ally. From his experience as director of the hospitals of the Grand Duchy and especially in the vulnerable port city of Leghorn, Betti defended the contagion theory. He favored targeted measures – even preventive ones – while recognizing that generalized sanitary cordons had proven ineffective because the population evaded them, and it was only activities and businesses that could be effectively blocked.[14] In short, in the latter half of the nineteenth century, this so to speak intermediate position between the two schools of thought sought to avoid the episodic, drastic measures typical of emergencies and of past centuries. But it also stressed the reluctance of governments to incur the damage that such measures caused to trade and human traffic in an increasingly connected European and Mediterranean space.

1867: A New Awareness?

Doctors specialized in epidemiology themselves often misunderstood the true seriousness of an epidemic, much less the population and local authorities. In August 1867, when a new wave of cholera aggravated by the summer climate was claiming victims from Northern to Southern Italy, a citizen of Pavia commented, "unfortunately this is almost always the case with the first invasion of contagious or epidemic diseases: first disbelief, then doubt. Lastly dismay."[15] Moreover, there had been outbreaks of the disease since the summer of 1865 in Egypt, Malta and later in Smyrna, to the point that some local administrations took several precautionary measures without fully committing themselves to prevention. One documented instance is that of Bergamo, in Lombardy, where some suspicious cases that appeared in the port city of Ancona caused "apprehension, albeit very remote and for now without any other foundation."[16] But it was the exchange of prisoners at the end of the 1866 war that brought cholera to the city in autumn, without doctors immediately recognizing the nature of the disease. Only after numerous cases, and under pressure from the city administration, "finally on November 9th the doctors decreed that 'cholera was in Bergamo.' "[17] Hence a belated decision, after hesitations and denials, that would be repeated during the wave of 1867, to the point that on May 31 the mayor, Giovanni Battista Camozzi Vertova, was so distressed that he wrote in his diary: "usual questions between doctors, disgusting matters at any time but even more disgusting with these poor sanitary conditions currently pouring into our city."[18] In this case, it was the mayor who urged transparency and speedy intervention, going so far as to use the economic incentive of a salary increase to motivate the doctors who were dealing with cholera. In 1869, Mayor Camozzi summed up the genesis of that tragedy as follows: "The uncertainties of the first cases came from the doctors, who were the technicians whose duty it was to ascertain its reality."[19] The city administration had to be careful in pronouncing the word "cholera" so as not to trigger panic, while "those who should have spoken plainly were the doctors, and the doctors only spoke when I forced them to."[20]

Not all mayors, however, were equal to the unusual task of directing and pressuring the local health machine, and the behavior of the inhabitants often contributed to delays in diagnosis and the activation of containment measures.[21] The reconstruction by Ermenegildo de' Cinque Quintili, general secretary of Rome's hospital commission, of what happened in the Latium countryside between August and September 1867 is a merciless account of how the fear of losing the summer vacationers led to concealing reality. This happened, for example, in Albano (population 3,500), which in the 39 days of the epidemic's peak recorded 677 cases and 443 deaths, with the cases passing from 2 to 63 in just a few hours. As the doctor explained, the inhabitants had concealed some cases "for fear of losing the revenue largely drawn from the unusual number of vacationers there."[22] Once the news spread that Albano was stricken by cholera, all the neighboring villages shut down in complete isolation, even under the protection of armed men, prohibiting any contact with people and objects from the infected locality. Those sanitary cordons, however, also combined with prophylaxis measures, had worked. It was a "new and effective test of the isolation system,"[23] which in truth had already been successfully practiced during the plagues of the mid-seventeenth century. The author of the pamphlet was therefore able to comment that it was not a matter of reintroducing a severity that could seem "excessive and even barbaric" in a progressive age like the nineteenth century, "of a milder civilization," but rather that it was necessary to learn the lesson of a past in which the legislators had put "the safety of the greatest number of citizens before any other consideration,"[24] and had achieved it.

The experience of another health supervisor regarding the situation in Voghera in Lombardy seemed to confirm how the lessons of the past could still repel the new epidemic scourge by reinstating the checks and quarantines so abhorred by the champions of free trade. At the same time, the health supervisor did not deny "the commercial needs, the needs of freedom of movement, the political exigencies"[25] that opposed the idea of a by now culturally unacceptable continental block. In addition to the emerging awareness of the need to reconcile market needs with those of public health, the various accounts of that epidemic wave tell of persistent popular superstitions and conspiracy theories at the local level, as well as a bungling generically attributed to the state. This is what emerges from various kinds of sources, such as Edmondo De Amicis's text *L'esercito italiano durante il coléra del 1867*,[26] an account of the Sicilian campaign in which the writer had served, or from the diary of the opposition parliamentarian Giorgio Asproni, who, on September 4, 1867, noted that according to "popular opinion," cholera was "caused by poisons, and this prejudice is the high price paid by the many who are killed, especially in Calabria, in the fury of the people."[27]

"So Everything Becomes Paralyzed"

In 1869, yet another wave of cholera gave new strength in Europe to those who contested the lockdown system, and in particular the quarantines in ports, the real target of the British government's strategy. The reports of the Privy Council's medical officer, published in 1875, were forthright in defining that instrument as "a mere irrational derangement of commerce," which at the continental level in 1865 had proved "utterly futile."[28] The real enemy, he seemed to feel, was the delay with which the various affected areas admitted the existence of outbreaks, thus allowing the contagion to spread to other locations in the meantime, in a lethal domino effect in the Mediterranean:

> Before Alexandria admitted to being infected, it had infected Marseilles; and through Marseilles it infected the rest of France. Then, before Marseilles admitted to being infected, Valencia had received a most disastrous infection from throughout it; and from Valencia all Spain was infected. . … Italy received its infection through the quarantine establishment of Ancona; which both infected the town of Ancona by sending infected things to be washed there, and also allowed an undiscovered case of cholera to pass on from its lazaret, after six days of detention, to infect the town of Pisa.[29]

Such a chain of contagion proved that only through joint international action, such as the one already called for at the 1866 Constantinople Sanitary Conference, could states block the spread of the disease from Asia by organizing a quarantine at the mouth of the Red Sea.[30] However, the measures taken in no particular order during the emergencies endured by individual European countries, joined by the United States, continued to hinder any coordinated policy. Once again, in the summer of 1875, during a debate in the Italian parliament, an opposition deputy, the Sardinian Salvatore Parpaglia, recalled that since the Paris Convention of 1852 left the powers free to establish quarantines or not, "it happened that Italy imposed quarantines, and France did not admit them, *because it was more concerned with trade than with the lives of its citizens.*"[31] In a political climate that was increasingly hostile to France – "this power, which is our closest rival"[32] – it was now clear that the contradictory attitudes of some governments ended up damaging everyone. As the parliamentarian recalled, there was no middle ground: "you must either apply quaratines seriously or be done with them, because if they are to be at all useful, it means total isolation."[33] And he went on: "I deem that quarantines, that precautions are not serious, that they are useless precautions that cost too much to commerce and are not beneficial to public health, and are reduced to a real hypocrisy, which a constitutional government should avoid."[34] The hypocrisy of governments arose from the dilemma of squaring the circle between defense of public health and defense of trade, which is the main point of this chapter. The blockage of goods in the lazarets, again the opinion that parliamentarian Parpaglia defended, caused serious damage: "So everything becomes paralyzed,"[35] while other vectors of contagion, such as dirty, tattered paper currency, circulated undisturbed.

After all, the Europe of the last decades of the nineteenth century was one now connected with the Red Sea as well as the Indian and Pacific Oceans thanks to the Suez Canal (opened in 1869). The first wave of emigration to the Americas posed new challenges to the policy of controls that were carried out in the ports of arrival, with medical inspections only conducted on clearly infected subjects, while asymptomatic individuals were allowed to freely circulate. Migrations and religious pilgrimages, such as those to and from Mecca, as well as the flow of goods, were now unstoppable. It was unthinkable "to immobilize the great tides of human life which convey it,"[36] as the health consultant of the English Privy Council noted with evident concern about the ability of epidemics to radiate from the Indian subcontinent. In short, restrictions on international traffic appeared ineffectual and even harmful, while it was prevention that took the brunt of curtailment to ensure more lasting results.

Progress and Hypocrisy between the Two Centuries

The public health/commerce dilemma did not disappear at the dawn of the "bacteriological era."[37] The scientific progress that at last paid tribute to Pacini's discoveries also embraced the opinions of Koch, the German delegate to the Venice health conference in 1892, where he defended his theory of overland rather than seaborne contagion. It was a theory confirmed by the epidemic wave of 1893, which arrived from Afghanistan via Persia and Baku, reached Moscow and St. Petersburg, and from there Paris and Hamburg, but which did not prevent the Dresden health conference held that same year from languishing without producing any useful results, with many countries, including Italy, being represented only by diplomatic delegates and not by medical experts.[38] In the 1880s, yellow fever, another invisible enemy, had raised concern above all over ships coming from the United States, while between 1889 and 1890 a wave of so-called Russian flu had hit Europe and in particular France. Here the warning signs of 1889 were denied or ignored, with authoritative experts such as Adrien Proust and Paul Brouardel attributing the disease to the winter season, while the press claimed the truth rather than doses of official line of optimism.[39]

In Italy, meanwhile, a generation of doctors working in the public health sector called attention to the fact that cholera was not the only problem.[40] In 1873, the Roman doctor Carlo Maggiorani asked to draft a bill for the Health Code in the Senate, painting a gloomy picture of the diseases that afflicted Italians: tuberculosis, scrofula, pellagra and syphilis circulated among the citizenry and the armed forces alike, while exotic infections spread easily: "smallpox raises its head; diphtheria increases daily."[41] To all this, malaria needed to be added.[42] It is therefore not surprising that at the beginning of the 1890s a pioneer in popular education on malaria such as the hygienist Angelo Celli felt dutybound to recall in parliament "the carnage caused by infectious diseases, with their more than 300,000 victims yearly, which could and should be saved."[43] According to the physician-parliamentarian, the hypocrisy of the medical establishment itself had favored what he called the doubletalk then prevalent in diagnoses to conceal infectious diseases, such as scarlet fever, in order to avoid the fines of up to 500 lire charged to those who failed to report them.

In 1896, Ferruccio Mercanti, a leading scientist and senator of the Kingdom of Italy, could still declare: "As for infectious diseases . . . in Italy there is only one disease that concerns us,"[44] namely cholera, which since 1865 had claimed 214,631 victims, while tuberculosis in just six years had claimed 341,410, almost 60,000 a year. Hence, while much had been done to combat cholera, "nothing has been done to combat the other [diseases] that plague us at home and cause so much carnage and so much ruin."[45] At the turn of the century, another voice denouncing invisible diseases, or those forgotten by politics, was Ausonio Zubiani's. He was a tisiologist and socialist from Valtellina who was engaged in the fight against tuberculosis, which he also considered to be a fight against poverty. Zubiani maintained that there were two kinds of tuberculosis: that of the rich, which sometimes healed, and that of the poor, which never healed. It is to him that we owe the first Italian sanatorium for patients with chest diseases, built in the pine forest of Sortenna above Sondalo in the early twentieth century.

Yet it was precisely cholera that came back to challenge the rationale of politics and trade. The sickness reappeared in Naples in the summer of 1910 after the severe epidemic of 1884, which had caused about 6,000 victims, two-thirds of the total Italian number. Among the first to perceive the seriousness of the situation was the American doctor Henry Downes Geddings, an official of the public health service, as well as an expert on yellow fever and a former American delegate to international health conferences. Geddings promptly communicated his assessments to his superiors in Rome but encountered a wall of resistance and denial. It was not cholera, they replied, but an unspecified Neapolitan fever, or Maltese fever. However, Geddings considered it his duty to warn the authorities in Washington of what the historian of medicine Frank M. Snowden has defined as "the secret epidemic."[46] The conspiracy of silence found its exponents at both the local and national level. In the month of June, the port workers of Naples, fearful of harmful closures, had already protested, putting pressure on the municipal government, which deluded itself into thinking it could control the epidemic before news of it reached outside the city. In the capital, Giovanni Giolitti's government, concerned about holding consensus against restrictive measures, declared an end to the epidemic as early as the fall. But that hasty move apparently did not convince everyone. On December 17 in the Chamber of Deputies, the parliamentarian Enrico De Nicola summoned the Minister of the Interior for questioning. De Nicola revealed the contradiction of travelers arriving from Naples to the Rome railway station, where they were subjected to sanitary measures, while the General Directorate of Health insisted on denying "absolutely the existence of an epidemic in the great Southern city."[47]

Fear of economic damage and a negative reaction from public opinion thus contributed to weaving a web of lies and contradictions. And as if that were not enough, in order to minimize the crisis that the nation was experiencing, the Statistics Office at the time directed by Giovanni Raineri only counted the victims whose cases had been "bacteriologically" confirmed by laboratory tests. This occurred while, as Snowden writes, "in all previous epidemics of Asiatic cholera in Italy, deaths were recorded on the basis of diagnoses provided by attending physicians or coroners."[48] The Italian state was thus only able to report 805 deaths in 1910 and 6,145 in 1911, while the number of victims was probably much higher. A further obstacle to a reliable picture of the emergency were the deliberately erroneous diagnoses demanded of doctors by the patients themselves, terrified of being quarantined against their will in hospitals. But the state also played its part in misdiagnoses. Snowden's judgment makes no concessions:

> Italy in 1911 is the only known example in which a Western nation succeeded both in concealing a substantial and widespread epidemic of the disease from its population during its course and in subsequently misleading posterity with regard to its magnitude and significance.[49]

Italy enforced a ban on medical knowledge and opposed any requests for transparency from abroad, such as those requested by America and France (the United States had a consulate in Naples, while France was engaged in protecting its Mediterranean ports). By doing so, Italy attempted to avoid fully applying the recommendations of the 1903 Sanitary Convention of Paris. But in the end, both the American Surgeon General and the French Public Service could not adequately protect their citizens who were traveling to Italy. Another isolated warning voice besides Geddings's was Surgeon General Walter Wyman, who only privately advised his correspondents to cancel their plans to visit the Italian peninsula.

Conclusion

The year 1911 was involved in celebrating the fiftieth anniversary of Italian Unity (called the *Giubileo della Patria*), with a big display of Italian grandeur in several cities, such as the three historical capital cities of Turin, Florence and Rome. This propaganda machinery obviously could not be compromised by a medical emergency and by such a cruel disease which, according to Professor Rocco Santoliquido, the Italian Director General of Public Health, delegate to the Paris Sanitary Conference of 1903, was now worse than the plague itself and struck the population with a kind of "atavistic terror."[50] This scenario explains the role played in that same year by some avant-garde literary magazines, such as the Florentine *La Voce*, which denounced the "great national lie" (*bugia nazionale*),[51] which the Jubilee efforts had concocted to promote the image of a united Italy both at home and abroad. On the contrary, the farcical Jubilee puppet show, (*la burattinata del cinquantenario*, as *La Voce* labeled it), was just a mask meant to hide a profoundly divided country: "The Two Italies" (*Le due Italie*), as Giustino Fortunato called it in his article on the Southern question published in *La Voce*'s special issue of March 16, 1911.[52]

In such a framework, a cholera-free Italy was therefore the hypocritical result of a political propaganda effort aimed at fighting medical truth by labeling it as sanitary defeatism. By this, it meant a kind of antipatriotic attitude that was banished from the official press and documents in the very year in which the country was coming of age, taking on its colonial military enterprise with the war for the conquest of Libya. During those same days, the Italian poet Giovanni Pascoli opened his public address in Barga on November 26, 1911, supporting the military expedition to Lybia, with the sentence: "The great proletariat has set itself in motion" (*La grande proletaria si è mossa*). Italy, the great proletarian nation, was now walking on its own legs and claiming for its children a land on the shore of its *Mare Nostrum*, the Mediterranean. According to the image chosen for the cover of the publication of his address, there, in a deserted land, the tools for colonization – shovels and picks – were waiting, wrapped in a national flag, for the Italian migrants to take up with their energies and vigor. Now more than ever, no space was left for talking about diseases and weaknesses.

As I have reconstructed in this chapter, minimizing if not outright denying the reality of contagions had been an early temptation for nineteenth-century Italy, particularly exposed through its ports, above all to the epidemic waves of cholera. The medical establishment, as a major interlocutor of international debate and scientific progress in the midcentury decades, attempted to contribute to preventing subsequent emergencies by relying on empirical data. Yet, as demonstrated in the devastating epidemic of 1867, hesitations and reticence prevailed, thus delaying the adoption of measures capable of containing the contagion in many areas. The economic interests linked to commerce and the increasingly connected human flow throughout the Mediterranean and Europe, which were evident to many doctors, often prevailed over concerns for public safety, delaying or attenuating institutional interventions. Moreover, the attention of the scientific community and the governing class was monopolized by cholera, leading the two sides to marginalize, when not ignoring, other infectious diseases that still affected the Italian population at the end of the century – a long list of illnesses that were denounced by those parliamentarian doctors who were sensitive to public health as a social issue.

However, it should not be forgotten that the lesson of the epidemics of the long nineteenth century was twofold: on the one hand, it increased efforts for international coordination on the subject of health emergencies, resulting in the creation of the International Health Office in Paris; on the other hand, it did not prevent the recurrence of egotism and national shortsightedness when the terrible typhus and so-called Spanish flu epidemics struck Europe as yet another human holocaust of the First World War.[53]

Notes

Epigraph: Alessandro Manzoni, *The Betrothed*, trans. Count O'Mahony (London, Bell and Bradfute, 1834), accessed December 11, 2022, www.gutenberg.org/files/35155/35155-h/35155-h.htm.

1 For an updated historiographic review on the topic of epidemics in the Mediterranean, see Benoît Pouget, "La Méditerranée et les grandes épidémies: Retour sur un demi-siècle de travaux historiques," *Cahiers de la Méditerranée* 103 (2021): 173–89, https://doi.org/10.4000/cdlm.15133.

   See also Benoît Pouget, *Un choc de circulations: La puissance navale française face au choléra en Méditerranée, 1831–1856* (Rennes: Presses Universitaires de Rennes, 2020).

2 On disease and infectious disease as a metaphor, see Susan Sontag's pioneering book, *Illness as Metaphor* (New York: Ferrar, Straus and Giroux, 1978); and Cynthia J. Davis, "Contagion as Metaphor," *American Literary History* 14, no. 4 (Winter 2002): 828–36. For its biopolitical aspects, see Emmanuel Betta, "Pandemia come metafora?" *Contemporanea: Rivista di storia dell'800 e del'900* 23, no. 4 (2020): 681–97.

3 Richard J. Evans, "Epidemics and Revolutions: Cholera in Nineteenth-Century Europe," *Past & Present* 120 (August 1988): 123–46, https://doi.org/10.1093/past/120.1.123.

4 On this topic, see Arianna Arisi Rota, "Prove di *Health Diplomacy*: Le conferenze sanitarie internazionali della seconda metà dell'Ottocento e il ruolo dei delegati italiani," in *Le istituzioni e le idee: Studi indisciplinati offerti a Fabio Rugge per il suo settantesimo compleanno*, ed. Elisabetta Colombo (Milan: Giuffré, 2022), 57–64, esp. 57 n3.

5 Frank M. Snowden, *Naples in the Time of Cholera, 1884–1911* (Cambridge: Cambridge University Press, 1995).

6 On the history of epidemics in nineteenth-century Russia, see Charlotte E. Henze, *Disease, Health Care and Government in Late Imperial Russia: Life and Death on the Volga, 1823–1914* (London: Routledge, 2011).

7 Norman Howard-Jones, *The Scientific Background of the International Sanitary Conferences, 1851–1938* (Geneva: World Health Organization, 1975), 18.

8 Giorgio Cosmacini, *Storia della medicina e della sanità in Italia: Dalla peste nera ai giorni nostri* (Rome: Laterza, 2010), chap. 1, pt. 3. See also Anna Lucia Forti Messina, "L'Italia dell'Ottocento di fronte al colera," in *Storia d'Italia*, vol. 7, *Malattia e medicina*, ed. Franco Della Peruta (Turin: Einaudi, 1984), 429–94.

9 See Alex Chase-Levenson, *The Yellow Flag: Quarantine and the British Mediterranean World, 1780–1860* (Cambridge: Cambridge University Press, 2020). See also Achille Spatuzzi, "La teoria di Max von Pettenkofer sul colera e le epidemie del 1873 e del 1884 in Napoli," *Il Morgagni: Giornale indirizzato al progresso della Medicina* 27 (1885): 138.

10 Spatuzzi, "La teoria di Max von Pettenkofer," 138.

11 *Giornale della Regia Accademia di Medicina di Torino*, 3rd ser., vol. 30, no. 3 (Turin: Regia Accademia di Medicina di Torino), 309.

12 Agostino Cappello, *Sul Sanitario Congresso Internazionale aperto a Parigi nel dì 23 luglio 1851 e chiuso nel dì 19 gennaio 1852: Cenni storici di Agostino Cappello, membro del medesimo e consigliere emerito del Supremo Romano Magistrato di Sanità* (Rome: Tipografia delle Belle Arti, 1852), 11. For a background analysis dedicated to the Papal States, see also Francesco Bartolini, "Salute pubblica e sicurezza dello stato: Il governo pontificio alle soglie della modernità biologica ottocentesca," *Contemporanea: Rivista di storia dell' 800 e del '900* 26, no. 1 (2023): 3–29.

13 Quoted in Jones, *The Scientific Background*, 20.

14 Martina Starnini, *L'uomo tutto intero: Biografia di Carlo Livi, psichiatra dell'Ottocento* (Florence: Firenze University Press, 2018), 91.

15 Giovanni Maria Bussedi, *Diario, 1864–1869*, ed. Mirko Volpi (Milan: Cisalpino, 2013), 150–51.

16 *Relazione amministrativa sulla invasione del cholera in Bergamo negli anni 1866 e 1867* (Bergamo: Tipografia Pagnoncelli, 1868), 20. On the situation in Ancona, see Andrea Pongetti, *Società e colera nell'Italia del XIX secolo: L'epidemia di Ancona del 1865–67* (Milan: Codex, 2009).

17 Fabrizio Costantini, *Dalle insurrezioni alle istituzioni: Giovanni Battista Camozzi Vertova a Bergamo tra 1848 e 1871* (Bergamo: Lubrina Bramani Editore, 2021), 98–99.

18 Ibid., 99n294.

19 Ibid., 104.

20 Ibid. In united Italy, municipal doctors were paid by the towns. The situation in Bergamo and its surroundings leads us to recall how in the COVID-19 pandemic the outbreak in Val Seriana ended up causing 6,000 deaths, making Bergamo the area where the containment machine dramatically jammed because of what journalists have defined as errors, omissions and underestimations. See, for example, Marco Imarisio, Simona Ravizza and Fiorenza Sarzanini, *Come nasce un'epidemia: La strage di Bergamo. Il focolaio più micidiale d'Europa* (Milan: Rizzoli, 2020).

21 Eugenia Tognotti, *Il mostro asiatico: Storia del colera in Italia* (Rome: Laterza, 2000), 231. See also Tognotti, "Storia dell'arrivo del colera negli anni Trenta dell'Ottocento: Lo shock e la cesura tra il 'prima' e il 'dopo,'" *Storicamente* 17, no. 15 (2021), https://doi.org/10.52056/9788833138732/15.

22 Ermenegildo de' Cinque Quintili, *Il colera di Albano nel 1867: Lettera di Ermenegildo de' Cinque Quintili al chiarissmo dottor Guglielmo Farr* (Rome: Tipografia Menicanti, 1869), 10–11.

23 Ibid., 13.

24 Ibid.

25 Giuseppe Poggi, *Il colera indico in Voghera nel 1867* (Voghera: Tipografia Giuseppe Gatti, 1868), 34. Poggi was a contagionist who supported isolation measures. He had deduced that in the area of Voghera the disease had been imported by gleaners, i.e., seasonal workers who arrived from the surroundings of Bergamo.

26 Edmondo De Amicis, *L'esercito italiano durante il coléra del 1867* (Milan: Bernardoni, 1869).

27 Giorgio Asproni, *Diario politico, 1855–1876*, vol. 4, *1864–1867*, ed. Tito Orrù (Milan: Giuffré, 1980), September 4, 1867.

28 *Reports of the Medical Officer of the Privy Council and Local Government Board*, n.s., vol. 5 (London: Her Majesty's Stationery Office, 1875), 6.

29 Ibid., 6–7.

30 Ibid., 7.

31 *Atti parlamentari, Camera dei Deputati, XII Legislatura, Sessione del 1874–75, Discussioni*, vol. 2 (Rome: Tipografia della Camera dei Deputati, 1875), February 17, session of 1875, 1373 (emphasis added).

32 Ibid., 1374.

33 Ibid.

34 Ibid., 1375.

35 Ibid.

36 *Reports of the Medical Officer*, 8.

37 Jones, *The Scientific Background*, 46.

38 Richard J. Evans, *Death in Hamburg: Society and Politics in the Cholera Years, 1830–1910* (Oxford: Oxford University Press, 1987).
39 Frédéric Vagneron, "Quand revient la grippe: Élaboration et circulation des alertes lors des grippes 'russe' et 'espagnole' en France (1889–1919)," *Parlement(s): Revue d'histoire politique* 25 (2017): 64–65.
40 On the health policies of united Italy, see Roberto Cea, *Il governo della salute nell'Italia liberale: Stato, igiene e politiche sanitarie* (Milan: FrancoAngeli, 2019).
41 *Rendiconti del Parlamento italiano, Discussioni del Senato del Regno, XI Legislatura, Sessione del 1871–72*, vol. 2 (Rome: Tipografia del Senato del Regno, 1873), 1895. See also Claudio Canonici and Giuseppe Monsagrati, eds., *Carlo Maggiorani: Politica e medicina nel Risorgimento* (Rome: Gangemi, 2004).
42 On the topic in English, see Frank M. Snowden, *The Conquest of Malaria: Italy, 1900–1962* (New Haven, CT: Yale University Press, 2006); for the Italian translation, see Snowden, *La conquista della malaria: una modernizzazione italiana, 1900–1962*, trans. Valentina Besi and Cinzia Di Barbara (Turin: Einaudi, 2008).
43 *Atti Parlamentari, Camera dei Deputati, XVIII Legislatura, Sessione del 1892–93, Discussioni*, vol. 4 (Rome: Tipografia della Camera dei Deputati, 1893), June 5, session of 1893, 4309–10.
44 *Atti Parlamentari, Camera dei Deputati, XIX Legislatura, Sessione del 1895–96, Discussioni*, vol. 4 (Rome: Tipografia della Camera dei Deputati, 1896), May 27, session of 1896, 4822. Already in May 1887, the Crispi government had created the Special Office of Health Police, a central body created precisely during a new cholera epidemic emergency to manage public health and the rehabilitation of Italian cities. Luigi Pagliani, an esteemed hygienist, was called on to lead the institution, to whom Prime Minister Agostino Depretis had entrusted the epidemiological investigation into the appearance of cholera in Sicily in 1885.
45 *Atti Parlamanetari, XIX Legislatura*, 4822.
46 Snowden, *Naples in the Time of Cholera*, 334–45. Snowden's account is based largely on Geddings's letters preserved in the Records of the Public Health Service at the National Archives in Washington, DC.
47 *Atti Parlamentari, Camera dei Deputati, XXIII Legislatura, Sessione del 1909–10, Discussioni*, vol. 9 (Rome: Tipografia della Camera dei Deputati, 1910), December 17, session of 1910, 10989.
48 Snowden, *Naples in the Time of Cholera*, 331.
49 Ibid., 333.
50 Jones, *The Scientific Background*, 90.
51 Emilio Gentile, *La Grande Italia: Il mito della nazione nel XX secolo* (Rome: Laterza, 2006), 66; for the English translation, see Gentile, *La Grande Italia: The Myth of the Nation in the Twentieth Century*, trans. Suzanne Dingee and Jennifer Pudney (Madison: University of Wisconsin Press, 2008).
52 The Southern question refers to the underdevelopment of the Southern regions (Mezzogiorno) of the Kingdom of Italy, namely the infrastructural, economic and cultural divide with respect to the more developed Northern areas of the peninsula.
53 On the Italian situation, see Eugenia Tognotti, *La "Spagnola" in Italia: Storia dell'influenza che fece temere la fine del mondo (1918–19)* (Milan: FrancoAngeli, 2015).

References

Arisi Rota, Arianna. "Prove di *Health Diplomacy*: Le conferenze sanitarie internazionali della seconda metà dell'Ottocento e il ruolo dei delegati italiani." In *Le *istituzioni e le idee: Studi indisciplinati offerti a Fabio Rugge per il suo settantesimo compleanno*, edited by Colombo Elisabetta, 57–64. Milan: Giuffré, 2022.

Asproni, Giorgio. *Diario politico, 1855–1876*, vol. 4, *1864–1867*, edited by Tito Orrù. Milan: Giuffré, 1980.

Atti parlamentari, Camera dei Deputati, XII Legislatura, Sessione del 1874–75, Discussioni. Vol. 2. Rome: Tipografia della Camera dei Deputati, 1875.

Atti parlamentari, Camera dei Deputati, XVIII Legislatura, Sessione del 1892–93, Discussioni. Vol. 4. Rome: Tipografia della Camera dei Deputati, 1893.

Atti parlamentari, Camera dei Deputati, XIX Legislatura, Sessione del 1895–96, Discussioni. Vol. 4. Rome: Tipografia della Camera dei Deputati, 1896.

Atti Parlamentari, Camera dei Deputati, XXIII Legislatura, Sessione del 1909–10, Discussioni. Vol. 9. Rome: Tipografia della Camera dei Deputati, 1910.

Bartolini, Francesco. "Salute pubblica e sicurezza dello stato: Il governo pontificio alle soglie della modernità biologica ottocentesca." *Contemporanea: Rivista di storia dell' 800 e del '900* 26, no. 1 (2023): 3–29.

Betta, Emmanuel. "Pandemia come metafora?" *Contemporanea: Rivista di storia dell'800 e del'900* 23, no. 4 (2020): 681–97.

Bussedi, Giovanni Maria. *Diario, 1864–1869*. Edited by Mirko Volpi. Milan: Cisalpino, 2013.

Canonici, Claudio, and Giuseppe Monsagrati eds. *Carlo Maggiorani: Politica e medicina nel Risorgimento*. Rome: Gangemi, 2004.

Cappello, Agostino. *Sul Sanitario Congresso Internazionale aperto a Parigi nel dì 23 luglio 1851 e chiuso nel dì 19 gennaio 1852: Cenni storici di Agostino Cappello, membro del medesimo e consigliere emerito del Supremo Romano Magistrato di Sanità*. Rome: Tipografia delle Belle Arti, 1852.

Cea, Roberto. *Il governo della salute nell'Italia liberale: Stato, igiene e politiche sanitarie*. Milan: FrancoAngeli, 2019.

Chase-Levenson, Alex. *The Yellow Flag: Quarantine and the British Mediterranean World, 1780–1860*. Cambridge: Cambridge University Press, 2020.

Cinque Quintili, Ermenegildo de'. *Il colera di Albano nel 1867: Lettera di Ermenegildo de' Cinque Quintili al chiarissimo dottor Guglielmo Farr*. Rome: Tipografia Menicanti, 1868.

Cosmacini, Giorgio. *Storia della medicina e della sanità in Italia: Dalla peste nera ai giorni nostri*. Rome: Laterza, 2010.

Costantini, Fabrizio. *Dalle insurrezioni alle istituzioni: Giovanni Battista Camozzi Vertova a Bergamo tra 1848 e 1871*. Bergamo: Lubrina Bramani Editore, 2021.

Davis, Cinthya J. "Contagion as Metaphor." *American Literary History* 14, no. 4 (Winter 2002): 828–36.

De Amicis, Edmondo. *L'esercito italiano durante il coléra del 1867*. Milan: Bernardoni, 1869.

Evans, Richard J. *Death in Hamburg: Society and Politics in the Cholera Years, 1830–1910*. Oxford: Oxford University Press, 1987.

______. "Epidemics and Revolutions: Cholera in Nineteenth-Century Europe." *Past & Present* 120 (August 1988): 123–46. https://doi.org/10.1093/past/120.1.123

Forti Messina, Anna Lucia. "L'Italia dell'Ottocento di fronte al colera." In *Storia d'Italia*, vol. 7, *Malattia e medicina*, edited by Della Peruta Franco, 429–94. Turin: Einaudi, 1984.

Gentile, Emilio. *La Grande Italia: Il mito della nazione nel XX secolo*. Rome: Laterza, 2006.

______. *La Grande Italia: The Myth of the Nation in the Twentieth Century*. Translated by Suzanne Dingee and Jennifer Pudney. Madison: University of Wisconsin Press, 2008.

Giornale della Regia Accademia di Medicina di Torino, 3rd ser., vol. 30, no. 3. Turin: Regia Accademia di Medicina di Torino, 1867.

Henze, Charlotte E. *Disease, Health Care and Government in Late Imperial Russia: Life and Death on the Volga, 1823–1914*. London: Routledge, 2011.

Howard-Jones, Norman. *The Scientific Background of the International Sanitary Conferences, 1851–1938*. Geneva: World Health Organization, 1975.

Imarisio, Marco, Simona Ravizza, and Fiorenza Sarzanini. *Come nasce un'epidemia: La strage di Bergamo. Il focolaio più micidiale d'Europa*. Milan: Rizzoli, 2020.

Manzoni, Alessandro. *The Betrothed*. Translated by Count O'Mahony. London: Bella and Bradfute, 1834. Accessed December 11, 2022. www.gutenberg.org/files/35155/35155-h/35155-h.htm.

Poggi, Giuseppe. *Il colera indico in Voghera nel 1867*. Voghera: Tipografia Giuseppe Gatti, 1868.

Pongetti, Andrea. *Società e colera nell'Italia del XIX secolo: L'epidemia di Ancona del 1865–67*. Milan: Codex, 2009.

Pouget, Benôit. *Un choc de circulations: La puissance navale française face au cholera en Méditerranée, 1831–1856*. Rennes: Presses Universitaire de Rennes, 2020.

———. "La Méditerranée et les grandes épidémies: Retour sur un demi-siècle de travaux historiques." *Cahiers de la Méditerranée* 103 (2021): 173–89. https://doi.org/10.4000/cdlm.15133.

Relazione amministrativa sulla invasione del cholera in Bergamo negli anni 1866 e 1867. Bergamo: Tipografia Pagnoncelli, 1868.

Rendiconti del Parlamento italiano, Discussioni del Senato del Regno, XI Legislatura, Sessione del 1871–72. Vol. 2. Rome: Tipografia del Senato del Regno, 1873.

Reports of the Medical Officer of the Privy Council and Local Government Board, n.s., vol. 5. London: Her Majesty's Stationery Office, 1875.

Snowden, Frank M. *Naples in the Time of Cholera, 1884–1911*. Cambridge: Cambridge University Press, 1995.

———. *The Conquest of Malaria: Italy, 1900–1962*. New Haven, CT: Yale University Press, 2006.

———. *La conquista della malaria: Una modernizzazione italiana, 1900–1962*. Translated by Valentina Besi and Cinzia Di Barbara. Turin: Einaudi, 2008.

Sontag, Susan. *Illness as Metaphor*. New York: Farrar, Straus and Giroux, 1978.

Spatuzzi, Achille. "La teoria di Max von Pettenkofer sul colera e le epidemie del 1873 e del 1884 in Napoli." *Il Morgagni: Giornale indirizzato al progresso della Medicina* 27 (1885): 137–54.

Starnini, Martina. *L'uomo tutto intero: Biografia di Carlo Livi, psichiatra dell'Ottocento*. Florence: Firenze University Press, 2018.

Tognotti, Eugenia. *Il mostro asiatico: Storia del colera in Italia*. Rome: Laterza, 2000.

———. *La "Spagnola" in Italia: Storia dell'influenza che fece temere la fine del mondo (1918–19)*. Milan: FrancoAngeli, 2015.

———. "Storia dell'arrivo del colera negli anni Trenta dell'Ottocento: Lo shock e la cesura tra il 'prima' e il 'dopo.'" *Storicamente* 17, no. 15 (2021). https://doi.org/10.52056/9788833138732/15.

Vagneron, Frédéric. "Quand revient la grippe: Élaboration et circulation des alertes lors de la grippe 'russe' et 'espagnole' en France (1889–1919)." *Parlement(s): Revue d'histoire politique* 25 (2017): 55–78.

4 Exporting Epidemics

The Cholera of 1910–11 from Southern Italy to Libya – Denial, Causes and Consequences

Gabriele Bassi

While in recent years the words "epidemic," "pandemic" and "infection" have become frequent in common parlance, they describe situations that have recurred for centuries in different forms and with different consequences. International studies devote attention to epidemics and their development throughout historical eras.[1] Cholera has struck Europe repeatedly, including in the past couple centuries, and has been studied in depth in medical, scientific and historical terms. An important point for historical research has been understanding how epidemics affect the social and economic systems of the countries afflicted by the disease and their political implications, such as those highlighted by Frank M. Snowden's study on Naples from 1884 to 1911.[2]

In contrast, the early twentieth-century cholera wave has long been neglected by scholars. This is not unexpected, however, as the government's desire to hide the epidemic's extent and severity – by means that I discuss below – was such that it came to influence later historiography. As Snowden has highlighted, this attempt to cover up the cholera outbreak compromised otherwise thorough studies with a general "amnesia" in historians like Richard J. Evans, Patrice Bourdelais and Jean-Yves Raulot.[3] Within Italy, studies are still scarce. Even in works covering several different periods, such as those by historian Eugenia Tognotti, the events of 1910–11 are not given adequate space and contextualization.[4] In 1980, Lorenzo Del Panta outlined the different epidemics more broadly and their demographic impact on society. He suggested one of the most plausible and well-developed estimates of deaths from cholera in the country.[5] But the epidemic is scarcely mentioned in Anna Lucia Forti Messina's chapter on cholera in the *History of Italy*, which considers the episodes of 1910–11 "numerically insignificant," ignoring the epidemic's extent and details.[6] Significantly, it fails to consider its consequences in the colonial context. In 2010, Guido Alfani and Alessia Melegaro identified common threads in their publication on Italian pandemics, but the history of cholera ends at the nineteenth-century waves.[7]

In addition to there being only a few works on the 1910–11 epidemic, there is another apparent shortcoming in scholarship on the topic – namely, the

DOI: 10.4324/9781003382805-4

lack of discussion regarding the impact the disease had in Italy when it was on the verge of making its approach to Libya in the middle of the two years within a quickly changing political, economic and social context. Although many studies now outline the stages of the Italian war for Tripolitania and Cyrenaica, few give more than a few lines to the epidemic's consequences in the trenches of Tripoli. While attentive historians, such as Angelo Del Boca and Nicola Labanca, mention the epidemic,[8] there are no references in many other publications to this significant aspect of the first months of Italians fighting on their future "fourth shore," as Italian Libya was termed. Surprisingly, the epidemic was noted in more limited works about local rather than national history. One is by Marcello Marcellini, who outlined Umbria's participation in the war in Libya and spent a short chapter on the epidemic, titled "In the Trenches with Cholera."[9]

What is still lacking is a reconstruction of the events that led to a considerable effort on the part of the military entities, health organizations (especially the Red Cross) and everyone directly or indirectly affected by the disease, including civilians and soldiers.[10] Although brief mentions appear in the army's official publications, the pandemic was downplayed in the descriptions of the operations or was considered something that affected the local population and had to be faced by the Italians on par with their Turkish-Arab enemies.[11]

From Naples to Tripoli

An attempt to reconstruct the events in Tripoli between September and December 1911 based on the events in Naples in 1884 and in 1910–11 might seem like a decontextualization of the topic, but I consider it appropriate for two reasons. First, Snowden's work is the most important specific study on cholera's spread in Italy. Though geographically circumscribed, it is a model of a multidisciplinary approach to the disease's impact on society and politics throughout Italy. Second, the disease's spread from Naples to Tripoli is how it was handled in terms of prevention; in both cities, the approach was to downplay the extent of the epidemic.

When what Snowden has called the "secret epidemic" of 1910–11 came to Italy, it was not exactly unexpected. As early as 1905, the General Health Directorate had prepared a dossier on prevention titled *Program of Preventive Measures against the Risk of a Cholera Epidemic in Italy*.[12] It included a report from the Ministry of the Interior from September 16, 1905. The epidemic came to Italian shores in 1910, to the coasts of Puglia. Some studies suggested it was brought by the fishermen of Trani and Barletta who had traveled far afield in their fishing expeditions.[13] The epidemic was enormously downplayed to the public, including with the help of American governmental authorities with which the Italian state was involved due to the high level of emigration to the United States at the time. This took on further significance in Libya, where authorities denied or talked down the extent of the disease to maintain the morale of the troops on the ground and public favor within the country.

Undoubtedly, the mobilization to occupy Tripolitania and Cyrenaica helped spread the disease. Naples was the primary repository of colonial troops and an essential dispatching center for men and equipment sent overseas. It has been theorized that Italian soldiers contracted cholera in Marseilles during a stopover before continuing to Tripoli. However, it would be incorrect to connect the health conditions of the city to the epidemic exported to Libya. Italian military health documents show that cholera had been in Tripoli at least since 1910, though not to the degree that it spread in the fall of 1911. It may have come from Constantinople or other parts of the Middle East under Ottoman control. However, the arrival of Italian troops could have contributed to the disease's spread due to the further introduction of the disease from Italy and by creating environments in Libya that fostered its growth and spread.

The motivations that prompted the authorities to downplay the epidemic (governmental authorities in Italy and military ones in Libya) were partially different in nature. Drawing attention to the seriousness of the situation in Tripoli could have undermined the morale of the troops who had been dragged into a complicated conflict and beset by many other obstacles besides the Arab Turks: heat, thirst, the *ghibli* wind and war techniques that often proved different from the army's standard ones. The considerable weakening of available forces would have worried officers stationed in Libya. Showing weakness in the eyes of Libyans and especially of the nation would have been something to avoid. As Labanca observed in his profile of the Spanish flu's influence in 1918–19 on World War I, the delay in dealing with cholera in the fall of 1911 could be attributed to a war-based priority. In 1918, the countries at war had to concentrate their efforts (organizational as well as health logistics) for victory. In the trenches of Tripoli, the Italians had to contain the enemy's reaction and effectively treat soldiers who fell ill. This led to a worsening of the epidemic, spreading contagion and delaying measures to contain it.[14]

While news of the epidemic was suppressed in Naples and Southern Italy in the most influential of national press outlets, it would have been even easier to hide what was happening in remote, unknown Tripolitania.[15] Military censorship was one of the most effective tools. As studies have examined, from the early days of arrival, the Press Office was directly under the command of the Libya Occupation Corps for war correspondent services and telegraph censorship.[16] In late October 1911, there were 56 correspondents from Italian newspapers and 30 from foreign ones in Tripoli. The Press Office was also in charge of censorship of the local newspapers, *L'Eco di Tripoli* and *La Nuova Italia*, "overseeing that they do not diverge from the realm of calm, objective criticism and do not hinder the Command's political and military action."[17]

The censorship imposed on journalists was strict and helped conceal the epidemic within the general war context. While the journalists' dispatches had to be submitted to the Troops Command for approval, we can see how the details of a disease they may have learned about could be censored and never reach Italy. Aldo Chierici, a war envoy who recounted his experience in a 1912 publication, recalled that "if we picked up any news on the way, it was useless to send it by telegraph. It would not get through due to the intense censorship. What about using coded language? That's hard, too. Censorship distrusts everything."[18] According to Del Boca, the silence of Italian journalists was not just imposed upon them but emerged from their patriotic sentiment, which inspired these journalists of their free will to avoid mentioning the problems that the Italian army faced, including issues with their health. "Cholera is raging and taking many victims," journalist Luigi Barzini wrote to the colleague Luigi Albertini on November 4, 1911. "All of us in the press are united in a patriotic understanding to which I myself have contributed no small amount. We try to avoid hurting the country by putting certain truths out there."[19]

Censorship was also applied to soldiers' letters. The rare references to illnesses were general or after the end of the cholera epidemic. "So many serious illnesses continue to hit here," Giuseppe Inverardi, a soldier stationed in Derna, wrote in 1913. "And a countless number of those inevitably end up in the cemetery."[20] In Cyrenaica, typhus was one of the worst plagues for the troops after 1912, hindering and straining the Italian health units. The soldier was, however, certainly referencing cholera in Tripolitania in the previous months, as he mentioned illnesses that "continued" and had taken countless victims.

Development and Spread of Disease

Several sources agree that cholera was in Tripoli before Italian navy sailors arrived in the city harbor. Still, Del Boca, who mentioned the disease's presence in Libya at least since 1910, called the disease an "adversary no one had foreseen,"[21] though it had been circulating for over a year in Southern Italy. This belief was echoed by other authors, such as historian Fabio Gramellini, who called cholera "an invisible enemy more insidious than bullets."[22] Part of the reason that the epidemic was so unexpected despite 30,000 soldiers being mobilized from areas in Italy afflicted by cholera is the way its origin was associated with the conditions of the city when the Italian troops arrived. Tripoli had already been struck by the disease, fed by the customs and conditions that Libyans lived in, especially in eastern Tripoli. The army's General Staff reiterated this assumption about its origin in 1913:

> But where we had to do most of our charitable works was in the health field in Tripoli, given the greater crowding of population and troops, and the cholera epidemic that was already spreading among the natives

at the time of our landing. The first measures sought to isolate and extinguish the dangerous infection; military health workers labored to these ends with great intelligence and self-sacrifice, first alone, and then with the help of civilian health workers; and despite the very great difficulty that they encountered and the scarcity of drinking water, the very poor hygiene of the homes and streets, the lack of sufficient and suitable means, they were able to quickly overcome the terrible epidemic.[23]

This idea regarding the epidemic's source undoubtedly influenced the historiography that followed. Historian Mariano Gabriele, who meticulously reconstructed the operations of the navy in Libya, in the few lines he gave to cholera attributes the disease's spread "to unsanitary conditions and crowding."[24] The first historical reconstructions of the war were published by the same General Staff of the army. Though they mentioned the difficulties of cholera, they attributed the origin of the disease to the environment and local population. Lauding the military's action, they noted how the army had shown its great skill both against the enemies and with "the energetic and enlightened efforts with which it managed to fight the severe cholera epidemic spreading among the natives; and that without having made such provisions, it could have spread widely among the troops, possibly compromising the success of the mission."[25]

Although an epidemic of such magnitude had not been predicted, the military took some precautions from the moment of their arrival. In September, the Health Inspectorate suggested that the Command of the General Staff buy at least "10 disinfection pumps from Dr. Gatteschi to be assigned to the Intendency,"[26] aware that local water, including in the shallow wells, could be a vehicle for gastrointestinal illnesses.

Nevertheless, a sailor died in Tripoli on October 13, 1911, with verified symptoms of cholera. Though this was the first officially recognized case it was not the absolute first. The day before, Dr. Repetti a medical officer accompanying the Italian army, had telegraphed from the boat called Solunto steamer reporting the serious state of health of a sailor, Garibaldi, who was disembarked as a precaution and admitted to the lazaret at the orphanage. On the same day, October 12, two Turkish soldiers were brought to the lazaret, identified as "suspected cases."[27] The same evening, Faravelli, another medical officer accompanying the Italian army, alerted General Caneva and started preparing early support measures. Admiral Borea Ricci informed Faravelli of the possibility of evacuating the Turkish hospital where cholera cases had spread. Caneva ordered the Surgeon Major Dr. Salinari to go to the area and arrange for the "complete isolation of the cholera patients."[28]

Many others followed the first victim, both in the army and among civilians and rescue workers. On October 27, the first aid worker was infected, a Red Cross worker of clinic no. 62 of Milan.[29] Starting that day, the hospital tent was transferred from the Umberto I barracks to the military hospital of the orphanage, where systematic treatment of infected patients began. The director was Dr. Oscar Campagnani, a doctor from Milan who had long experience with epidemics, having seen cholera in 1910 in Puglia during the most virulent phase of the disease's spread through the region. On October 30, as the number of infections rose quickly, he planned to move hospital tent no. 27 of Milan near the Bab el Gedil plateau, outside Porta Nuova, for use in the specialized treatment of cholera patients. Hospital tents no. 19 and no. 64 were then turned into centers to treat infected Libyans.

On October 31, "given the worsening health conditions in terms of cholera of the expedition corps in Tripolitania,"[30] according to a telegram from the Military Health Inspectorate, efforts were intensified to get equipment to contain the contagion. Two additional Giannolli disinfection locomotive stoves were requested from the Ministry of War, in addition to the four sent to Tripoli earlier. The request for medical supplies attests to how the epidemic had spread quickly enough to arouse concerns of the Military Health Department. Three days later, on November 3, Dr. Cavallerleone, chief inspector in Tripoli, maintained that "given the considerable increase in cholera in recent days in Tripoli, there is reason to believe that six Giannolli disinfection stoves will be insufficient for their purpose."[31] The request was upped to another six units, suggesting that those in the Italian military hospital's equipment be sent urgently to Libya.[32] On November 10, additional stoves were at the colonial troops' depot in Naples, ready to be sent to Tripoli with specialized machinists to operate them.

The Red Cross worked to prevent the continuous rise of the epidemic's numbers. Its efforts were recognized by the General Staff, who the next year would laud "the work of the Red Cross during the Italo-Turkish conflict, including its service to combat the spread of disease in the colony."[33] In the aforementioned report of the Command of the General Staff on October 1912, which mentioned the "outbreak of cholera in Tripoli," the Red Cross is said to have created aid stations that could provide prophylaxes and "anti-cholera services."[34]

Dispatching additional doctors to Tripoli, though in inadequate numbers for the severity of the situation, was intended to boost the preventive service there. They inspected infected houses and organized transportation of corpses that were often hidden by family members for fear of being quarantined. They also planned to transfer the sick to the infirmaries ready to treat cholera.

The progression of contagion among the troops can be partly reconstructed through the *Historical-Military Journal of the Occupation Corps of Libya*, which gave a daily record of the health conditions of forces in the colony.[35] The rather low numbers compared to overall estimates and the prevalence of classifying the disease as "gastroenteritis," alongside those defined as cholera patients, nonetheless suggest that there were many more cases than those reported. The official nature of the sources and their superficial compilation make the *Journal* a source of interest to support understanding at least the general pattern of troop contagions. The historical-military journals of individual regiments failed to report the disease with only a few exceptions.[36] For example, the major general wrote in the *Journal* on October 23, 1911, "One new case of cholera in the population, two in the troops. Two of those cases died. There are a total of fourteen cholera patients now in treatment."[37] The journal of the 6th Infantry Regiment made no mention of the soldiers' health situation until July 1912, when it began to describe it as "normal." The journals of the 6th Regiment were compiled again in July 1913 due to incomplete sections and errors in the previous ones that had been delivered. This notwithstanding, it was a choice to neglect the matter of cholera and other diseases. From 1913, when typhus had not yet disappeared from Cyrenaica, the regiment's state of health was deemed "excellent." There is no reference to cholera in the journals of the 16th and 11th Regiments. The writer of the 18th Regiment referred to it but reported the illness starting in November 1911 without mentioning cholera. An increasing number of military personnel were reported as suffering from gastroenteritis, up to thirty per day.

In the last week of October, infections rose rapidly in the army ranks. On October 29, there were thirty new cases in the troops and a "considerable resurgence in the Arab population."[38] It was noted that they had "taken all possible measures."[39] On November 5, forty-nine soldiers and nine officers fell ill, bringing the total number of military men infected and under treatment men to 347. The unavailability of many men led Caneva to request that new battalions be sent from the 52nd Regiment. A telegram mentions "the continuous loss of forces due to health reasons."[40] The peak was reached around mid-November, when in the *Journal*, 52 new cases in the army were recorded in one day with 12 deaths on November 14 alone. The next day another eleven soldiers died, but this was the start of an inverse trend with declining infections and deaths. The first days without any cases were reported at the end of the month. Starting in mid-December, cholera was no longer mentioned in the *Journal*. There were many cases of other infectious diseases like typhus, which would continue through the Italian military operations in Libya, but cholera could be considered eradicated.

Prevention and Organization

The intensive correspondence between the Health Inspectorate and the Command of the Occupation Corps of Tripolitania during the epidemic's months allows us to reconstruct how prevention and treatment of the disease were carried out on-site. This aspect has been lost in the historical accounts of the enterprise in Libya, which has focused on military operations and the war's political implications.

The units of the Italian Red Cross, which led in organizing aid, were coordinated by a medical inspector whose goal was to standardize preventative operations and the internal organization of hospital tents specialized in treatment of cholera patients. The tents were equipped with a floor in modular wooden boards for easy cleaning. Separate latrines were installed with recurrent disinfections. Isolated housing was built for nurses and medical staff. The water needed to prepare food and for the health workers and patients to drink was boiled or treated with hydrochloric acid.

A camp was set up in the western part of Tripoli, serving as a filter for those planning to enter the city. The Arabs were placed under observation by the medical staff led by the Red Cross medical officer. During its peak use, the center accommodated up to two thousand people at a time, itself a potential risk for the spread of contagion. The water supply, a potential vehicle of infection, was filtered through purifiers, which were not enough for the needs of civilians and military personnel, or it was transported directly from Italy on "water-bearing" steamers.

> These provisions aimed to protect hygiene and preserve the troops' health. Large shipments of mineral water, lemons, and water treatment products were also made, serving the same purpose. The garrisons were provided with modern equipment to prevent the onset and stop the spread of infectious diseases. The best equipment for treating and caring for patients came with large shipments of medicine, which with they built the latest style barracks hospitals.[41]

Indeed, a soldier from Terni stationed in Tripoli wrote to his family back in Italy, "We drink San Faustino water in Tripolitania."[42] Unfortunately, though these were useful and necessary precautions, they were still insufficient to stop the major outbreak between October and November 1911.

A report by the Health Inspector to General Caneva laid out the measures to be taken both within the army and to govern civilian life in the occupied city. The report highlighted the most critical issues, starting with the lack of personnel, and evaluated the limitations of the organization should the epidemic spread further.

> The civil health administration does not meet its purpose adequately due both to personnel and space shortages [. . .] the current location of the lazaret, where several cholera patients are hospitalized, is dangerous and ill-suited in many respects; it suffices to mention one, which is that it prevents the practice of all the maritime health procedures that would be necessary if an infected ship should come in. How could we disembark high numbers of passengers if that lazaret is already filled with cholera patients as well as inadequate in hygienic terms for this service if there were many incoming patients? It would in that case be necessary to reserve that lazaret for the sole needs of the maritime service and provide for a new hospital for cholera patients of the city.[43]

Although the Red Cross and the Health Inspectorate were working to provide facilities and prepare effective practices for isolating the sick, they were unable to give a tangible answer to the critical issues, according to Caneva's report:

> To avoid crowding the lazaret, most of the cholera patients were treated at home. However, there was inadequate personnel to ensure true oversight to prevent the disease's rapid spread and provide disinfection. Yesterday, I was informed of the case of a woman infected with cholera who was found in a pitiable condition lying on a bit of straw in a hut. This fact is enough to see the risk this population is running and, consequently, the Occupation Corps troops, as well. Therefore, we request that twelve new surveillance workers be recruited urgently, with a greater number in reserve in the unfortunate case that the epidemic should spread.[44]

The general then addressed the issue of where to put corpses as delay in their burial could create a serious risk of contagion. This issue was addressed by the Health Inspectors, who on several occasions recommended burning the corpses. Chief Inspector Cavallerleone wrote to the Directorate of the Army Corps of Tripoli with a "highly confidential" communication on November 1911, "To avoid the danger of infection, it would be advisable to practice the cremation of Turkish-Arab corpses with the Japanese method if the necessary means are available, and if it does not offend Muslim religious sentiment."[45]

In a subsequent appeal to the Command of the Occupation Corps, Cavallerleone called for the utmost caution and strict adherence to all standards set to stem the disease's spread. He implored them to not spread alarm and mention cholera only when it had been completely verified.

> This should be kept in mind while taking all the immediate measures of strict isolation and disinfection, as a general requirement. It should not be considered appropriate other than when the main clinical symptoms make it so, and when the clinical symptoms are supported by bacteriological evidence. Great accuracy will be needed in the bacteriological exam, when it can be performed and with complete certainty, before reporting a soldier as positive for the current contingencies, though not recognizing an actual case could be fatal, reporting a case of cholera that did not exist would be a no less serious mistake due to the repercussions it could have on the troop morale.[46]

While the inspector emphasized the need for bacteriological tests to identify certain cases of disease, he also suggested isolation of suspected cases: "it would be advisable if they were numerous to remove them from the forces in battle."[47] This risk was limited to their excretions in less severe cases but could be more dangerous if the soldiers had gastroenteritis disturbances, "which would heighten the virulence of their vibrions."[48] Cavallerleone still considered it an "excessive measure to remove [the soldiers] from their troop units and force them into inactivity in large isolation rooms"[49] when the war was already straining military operations beyond the disease.

Among the greatest problems encountered by the Occupation Corps in addition to the shortage of military force was managing the sick. The theory of preventive isolation, which we have seen was considered important but feared if too rigid, was not always complete or did not alone resolve the problems of the risk of contagion. Since it was soon apparent that the Italian facilities in Tripoli were insufficient to accommodate and manage civilian and military cholera patients, they started to look elsewhere. The most practical ideas were to set up a lazaret ship to be moored in the city port or to transfer them to Italian military hospitals.

Four large steamers brought aid to the wounded and sick during the Italo-Turkish War.[50] The idea of accommodating cholera patients on board was rejected for safety reasons with the intention of preventing hotspots from developing. The transport of wounded and noncontagious patients was the priority for the Occupation Corps. This was a primary reason for rejecting the plan to transfer contagious patients to Italy. That choice did not mean there would be no cases on board because many wounded soldiers or those with a diagnosis that had not detected cholera could have been repatriated without knowing they had the disease. Their awareness of this is shown by the invitation to be prepared in the telegram from the Occupation Corps to the Directorate of Military Health of the 10th and 12th Corps of Naples and Palermo. Cavallerleone wrote,

> As wounded and sick starting to arrive from Tripolitania, we request this directorate to issue exact orders to strictly observe prophylactic measures against cholera, prescribing individual health checks to all patients on the boat before disembarkation to isolate in special recovery rooms all individual suspected cases and those who had contact with such cases.[51]

The risk of outbreaks on board hospital ships was always considered high. In a memo from November 1911, Cavallerleone suggested that the Ministry of War prepare a fifth unit to transport the ill and wounded, considering the four units in use not sufficient.

> If some cholera cases were to develop on board, it could happen that the infected ship would have to be quarantined. In this eventuality, given the current expeditionary force in Tripolitania and Cyrenaica, the three remaining hospital ships would be insufficient to perform the

service. As such, we consider it necessary to prepare a fifth hospital ship that would be equipped for the special service by the Ministry of War with its own personnel and material.[52]

During the occupation of Libya, many Italian health institutions declared themselves available to accommodate the sick and wounded of the war, writing to the Command of the General Staff to offer service staff and beds in their hospitals. In this context, it is interesting to see how fear of cholera had developed as it spread in Tripoli. Though little came out of the health condition of the army on a public level, none of these institutions mentioned the possibility of treating the cholera patients or taking in the epidemic's victims. In one case, the opposite happened; the prefect of Messina implored the Ministry of War to not send potential cholera patients to his jurisdiction.

As these hospitals had no isolation rooms, should the wounded or sick come from Africa, not being able to place them for an observation period in the cholera hospital, it would be inconvenient and a problem given the unfortunate location of the lazaret in the moats of the citadel and far from the hospital. If it should then happen that we had to isolate some cholera patients in the lazaret, the two services would no longer be compatible. As a result, I ask the Honorable Minister to avoid sending us the wounded from Tripolitania and Cyrenaica, since Messina is not a suitable place to receive outside patients; in the best case, they would have to suffer from transport first to a remote lazaret then from the lazaret to the hospital buildings.[53]

In November 1911, when military hospitals were being prepared to receive the wounded and sick from Libya in Naples, Palermo and Catania,[54] General Marini said he reserved the Lazaret at the Plaia di Palermo for cholera patients, again demonstrating that, regardless of the choice not to bring symptomatic cholera patients to Italy, there were numerous cases found upon arrival in Italy.[55]

The same fears of giving rise to outbreaks were partly behind the choice to not prepare a hospital ship as a lazaret in Tripoli. In early November 1911, Cavallerleone, the medical lieutenant general, reported through a confidential protocol to General Inspector Claudio Sforza that the port of Tripoli "was not large enough to allow a lazaret ship that would be stationed there to have a free area large enough for isolation."[56] The logistical factor was also considered, in that the continuous transit of sick would have to happen within the port, entailing a high risk of spreading the epidemic. This contagion was considered "so much more dangerous . . . in the water of the harbor, where the freshwater and city waste join with the seawater, vibrions find ideal breeding grounds."[57] The investigation found that it was not suitable to "establish a lazaret ship to isolate and treat cholera patients."[58] The inspector suggested considering such a possibility only for the sick who had already emerged from the illness's acute phase, and for the ship to be anchored outside of the port in the open sea and to be reached by boats only once a day to transport soldiers suffering from the disease. However, this suggestion was also not pursued.

Context and Total Numbers

Italian losses from the war totaled 3,431 dead (1,483 in combat and 1,948 from illness) and 4,220 wounded; Turkish-Arab losses were estimated at 14,800 men.[59] Cholera was not the only disease that spread to Tripolitania and Cyrenaica but it was undoubtedly responsible for a substantial number of the victims.

Various factors make it difficult to give an accurate estimate of infections. The diverse measures taken to contain contagion did not prevent up to 80 admissions per day in the Tripoli area during the period of the epidemic's greatest spread – a number that does not consider the high number of sick admitted with gastroenteritis or general diseases, a substantial number of which were actually cholera. Moreover, available sources offer partial data and various omissions of the illnesses of soldiers, sometimes intentionally to downplay the disease within the units and sometimes due to the superficial completion of the historical-military journals. General classifications such as "gastroenteritis" or "infectious diseases" concealed undetected cholera infections or cases that were intentionally recorded as other illnesses. The decision to transport the wounded and sick to Italian hospitals led to many infected patients not yet being declared as having cholera while in Tripolitania; they were admitted to the hospitals of Naples or Palermo and therefore were likely included in the statistics of the kingdom of Italy rather than in Libya.

Officially, 376 people died from cholera in the colony in the three months of the epidemic, including seven officers. This number was about a quarter of those who contracted the disease and not far from the number of those are died in battle in the same period: 34 officers and 432 soldiers.

Although historical accounts of this period have ignored or unduly neglected the wave of cholera that hit Tripoli during the early months of occupation, it would be inaccurate to consider cholera the only disease within the health and epidemic situation in the early years of the Italian presence in Libya. Health reports, historical-military journals and testimonies of soldiers regularly refer to infectious diseases, gastroenteritis, fevers and other diseases considered "general" or "common." Typhus also seems to have been present alongside all the Italian military operations for months, including in the eastern part of the country.

In the context of a war, where censorship always plays a key role, the cholera epidemic that broke out in Tripoli in the fall of 1911 was a further obstacle to the military action at that time, which was going far from smoothly. The few outside testimonies of the epidemic, written by journalists and soldiers not involved in health services, offer a different view, conflicting with what can be gathered from military sources. While the Occupation Corps did not underestimate the extent of the disease but thought it had prepared everything needed to fight contagion, providing expertise, equipment and men, the few available external accounts of this period present a different version.

Edoardo Caretta, a journalist who had returned to Italy perhaps because of his skepticism about the epidemic, argued that after arrival in Tripoli, "everything had been thought of, except for the possibility of disease."[60] According to what he wrote in 1913, denouncing the military health unit's conduct and that of the medical personnel sent to the colony, "a major of the 1st Grenadier Regiment and his adjutant general died on the third day after their arrival; others suffered much more and met an equally tragic death, poorly cared for, poorly comforted, almost abandoned."[61] For the first two victims, it seems likely that the disease incubated in Italy, but many other soldiers certainly caught it in Tripoli, where the means of support were not enough to stem the disease's spread. Caretta also wrote, "When the epidemic broke out, there was nothing that was specifically needed for the special circumstances in the Occupation Corps."[62] While it is true that the disease's speed and virulence surprised troops mobilized in Libya, some provisions were quickly taken, such as preparing hospital tents specifically to treat cholera, setting up lazarets and preparing regulations for containing contagion. The factor that emerges from Caretta's accounts is rather the treatment given to the sick, which he saw as without particular attention or care. This was likely partly due to the need to avoid showing the public and troops how serious the epidemic was.

> The afflicted were transported to the orphanage by the Franciscan mission . . .. The few available doctors did what they could, but they had the equipment to treat the war wounded, not cholera patients; there were no nurses or aides to speak of.[63]

While these descriptions differ from the Military Health Service's documents and those of the Red Cross, which provided manpower and equipment to Libya, Caretta's report is still significant, showing how the perception of the few Italian civilians in Tripoli in those weeks was that there was a neglected, downplayed and concealed epidemic. Gustavo Tanfani, a volunteer psychiatrist for the Red Cross, remembered "men who have been stuck within those few square meters for six months, decimated by cholera. They have fought many times, and every night they are ready for an attack, always fully dressed."[64] In some publications of the time, mostly accounts by doctors, the epidemic was described, but their limited circulation did not contribute to making the matter broadly known.[65] Though the Occupation Corps' documents show that it was being combated in some ways, the actions taken were not obvious to the soldiers and the few civilians there. This impression of being neglected was confirmed by Felice Piccioli, a rifleman hospitalized in the lazaret:

> The doctors discussed among themselves, and then the captain said to me: 'There is little left to still try for you. There's an injection, but I can't do it without your consent because after five minutes you find out the outcome: either it goes well or it goes badly. Think about it and give me your answer.[66]

These details do not come from the documents of the Military Health Service, which discuss vaccinations frequently but never mention their possible lethal consequences.

Another conflicting element between the propaganda and local reality was in the application of prophylactics and preventive measures. The official publications that lauded the work by the military and the Red Cross compare with testimonies that contradict the dedication in applying these recommendations. A Health Service report from December 1912 did not conceal disappointment in the neglect found in the health facilities. It noted that only during cholera, a disease wrongly more feared than any other, did they give it the necessary attention:

> "Breaking the chain" of contagion would be easier if "conscientious hygiene" were truly widespread among our people and in the educated classes; for now, this emerges, due to a powerful psychological phenomenon, only when cholera threatens, a disease that is essentially less fearsome in terms of health than typhus. Because of the nature of cholera, it is quickly recognized and isolated, and the infection is not as protracted as others, such as typhus. Out of fear of cholera, the most meticulous individual hygiene is observed, which makes it not too difficult to combat. The results were clear for the army as well in the recent epidemics in our Italy.[67]

The numbers discussed above, the broader health context and the mobilization that happened in those frenetic months of battle suggest a new dimension to a lesser-known aspect of the war. If the epidemic was clear and recurring in military correspondence, it was suppressed or dramatically downplayed in the colony and the motherland, not unlike what had happened in 1910 in Naples in Southern Italy. Considering the accumulation of the many other illnesses that struck Libya during the early years of the Italian occupation, we should seriously reconsider the conclusion the Army General Staff made of its action during the 1911–12 conflict:

> The dominant illnesses among our soldiers were for the most part intestinal and rheumatic diseases in the rainy season. In relationship to the

average force present, the daily proportion of admissions to treatment places ranged from a minimum of 1.30 a month in March to a maximum of 2.10 a month in October per 1,000 men. Overall, therefore, the health conditions of the troops were more than satisfactory, and the medical corps . . . can rightly be proud of the results.[68]

While such drastic downplaying might have been understandable, if not justifiable, in 1913, it is not acceptable in current times that the management of cholera in Tripoli in the fall of 1911 has been so understudied (with the few exceptions mentioned) in today's historiography.

Notes

1 In contrast to the few Italian studies, there are many important works on other countries. See, e.g., Roderick E. McGrew, *Russia and the Cholera, 1823–1832* (Madison: University of Wisconsin Press, 1965); Michael Durey, *The Return of the Plague: British Society and the Cholera, 1831–2* (Dublin: Gill and Macmillan, 1979); Peter Baldwin, *Contagion on the State of Europe, 1830–1930* (Cambridge: Cambridge University Press, 1999); and Pamela K. Gilbert, *Cholera and Nation: Doctoring the Social Body in Victorian England* (Albany: State University of New York Press, 2008).
2 Frank M. Snowden, *Naples in the Time of Cholera, 1884–1911* (Cambridge: Cambridge University Press, 1995). While it might seem surprising that this book has never been translated into Italian, despite it being a fundamental study related to the two cholera epidemics in Italy, the lack of interest by Italian publishers and by extension the Italian public might be a result of the Italian denial of diseases that has persisted until our times, downplaying their extent and significance.
3 Patrice Bourdelais and Jean-Yves Raulot, *Une peur bleue: Histoire du choléra en France, 1832–1854* (Paris: Payot, 1987); Richard J. Evans, "Epidemics and Revolutions: Cholera in Nineteenth-Century Europe," *Past & Present* 120 (August 1988): 123–46; Bourdelais, *Epidemics Laid Low: A History of What Happened in Rich Countries* (Baltimore, MD: Johns Hopkins University Press, 2006); Patrice Bourdelais, "The COVID-19 Pandemic in Historical Perspective," in *Epidemics and Pandemics – The Historical Perspective*, supplement, ed. Jörg Vögele, Luisa Rittershaus and Katharina Schuler, *Historical Social Research/Historische Sozialforschung* 33 (2021): 302–15;
4 Eugenia Tognotti, *Il mostro asiatico: Storia del colera in Italia* (Rome: Laterza, 2000).
5 Lorenzo Del Panta, *Le epidemie nella storia demografica italiana (secoli XIV–XIX)* (Turin: Loescher, 1980).
6 Anna Lucia Forti Messina, "L'Italia dell'Ottocento di fronte al colera," in *Storia d'Italia*, vol. 7, *Malattia e medicina*, ed. Franco Della Peruta (Turin: Einaudi, 1984), 431–94. The author has also written a highly analytical book about the 1836 pandemic: Forti Messina, *Società ed epidemia: Il colera a Napoli nel 1836* (Milan: FrancoAngeli, 1979).
7 Guido Alfani and Alessia Melegaro, *Pandemie d'Italia: Dalla peste nera all'influenza suina; L'impatto sulla società* (Milan: Egea, 2010). As the text explains, cholera took about 7,000 victims in 1910–11 compared to more than half a million deaths in the nineteenth century, but such specialist treatment could have given it at least a few words. Mortality from the disease in the Italian context

was discussed in Alfani, "Le stime della mortalità per colera in Italia: Una nota comparativa," *Popolazione e storia* 15, no. 2 (2014): 77–85.

8 Angelo Del Boca, *Gli italiani in Libia: Tripoli bel suol d'amore, 1860–1922* (Rome: Laterza, 1986); and Nicola Labanca, *La guerra italiana per la Libia, 1911–1931* (Bologna: Il Mulino, 2012).

9 Marcello Marcellini, *L'Umbria e la Guerra di Libia (1911–1912)* (Terni: Kion Editrice, 2016), 29.

10 The only study on the Red Cross in Tripoli is Alberto Galazzetti and Filippo Lombardi, *L'opera della Croce Rossa Italiana nella guerra di Libia (1911–1912)* (Piacenza: Grafiche Lama, 2010).

11 Army Staff, Colonial Office, *L'azione dell'Esercito italiano nella guerra italo-turca (1911–1912): Relazione* (Rome: Command of the General Staff; Ministry of War, 1913); and General Staff of the Royal Army, *Campagna di Libia, vol. 1, Parte generale: Operazioni in Tripolitania dall'inizio della campagna alla occupazione di Punta Tagiura (Ottobre–Dicembre 1911)* (Rome: Stabilimento poligrafico per l'amministrazione della guerra, 1922).

12 Archivio Centrale dello Stato (ACS), Ministero dell'Interno (MI), Rome, Direzione Generale della Sanità, b. 176, fasc., *Colera: Istruzioni per prevenire lo sviluppo del colera, 1901–1906*.

13 According to Galazzetti and Lombardi, *L'opera della Croce Rossa Italiana*, 53, it was gypsies who brought the disease to the coasts of Puglia, and then it went through the Caucasus and Eastern Europe and arrived in Brindisi in the summer of 1910.

14 Nicola Labanca, "L'influenza spagnola: Allora e oggi," Associazione Aula 1240 Siena, April 30, 2020, *YouTube Video*, www.youtube.com/watch?v=u YZEQjMZP5Q.

15 See Snowden, *Naples in the Time of Cholera*, 307.

16 Aldo Chierici, *A Tripoli d'Italia: Diario di un corrispondente di guerra* (Pistoia: Simonti, 1912); Mario Caracciolo, "L'ufficio stampa e la censura a Tripoli durante la guerra," *Nuova antologia*, March 1, 1914; Antonio Fiori, "La censura durante la guerra di Libia," *Clio* 26, no. 3 (1990): 483–511; and Lorenzo Benadusi, "Giornali e giornalisti nella guerra italo-turca," in *L'Italia e la guerra di Libia cent'anni dopo*, ed. Luca Micheletta and Andrea Ungari (Rome: Studium, 2013), 186–215.

17 Luigi Tuccari, *I governi militari della Libia (1911–1919), vol. 2, Documenti* (Rome: Ufficio Storico Stato Maggiore dell'Esercito, 1994), 47.

18 Chierici, *A Tripoli d'Italia*, 8.

19 Luigi Albertini, *Epistolario, 1911–1926*, vol. 1 (Milan: Mondadori, 1968), 28.

20 Gianpietro Belotti and Giovanni Santi, *Dalla Libia all'Isonzo: Diari e lettere dei caduti di Calino e Cazzago* (Brescia: Fondazione Civiltà Bresciana, 1998), 39.

21 Del Boca, *Gli italiani in Libia*, 105.

22 Fabio Gramellini, *Storia della guerra italo-turca, 1911–1912* (Forlì: Acquacalda Editore, 2005), 98.

23 Army Staff, Colonial Office, *L'azione dell'Esercito italiano*, 119.

24 Mariano Gabriele, *La Marina nella guerra italo-turca: Il potere marittimo strumento militare e politico (1911–1912)* (Rome: Ufficio Storico delle Marina Militare, 1998), 200–01.

25 Army Staff, Colonial Office, *L'azione dell'Esercito italiano*, 95.

26 Archivio dell'Ufficio Storico dello Stato Maggiore dell'Esercito (AUSSME), Rome, *Libia* L-8, b. 207, September 19, 1911, Military Health Inspectorate, Chief Inspector Office in Command of the General Staff – Operations Department Services Office.

27 Ibid., October 12, 1911, copy of telegram signed Dr. Repetti.
28 Ibid, handwritten on copy of telegram signed Dr. Repetti.
29 "On October 27 – the report of the Command of the Occupation Corps of Tripolitania of December 6, 1912, stated that Hospital Tent 62 reported a case of cholera among its personnel and is deployed by the Imperial Barracks to the military lazaret of the Orphanage, where it continued to provide charitable work during the cholera epidemic" (AUSSME, *Libia* L-8, b. 208, f. December 5, 6, 1912, Deputy Commissioner of the Italian Red Cross to Occupation Corps Command of Tripolitania, *La Croce Rossa italiana in Libia sino al giorno della pace*).
30 AUSSME, *Libia* L-8, b. 207, October 31, 1911, Military Health Inspectorate under the Command of the General Staff Corps.
31 Ibid., November 3, 1911, Military Health Inspectorate under the Command of the General Staff Corps.
32 Ibid., November 4, 1911, Command of the General Staff Service Office to the Ministry of War: "In response to the proposal by the military health chief, this command extends the request to this ministry to be able to arrange that as soon as possible 6 locomotive Giannolli stoves be sent to Tripoli, which should be provided to the following hospitals along with licensed machinists for each. Bologna 1, Piacenza 2, Verona 1, Milan 1, Brindisi 1."
33 Ibid., October 29, 1912, Command of the Staff Corps, Memo to SE, the Chief of Staff of the Army.
34 Ibid.
35 AUSSME, *Libia* L-8, b. 12, Military-Historical Journal of the Command of the Libyan Occupation Corps, 1st dossier: from October 1, 1911, to December 22, 1911.
36 The Command of the General Staff pointed out to the Commander of the Occupation Corps, among other matters, the drafting of the journals: "Many of the Commands do not give the completion of these documents the importance they actually merit" (AUSSME, *Libia* L-8, b. 12, March 12/16, 1912, Command of the General Staff to the Commander of the Occupation Corps). Omissions mentioned included the orders received and those given, superficial descriptions of the operations, schedules and even the locations in which they took place.
37 Ibid., Military-Historical Journal of the Command of the Libyan Occupation Corps, 1st dossier: from October 1, 1911, to December 22, 1911.
38 Ibid.
39 Ibid.
40 Ibid., Annex No. 53 to the Journal of the Libyan Occupation Corps. Telegram, November 6, 1911, Caneva to Chief of Staff Rome.
41 AUSSME, *Libia* L-8, b. 207, October 29, 1912, Command of the Staff Corps, Memo to SE, the Chief of Staff of the Army.
42 Marcellini, *L'Umbria e la Guerra di Libia*, 30.
43 AUSSME, *Libia* L-8, b. 207, undated, Report to S.E. General Caneva, Governor General of Tripolitania and Cyrenaica.
44 Ibid.
45 AUSSME, *Libia* L-8, b. 207, undated, Chief Inspector Cavallerleone for the Health Directorate of the Tripoli Army Corps.
46 Ibid., n.d., Regulations for the health service in Tripolitania.
47 Ibid.
48 Ibid.
49 Ibid.
50 These were the *Re d'Italia*, *Regina d'Italia*, *Memfi* and *Regina Margherita*. In late February 1912, the *Re Umberto* steamer was also identified, which already had isolation rooms for which rental had been planned. See ibid., February 29, 1912, Authorities of the Libyan Occupation Corps at the Command of the General Staff Corps.

51 Ibid, n.d., Ferrero di Cavallerleone to the 10th and 12th Military Health Directorate of the Naples-Palermo Army Corps.
52 Ibid, November 17, 1911, "Memo" Addressed to the Inspectorate of Military Health, Colonial Office, Command of the R. Marine Corps, Transport, Minister of War.
53 AUSSME, *Libia* L-8, b. 73, December 15, 1911, Prefecture of Messina in Ministry of War, Inspectorate of Military Health.
54 Ibid, October 10, 1911, Command of the General Staff Department, memo to the Office of S.E, the Chief of Staff of the Army, Military Reserve Hospitals for the Special Army Corps Operating in Tripolitania.
55 Ibid., November 11, 1911, Directorate of Health Palermo at the Command of the General Staff of the Army.
56 Ibid, November 3, 1911, Military Health Inspectorate to Medical General Inspector Claudio Sforza.
57 Ibid.
58 Ibid.
59 For these numbers, which are supported by historians, see Gabriele, *La Marina nella guerra italo-turca*, 201. See also Army Staff, Colonial Office, *L'azione dell'Esercito italiano*, 70.
60 Edoardo Caretta, *Nove mesi a Tripoli, Settembre 1911–Giugno 1912* (Rome: EditriceAgenzia Coloniale, 1913), 19–20.
61 Ibid., 20.
62 Ibid.
63 Ibid.
64 Gustavo Tanfani, Lettera da Tripoli (23 marzo 1911), *Quaderni di psichiatria* 1, no. 3 (1911): 84.
65 Luigi Dozzi, *Lettere sanitarie da Tripoli* (Milan: Vallardi, 1911); Camillo Barba Morrihy, *Notizie sulle malattie predominanti a Tripoli* (Tripoli: Stabilimento Arti Grafiche Tripoli, 1911); and Dozzi, *Su alcuni casi di colera osservati a Tripoli* (Milan: Vallardi, 1912).
66 Felice Piccioli, *Diario di un bersagliere* (Milan: Il Formichiere, 1974), 29.
67 Ibid.
68 Army Staff, Colonial Office, *L'azione dell'Esercito italiano*, 95.

References

Albertini, Luigi. *Epistolario, 1911–1926*. Vol. 1. Milan: Mondadori, 1968.
Alfani, Guido, and Alessia Melegaro. *Pandemie d'Italia: Dalla peste nera all'influenza suina; L'impatto sulla società*. Milan: Egea, 2010.
______. "Le stime della mortalità per colera in Italia: Una nota comparativa." *Popolazione e storia* 15, no. 2 (2014): 77–85.
Army Staff, Colonial Office. *L'azione dell'Esercito italiano nella guerra italo-turca (1911–1912): Relazione*. Rome: Command of the General Staff; Ministry of War, 1913.
Baldwin, Peter. *Contagion on the State of Europe, 1830–1930*. Cambridge: Cambridge University Press, 1999.
Barba Morrihy, Camillo. *Notizie sulle malattie predominanti a Tripoli*. Tripoli: Stabilimento Arti Grafiche Tripoli, 1911.
Belotti, Giampietro, and Giovanni Santi, *Dalla Libia all'Isonzo: Diari e lettere dei caduti di Calino e Cazzago*. Brescia: Fondazione Civiltà Bresciana, 1998.
Benadusi, Lorenzo. "Giornali e giornalisti nella guerra italo-turca." In *L'Italia e la guerra di Libia cent'anni dopo*, edited by Luca Micheletta and Andrea Ungari, 186–215. Rome: Studium, 2013.

Bourdelais, Patrice. *Epidemics Laid Low: A History of What Happened in Rich Countries*. Baltimore, MD: Johns Hopkins University Press, 2006.

______. "The COVID-19 Pandemic in Historical Perspective," In "Epidemics and Pandemics – The Historical Perspective." Supplement, edited by Jörg Vögele, Luisa Rittershaus, and Katharina Schuler. *Historical Social Research/Historische Sozialforschung* 33 (2021): 302–15.

Bourdelais, Patrice, and Jean-Yves Raulot. *Une peur bleue: Histoire du choléra en France,1832–1854*. Paris: Payot, 1987.

Caracciolo, Mario. "L'ufficio stampa e la censura a Tripoli durante la guerra." *Nuova antologia*, March 1, 1914.

Caretta, Edoardo. *Nove mesi a Tripoli, Settembre 1911–Giugno 1912*. Rome: Editrice Agenzia Coloniale, 1913.

Chierici, Aldo. *A Tripoli d'Italia: Diario di un corrispondente di guerra*. Pistoia: Simonti, 1912.

Del Boca, Angelo. *Gli italiani in Libia: Tripoli bel suol d'amore, 1860–1922*. Rome: Laterza, 1986.

Del Panta, Lorenzo. *Le epidemie nella storia demografica italiana (secoli XIV–XIX)*. Turin: Loescher, 1980.

Dozzi, Luigi. *Lettere sanitarie da Tripoli*. Milan: Vallardi, 1911.

______. *Su alcuni casi di colera osservati a Tripoli*. Milan: Vallardi, 1912.

Durey, Michael. *The Return of the Plague: British Society and the Cholera, 1831–2*. Dublin: Gill and Macmillan, 1979.

Evans, Richard J. "Epidemics and Revolutions: Cholera in Nineteenth-Century Europe." *Past & Present* 120 (August 1988): 123–46.

Fiori, Antonio. "La censura durante la guerra di Libia." *Clio* 26, no. 3 (1990): 483–511.

Forti Messina, Anna Lucia. *Società ed epidemia: Il colera a Napoli nel 1836*. Milan: FrancoAngeli, 1979.

______. "L'Italia dell'Ottocento di fronte al colera." In *Storia d'Italia, vol. 7, Malattia e medicina*, edited by Della Peruta Franco, 431–94. Turin: Einaudi, 1984.

Gabriele, Mariano. *La Marina nella guerra italo-turca: Il potere marittimo strumento militare e politico (1911–1912)*. Rome: Ufficio Storico delle Marina Militare, 1998.

Galazzetti, Alberto, and Filippo Lombardi. *L'opera della Croce Rossa Italiana nella guerra di Libia (1911–1912)*. Piacenza: Grafiche Lama, 2010.

General Staff of the Royal Army. *Campagna di Libia. Vol. 1, Parte generale: Operazioni in Tripolitania dall'inizio della campagna alla occupazione di Punta Tagiura (Ottobre – Dicembre 1911)*. Rome: Stabilimento poligrafico per l'amministrazione della guerra, 1922.

Gilbert, Pamela K. *Cholera and Nation: Doctoring the Social Body in Victorian England*. Albany: State University of New York Press, 2008.

Gramellini, Fabio. *Storia della guerra italo-turca, 1911–1912*. Forlì: Acquacalda Editore, 2005.

Labanca, Nicola. *La guerra italiana per la Libia, 1911–1931*. Bologna: Il Mulino, 2012.

______. "L'influenza spagnola: Allora e oggi." Associazione Aula 1240 Siena. *YouTube Video*, April 30, 2020. www.youtube.com/watch?v=uYZEQjMZP5Q.

Marcellini, Marcello. *L'Umbria e la Guerra di Libia (1911–1912)*. Terni: Kion Editrice, 2016.

McGrew, Roderick E. *Russia and the Cholera, 1823–1832*. Madison: University of Wisconsin Press, 1965.

Piccioli, Felice. *Diario di un bersagliere*. Milan: Il Formichiere, 1974.

Snowden, Frank M. *Naples in the Time of Cholera, 1884–1911*. Cambridge: Cambridge University Press, 1995.

Tanfani, Gustavo. "Lettera da Tripoli (23 marzo 1911)." *Quaderni di psichiatria* 1, no. 3 (1911): 3–5.
Tognotti, Eugenia. *Il mostro asiatico: Storia del colera in Italia.* Rome: Laterza, 2000.
Tuccari, Luigi. *I governi militari della Libia (1911–1919).* Vol. 2, *Documenti.* Rome: Ufficio Storico Stato Maggiore dell'Esercito, 1994.

5 Medical Mistrust and Contagious Disease in the Italian 1860s

Professor Angelo Scarenzio's Neglected Therapy for Syphilis

Paolo Mazzarello

A New Disease

Before the advent of AIDS, syphilis was the morbid condition that most represented a metaphor for culpable and subversive behavior to be stigmatized on a religious and social level. The disease had suddenly exploded to epidemic proportions following the September 1494 military expedition led by King Charles VIII of France along the Italian peninsula.[1] The French sovereign crossed the Alps at the head of a cosmopolitan army of some thirty-six thousand mercenaries – Swiss, Gascon, Flemish, Spanish – whose ranks gradually swelled to sixty thousand with Italian militias. With them were cooks, supply officers, medical assistants and many prostitutes. The expedition reached Rome and then Naples, where Charles VIII entered on February 22, 1495, to claim dynastic rights over the city and make it a base from which to launch a crusade. Several Italian states, in addition to the king of Spain, the Pope and Maximilian I of Habsburg, gathered to fight him. The French expedition soon failed, and on the way back, the king had to face the alliance of powers aiming to oust him.

The most important war episode was the Battle of Fornovo, in the province of Parma, fought on July 6, 1495, between an exhausted retreating French army and the league of its opponents. It was while treating the wounded from the armed clash that a Venetian military surgeon, Marcello Cumano, described the presence of strange pustules on the genitals – particularly glans and foreskin – of soldiers. It was the first clinical manifestation of syphilis, which was followed within a few weeks by a generalized and devastating rash over the entire body of the affected individual, together with fever, muscle pain – especially at night – followed by foul-smelling abscesses, ulcers that eroded deep into the bones, destroying and deforming the face, especially the nose, eyes and lips. Frequently, the generalized infectious state was followed by the death of the patient.

About twenty days earlier, an almost overlapping description of the disease had been outlined in a letter by the Sicilian physician Nicolò Scillacio, who observed it in Barcelona in early 1495. Reports of this new epidemic accumulated rapidly over the following decades as it spread through France,

DOI: 10.4324/9781003382805-5

Swiss and German territories, then England, Scotland and Eastern Europe, eventually becoming a pandemic that penetrated Asia, Africa and Oceania. Early on, the strange clinical entity was recognized as the consequence of promiscuous sexual intercourse. The lack of clear descriptions of the disease in ancient medical texts soon suggested that it was a new disease that had appeared after the return of the first Spanish expeditions led by Christopher Columbus to the New World. It was suspected that the disease was due to Iberian sailors' sexual contact with natives; repatriates would then spread it to the mother country. Moreover, Christopher Columbus returned to Spain from his first voyage bringing back some natives (he reached Seville on March 31, 1493, and Barcelona the following April 20). Over the next two years, other Native American men and women (some of them almost certainly led into prostitution) were brought to Spain by his friend Antonio de Torres. According to this interpretation, however, syphilis spread into the Italian peninsula because of the concentration of prostitutes around the armies – in particular, there were many Spanish soldiers – who fought each other in Naples. The American theory of the origin of syphilis has been variously disputed but has received increasing – though not conclusive – confirmation in recent years thanks to studies in molecular biology and genetics.[2]

The disease took several names, and in order to identify it with an external enemy, the different peoples in which it spread tended to label it with the name of their own rival or adversary – hence the designation of French or Gallic disease for the Italians, Neapolitan or Italian disease for the French, Castilian disease for the Portuguese, German disease for the Poles and so on. For more than two centuries, however, the most common designation was Gallic disease, linked to the event from which it arose: the descent of the French into Italy.

In 1530, the Veronese physician Girolamo Fracastoro published the work *Syphilis sive de morbo gallico*, which would have dozens of editions and translations. It was an elegant poetic description of the disease in Latin hexameters, but not only that. For Fracastoro, it was also a true medical study in literary form. The shepherd Syphilus was struck down by a cruel disease as a punishment for offending the god Apollo. The poor man's skin filled with pustules, his teeth fell out, his breath became fetid and sores plagued his body. The disease was called syphilis by the inhabitants of the surrounding countryside described in the poem. The term did not enter medical usage until about two centuries after the publication of Fracastoro's poem, replacing the more common name Gallic disease.

Treatment Attempts

The epidemic outbreak of syphilis presented physicians with a therapeutic dilemma because there was no idea of how to treat it. Based on the assumption that the disease was caused by an imbalance of flowing humors in the body (in accordance with ancient Galenic-Hippocratic theories), attempts included the classic paraphernalia of cures: bloodletting, diet, purgatives and drugs that induced sweating and salivation. In 1519, Ulrich von Hutten, a German poet who contracted syphilis (of which he died four years later), described a treatment with Guaiacum or holy wood, a vegetable from Central America, particularly Santo Domingo, used in powder or decoction form for its diaphoretic, diuretic and depurative properties. Benvenuto Cellini told of getting rid of syphilitic symptoms thanks to the plant's properties.[3] However, the therapy was later deemed ineffective and abandoned; in parallel, other diets were introduced, although with dubious results: sarsaparilla, sassafras, cinchona and even viper venom and turtle meat.[4]

Ever since the epidemic outbreak of syphilis, an alternative therapy quickly became dominant: mercury.[5] There was an ancient tradition of using this metal for the treatment of skin diseases by the Greeks and Arabs, and the use of mercury had also been advocated in the twelfth century by – among others – the influential surgeon Roger of Salerno and in 1363 by the physician Guy de Chauliac in his work *La grande chirurgie*.[6] Early treatments of the disease were carried out with the use of mercurial ointments advocated by, among others, the famous Swiss physician Paracelsus. Fumigation was later introduced and became popular in the first half of the sixteenth century. Patients were placed in heated, enclosed and suffocating rooms, or in tents or large barrels (mercurial stoves), where the sweating body was forced to absorb, from the skin or by inhalation, vapors of cinnabar (mercury sulfide, HgS), mercury dichloride (corrosive sublimate, $HgCl2$) or metallic mercury (which, however, was quickly abandoned in vapor form due to its high toxicity). The treatment lasted for weeks and was repeated if imposing signs of the disease persisted. As it was said, "A night with Venus and a life with mercury."[7]

Such heroic treatments with the metal caused severe toxic effects that included ulcerative stomatitis with loss of teeth, personality alterations with mental disorders up to psychosis, neuropathy, gastroenteritis and kidney damage. This often caused the patient's death. Mercury was also taken orally – for example, in the form of corrosive sublimate and metallic mercury. From the seventeenth century, the dosage of mercury was lowered, and calomel (mercurous chloride, $Hg2Cl2$), which is less toxic and naturally occurring as a mineral, was introduced. However, regardless of the chemical form of the metal taken, the effectiveness of the treatment was highly variable and not without side effects. In 1864, a thirty-three-year-old professor of the Clinic of Dermatological and Syphilitic Diseases at the University of Pavia, Angelo Scarenzio, published an article with a new therapeutic proposal for the treatment of syphilis: subcutaneous injection of calomel. The route of administration seemed to provide significant efficacy, although there were side effects.

Angelo Scarenzio: The New Way

Born in Pavia on February 1, 1831, Scarenzio was the son of a physician and professor at the University of Pavia.[8] In 1846–47, he enrolled in Pavia's medical school and made an early name for himself by publishing three scientific papers before obtaining his medical degree in April 1854. In the meantime, he strongly felt the academic influence of the famous surgeon Luigi Porta (who would later be called upon to treat Giuseppe Garibaldi wounded in the leg by a gunshot), orienting himself professionally in the practice of surgery. In 1857, he obtained the post of chief surgeon at the hospital of Mantua, and in June and July 1859, he treated the wounded from the battles of San Martino and Solferino during the Second Italian War of Independence. He returned to Pavia in 1860, at Porta's request, and obtained the new teaching position of *Clinica sifilitica* (syphilitic disease) entirely devoted to the clinical aspects and complications of syphilis.[9]

Scarenzio then began to take an interest in the study of venereal diseases and their treatment. The results of this research included a work on the cauterization of ulcerative syphilitic lesions as a prophylactic means in the development of the disease, two essays on the involvement of the nervous system in luetic pathology (from the Latin *lues*, "pestilence," a term that became synonymous with syphilis) and an extensive review of the syphilographic literature. By analyzing the scientific studies on venereal diseases in depth, Scarenzio understood that the treatments used until then for syphilis (ointments, fumigations, pills and oral solutions of mercurial preparations) imposed long periods of administration with many and prolonged side effects and inconstant therapeutic results due to the variability of drug assimilation.

Scarenzio then had the idea of using a mercurial preparation by the hypodermic route – in predetermined quantities – "for the purpose of facilitating and regulating its absorption,"[10] making it "slow and graduated."[11] From the hypodermal cell tissue, the drug suspension would be absorbed gradually but steadily. Of all the mercurial compounds available, he then thought of employing calomel, which was certainly less immediately toxic than the corrosive sublimate known for its gangrenous effects on the tissues. Calomel was vaporized and suspended in glycerin – the fluid took on the appearance of a "mucilaginous liquid" – which because of its viscosity was "less readily absorbed."[12] In the body, the mercurial compound would then gradually turn into corrosive sublimate, thus reducing its necrotizing impact.

The opportunity to try the new route of administration took place on April 4, 1864, when a thirty-year-old peasant woman suffering from luetic lesions on her face and left arm was admitted to the small Clinic of Syphilitic Diseases that Scarenzio was directing in Pavia. The patient was an old acquaintance of the ward, where she had already been admitted about a year earlier because of a syphilitic sore around her nostrils, another at the root of her nose (glabella) and others on the inner side of her arm and on her external genitals. The woman had contracted the disease after having breast-fed a child with congenital syphilis for pay (i.e., transmitted to the fetus via the placental route). At the time of her initial hospitalization, she had been treated with mercurial frictions to her lower extremities, with apparently positive results. However, the syphilitic lesions had reappeared; the sore at the glabella had spread, invading and corroding the forehead for a length of three centimeters, especially expanding into the nose which appeared entirely consumptive, leaving in its place a vast and deep ulcer. Meanwhile, the sore on her left arm had also reopened. "The woman, eighth month pregnant, was very thin and her general state was wasted."[13]

Scarenzio thought that the treatment that had already been tried was not repeatable, as it had failed; moreover, symptoms of "atony" of the digestive tract led him to avoid an attempt to administer a mercurial preparation by the "stomach route."[14] It seemed plausible to him to attempt in this case a "new route of entry by subcutaneous injection."[15] On April 7, using a Pravaz syringe (invented by the French surgeon Charles-Gabriel Pravaz in 1853) inserted into the middle inner part of her left leg, he injected 20 centigrams of vaporized calomel suspended in 1.5 grams of glycerin. The next day he repeated the administration in the symmetrical position of her right leg. On April 13, the patient gave birth to an apparently healthy baby, who was immediately entrusted to the Pio Luogo degli Esposti (the Pavia orphanage that admitted abandoned infants or those from difficult families) for artificial feeding, but after fifteen days, the baby died "in the grip of a pustular syphilitic rash."[16] Meanwhile, almost two weeks after the start of the treatment, the woman's dermatological lesions began to heal, and by August they were substantially gone. The most dramatic outcome was the mutilation of her nose, which Scarenzio tried to remedy with an "artificial nose."[17]

The second patient treated – a thirty-five-year-old man – received the calomel injection on June 9, 1864. He was a "shoe-shiner, dwarf, hunchbacked, crippled and suffering from scurvy, already ill with syphilis several times."[18] The patient had been admitted to the clinic on February 23 with a primary syphilitic ulceration in his glans, and after about ten days, a papulo-squamous eruption had appeared, sprinkling the entire body. The man's general condition had deteriorated, partly due to scurvy, so he was initially treated mainly with a "good and lavish diet."[19]

An injection of calomel, in the same dose as in the previous case, was given to the middle outer part of his left arm, followed five days later by a second one to his right arm. Two small abscesses formed at the site after eight to ten days, and pus analysis showed no trace of mercury, which meant complete reabsorption. On the twelfth day after the first injection, the skin manifestations quickly began to heal, and the patient was discharged "in perfect health" the following July 14.[20]

On June 9, Scarenzio treated a third patient (who in the preceding years had suffered from several eruptive recurrences of syphilitic nature treated with mercurial skin frictions and other treatments) with an injection of calomel, but the results were inconsistent. The injection was repeated the following June 14, and the new treatment quickly made the manifestations of syphilis disappear; the patient was discharged the following August 15. By the end of August, a total of eight patients had been treated with calomel injection therapy, among them two twenty-one-year-old women who had contracted syphilis from their husbands shortly after marriage. In seven cases, the treatment had given largely positive results, although one patient had not responded. As Scarenzio wrote, the diagnosis was not certain, and "perhaps there were some hidden diseases that always prevented the necessary improvement of the general health."[21] The main side effect of the treatment was the formation of abscesses at the injection point, which, however, "healed very quickly with pus evacuation."[22]

Such important results had to be publicized immediately, so the August – September issue of the influential medical journal *Annali universali di medicina* reported a detailed description of the eight cases in which the treatment had been attempted.[23] The new route of administration of mercury salt, despite the very positive results present in Scarenzio's report, was received "with much distrust."[24] The reason that made physicians dubious about applying that method was the constant formation of abscess at the injection point. However, as mentioned, the problem was alleviated by surgically opening the abscess and draining the pus. Scarenzio consistently noted the absence of mercury in the purulent material, which meant complete absorption of the drug.

After the publication of his work, Scarenzio learned that since 1860 the English physician Charles Hunter and the Austrian dermatologist Ferdinand Hebra had treated a few syphilitic patients with hypodermic injections of corrosive sublimate, but the method had raised doubts.[25] However, this therapy had been taken up on a large scale by Georg Lewin, who worked in the Charité Hospital in Berlin and wrote an impressive monograph on the subject.[26] The work contained the history of more than five hundred cases of syphilis treated with subcutaneous injections of sublimate and other substances. Lewin used an average of twenty-three injections for males and eighteen injections for females because the former generally had more severe forms than the latter. The direct administration of sublimate produced many side effects, such as the formation of gangrenous abscesses and frequent excessive salivation, so doses of the drug per injection had to be kept very low (although in the end the overall mercurial administration was much greater), but recurrences were very frequent.

Scarenzio became convinced that calomel was a much better treatment. Confident in the belief that he had found something new for syphilis therapy and despite the cold reception of his new therapeutic proposal, he was not discouraged and continued to treat his syphilitic patients. Meanwhile, the results of Scarenzio's clinical experiments were mentioned early on in the international scientific literature and found confirmation in Italy, though criticized in France.[27]

Success and Oblivion

Scarenzio found in surgeon Amilcare Ricordi – who worked in the Special Department of Venereal Diseases at the Ospedale Maggiore of Milan – an enthusiastic collaborator. The two doctors began to combine efforts with the aim of collecting a large series of case reports on the effects of hypodermic calomel injection. The collaboration began in September 1864, and by June 1868, the two clinicians had treated eighty-six patients with hypodermic injections of calomel and eighty-six patients with syphilis in various stages of the disease (primitive – that is, congenital – early and late). They then treated a second group of patients consisting of eighteen similar cases by employing corrosive sublimate and various other mercury salts (phosphate, cyanide, bisulfate, protoxide), as well as other mercurial preparations. In the first group, most patients were given two administrations, some three, and others one injection, with doses ranging from 10 to 40 centigrams, depending on clinical severity. The patients were of both sexes, of all ages (even many children, one born forty days early and suffering from congenital syphilis) and all categories of workers were represented – for example, peasants (the largest category), landowners, prostitutes, professionals, military personnel, students, artisans, porters, customs guards, shopkeepers, clerks, nurses and so on.

Among those patients was Scarenzio himself, who had become infected while treating patients in the venereal disease ward of the Pavia Military Hospital. The doctor therefore experimented on himself with entirely positive results using the cure he had invented, administering calomel subcutaneously three times (two first injections at a dose of 10 centigrams and a third of 7 centigrams). Out of eighty-five cases treated with calomel alone, Scarenzio and Ricordi recorded seventy-nine healed syphilitic subjects; in three cases, there were incomplete recoveries, and in another three cases, the death of the patients was due to their severe wasting or intercurrent affections. Although the second group did not appear easily comparable, due to the heterogeneity of treatments it was evident that the efficacy of the various preparations was lower and the side effects greater than when calomel was used. But the advantages obtained by comparing the results with those of Lewin were great. The method appeared especially suitable for treating children, pregnant women and all those who could not take mercury by mouth or through skin rubs.

Scarenzio and Ricordi then decided to submit an essay containing the detailed description of their cases to the scientific competition opened by the Royal Society of Medical and Natural Sciences in Brussels. The paper, received by the Society in July 1868, immediately aroused great interest, so much so that the treatment suggested by the two Italian doctors was immediately tried in various hospitals in the Belgian city.[28] The results were deemed so positive that Scarenzio and Ricordi's paper was translated into French, published in the Royal Society's journal and received the prize consisting of a gold medal.[29] After this success, the two doctors continued to collaborate, and in 1871 they published the original long Italian article sent to the competition together with an appendix that further extended the case history of patients treated and confirmed the results already obtained.[30]

With such an authoritative viaticum, all indications were that the method would quickly establish itself internationally. Instead, as early as 1870, *The Lancet*, the leading British medical journal, while pointing out that Scarenzio and Ricordi's method "seems to present, at any rate, many advantages over corrosive sublimate, which is much too violent in its action even in small doses,"[31] also stated that "the constant or almost constant production of an abscess will, we think, militate against its general introduction into English surgery."[32] This point of view was quickly shared. As dermatologist Mario Truffi wrote:

"Even in Italy, except for a small circle of practitioners, who reported almost exclusively to the Pavia school, ancient means or injections of soluble salts [i.e., especially corrosive sublimate] were preferred in the treatment of syphilis. Abroad, calomel injection found only very few stern advocates,"[33] becoming a neglected therapy.

Dermatologists "with a few, rare, praiseworthy exceptions, either did not recognize it as a right of citizenship in the therapeutic arsenal, pointing to it as a barbaric and dangerous method, or merely gave it a vague mention."[34] On the one hand, the main reason that kept physicians from employing subcutaneous injections was the problem of abscesses, although Scarenzio and Ricordi had demonstrated their substantial harmlessness. On the other hand, the formation of abscesses was the problem that sublimate administration also presented on a larger scale. Yet this drug continued to be used, perhaps because sublimate had been introduced earlier and backed by health centers and names of greater international prestige. Things would not change until 1883, when the method was revived and became popular through a small but substantial change.

Resurrection and Definitive Overcoming of the Method

In 1883, a forty-three-year-old Finnish physician, Georg Smirnoff (a professor at the University of Helsinki), proposed a modest modification of Scarenzio's procedure with the intention of making the local irritation phenomena of calomel injection more easily tolerable, while also favoring the gradual and prolonged assimilation of the drug.[35] After a long series of attempts, he succeeded in demonstrating "how there was a point on the skin surface, the retro-trochanteric region, in which the injection was better tolerated by the patient."[36] Perhaps this fact was the consequence of the particular subcutaneous cell conformation of the affected area. In short, the new injection site proved capable of reducing the incidence of abscesses formation by 35 percent. In subsequent treatments, this result was further improved, partly because Smirnoff used lower doses of calomel. In a final memoir published in 1886, he was adamant about affirming the superiority of Scarenzio's method (modified according to his suggestions) over the therapies used up to that time because of its applicability at every stage of the disease, its efficacy, controllability and the reduced extent of the side effects.[37]

Smirnoff's proposal immediately caught the general attention of dermatologists and became a great success, beginning a rapid international "triumphant spread."[38] Having drastically reduced or "eliminated the inconvenience of abscess formation, physicians [became] more confident in experimenting and adopting it. The distrust that had lasted for so many years gradually faded."[39] Further small methodological changes improved the treatment. These included intramuscular injections of calomel, suggested by Scarenzio himself, and the use of oily excipients that were less irritating to tissues.

In sum, the method introduced by Scarenzio, in one or another of its variants, became the most widely used therapy for syphilis until the spring of 1909, when Paul Ehrlich identified an arsenical compound, arsphenamine, also known as Salvarsan (the famous compound 606), which proved to be superior to every other drug for the treatment of syphilis. The disease then entered a new therapeutic era.

Notes

1 On the concept of disease as metaphor, see Susan Sontag, *Illness as Methaphor* (New York: Ferrar, Straus and Giroux, 1978). On the emergence of syphilis, see the general works: Claude Quétel, *Le mal de Naples: Histoire de la syphilis* (Paris: Robert Laffont, 1986); and Eugenia Tognotti, *L'altra faccia di Venere: La sifilide dalla prima età moderna all'avvento dell'Aids (XV–XX sec.)* (Milan: FrancoAngeli, 2006).

2 See, e.g., three recent papers: Kristin N. Harper et al., "On the Origin of the Treponematoses: A Phylogenetic Approach," *PLoS Neglected Tropical Diseases* 2, no. 1 (2008): e148, https://doi.org/10.1371/journal.pntd.0000148; Lorenzo Giacani and Sheila A. Lukehart, "The Endemic Treponematoses," *Clinical Microbiology Reviews* 27, no. 11, https://doi.org/10.1128/cmr.00070-13; and Kerttu Majander et al., "Ancient Bacterial Genomes Reveal a High Diversity of Treponema Pallidum Strains in Early Modern Europe," *Current Biology* 30, no. 19 (October 2020): 3788–803.

3 Benvenuto Cellini, *Vita di Benvenuto Cellini scritta da lui medesimo*, vol. 1 (Florence: Tipografia all'Insegna di Dante), 159.

4 Marco Zini, "Medicamenti mercuriali nella farmacologia risolvente secondo il trattato pratico di farmacoterapia di Giovanni Bufalini dell'Istituto di studi superiori in Firenze (1896)," *Atti e memorie rivista di storia della farmacia* (December 2018): 225–31.

5 On this topic, see J. G. O'Shea, "Two Minutes with Venus, Two Years with Mercury–Mercury as an Antisyphilitic Chemoterapeutic Agent," *Journal of the Royal Society of Medicine* 83, no. 6 (June 1990): 392–95; John Firth, "Syphilis – Its Early History and Treatment until Penicillin, and the Debate on Its Origin," *Journal of Military and Veterans Health* 20 (November 2012): 49–58; and Charles T. Ambrose, "Pre-Antibiotic Therapy of Syphilis," *Journal of Infectious Diseases and Immunology* 1, no. 1 (2016): 1–20.

6 Guy de Chauliac, *La grande chirurgie* (Paris: Alcan, 1890), 421–22.

7 Mary Dobson, *Disease: The Extraordinary Stories behind History's Deadliest Killers* (London: Quercus History, 2007), 140.

8 Giacomo Rabbiosi and Giovanni Borroni, "Storia della Clinica dermatologica dell'Università di Pavia," in *Storia della dermatologia e della venereologia in Italia*, ed. Gelmetti Carlo (Milan: Springer-Verlag Italia, 2015), 239–46; and Valentina Cani, "Scarenzio, Angelo," *Dizionario Biografico degli Italiani* 91 (2018), www.treccani.it/enciclopedia/angelo-scarenzio_%28Dizionario-Biografico%29/.

9 *Annuario della Regia Università di Pavia: Anno Scolastico, 1860–61* (Pavia: Tipografia degli eredi Bizzoni, 1861), 9. The following academic year (1861–62) the course will be renamed: Clinic of Syphilitic Diseases. In 1866–67, it will become the Clinic of Skin Diseases and Syphilitic Diseases, and in 1875–76 Clinic of Dermopathy and Syphilopathy.

10 Mario Truffi, "Il metodo Scarenzio dalla sua origine ai nostri giorni," in *Ad Angelo Scarenzio in occasione del XL anniversario della prima iniezione di calomelano* (Milan: Tipografia degli operai, 1904), 30.

11 Angelo Scarenzio, "Primi tentativi di cura della sifilide costituzionale mediante la injezione sottocutanea di un preparato mercuriale," *Annali universali di medicina*, 4th ser., 53 (September 1864): 606.

12 Ibid., 604.

13 Ibid., 606.

14 Ibid.

15 Ibid.

16 Ibid.

17 Ibid., 607. Scarenzio does not provide details about the "artificial nose" adopted. Nasal prostheses for cosmetic purposes had been introduced since ancient times. One of the best-known examples was that of the astronomer Ticho Brahe, who lost his nose in a duel, and it was replaced by a prosthesis perhaps made of gold or silver.

18 Ibid., 608.

19 Ibid.

20 Ibid., 609.

21 Ibid., 620.

22 Ibid., 621.

23 Ibid., 602–22.

24 Mario Truffi, "Angelo Scarenzio," in *Annuario della Regia Università di Pavia: Anno accademico, 1904–05* (Pavia: Tipografia degli eredi Bizzoni, 1905), 267.

25 Hermann Zeissl, *Lehrbuch der constitutionellen Syphilis* (Erlangen: Verlag von Ferdinand Enke, 1864), 380–81; Angelo Scarenzio, "Rivista sifilografica," *Annali universali di medicina*, 4th ser., 56 (1865): 666; Truffi, "Il metodo Scarenzio dalla sua origine ai nostri giorni," 44; and Scarenzio and Amilcare Ricordi, "Il metodo ipodermico nella cura della sifilide," *Annali universali di medicina*, 4th ser., 79 (1871): 21–22.

26 Georg Lewin, "Ueber Syphilis-Behandlung mit hypodermatischer Sublimat-Injection nebst epikritischen Bemerkungen," *Annalen des Charité-Krankenhauses und der übrigen Königlichen medicinisch-chirurgischen Lehr- und Kranken-Anstalten zu Berlin* 14 (1868): 122–762.

27 In the April 7, 1866, issue of the influential British medical journal *The Lancet*, Scarenzio's article was briefly summarized, and his clinical experiments were cited in a letter to the same journal by Matthew Berkeley Hill, "Subcutaneous Injection of Mercury in Constitutional Syphilis," *Lancet* 87, no. 2227 (May 1866): 498, and in Georg Lewin's article, "Ueber Syphilis-Behandlung," 136. See also Carlo Ambrosoli, "Sul modo di curare la sifilide costituzionale colle iniezioni sottocutanee di un preparato di mercurio," *Giornale italiano delle malattie veneree e delle malattie della pelle* 1 (1866): 97–116; and Charles Lasègue, "De la médication

hypodermique," *Archives générales de médecine* 6th ser., 7, no. 1 (January 1866): 80–96, esp. 86–87.

28 At the July 6, 1868, meeting of the Royal Society, an account was given of the arrival of the work submitted in the competition for the prize; see *Journal de médicine de chirurgie et de pharmacologie* 47 (1868): 69. Scarenzio's method was first applied in Brussels on November 11, 1868; see *Journal de médicine de chirurgie et de pharmacologie* 48 (1869): 570. On therapeutic trials carried out in Brussels, particularly in Saint Pierre Hospital, see *Journal de médicine de chirurgie et de pharmacologie* 49 (1869): 62–74, 174–82, 290–97, 431–58, 538–43, 639–47.

29 Angelo Scarenzio and Amilcare Ricordi, "La méthode hypodermique dans la cure de la syphilis," *Journal de médicine de chirurgie et de pharmacologie* 49 (1869): 105–18, 232–39, 360–67, 482–89, 578–85; and 50 (1870): 139–46, 224–32, 332–40, 425–30, 530–35. For the awarding of the gold medal, see *Journal de médicine de chirurgie et de pharmacologie* 48 (1869): 571.

30 Angelo Scarenzio and Amilcare Ricordi, "Il metodo ipodermico nella cura della sifilide".

31 *Lancet* 2 (1870): 716. No title or author is listed.

32 Ibid., 716.

33 Truffi, "Il metodo Scarenzio," 46.

34 Ibid.

35 Georg Smirnoff, *Om behandling af syfilis medelst subkutana Kalomelinjektioner* (Helsingfpres: J. C. Frenckell, 1883).

36 Truffi, "Il metodo Scarenzio, 46–47.

37 Georg Smirnoff, *Dévelopment de la méthode de Scarenzio* (Helsingfors: Verlag nicht ermittelbar, 1886).

38 Truffi, "Il metodo Scarenzio," 47.

39 Ibid., 47.

References

Ambrose, Charles T. "Pre-Antibiotic Therapy of Syphilis." *Journal of Infectious Diseases and Immunology* 1, no. 1 (2016): 1–20.

Ambrosoli, Carlo. "Sul modo di curare la sifilide costituzionale colle iniezioni sottocutanee di un preparato di mercurio." *Giornale italiano delle malattie veneree e delle malattie della pelle* 1 (1866): 97–116.

Annuario della Regia Università di Pavia: Anno scolastico, 1860–61. Pavia: Tipografia degli eredi Bizzoni, 1861.

Berkeley Hill, Matthew. "Subcutaneous Injection of Mercury in Constitutional Syphilis." *Lancet* 87, no. 2227 (1866): 498.

Cani, Valentina. "Scarenzio, Angelo." *Dizionario biografico degli italiani* 91 (2018). www.treccani.it/enciclopedia/angelo-scarenzio_%28Dizionario-Biografico%29/.

Cellini, Benvenuto. *Vita di Benvenuto Cellini scritta da lui medesimo.* Vol. 1. Florence: Tipografia all'Insegna di Dante, 1832.

de Chauliac, Guy. *La grande chirurgie.* Paris: Alcan, 1890.

Dobson, Mary. *Disease: The Extraordinary Stories Behind History's Deadliest Killers.* London: Quercus History, 2007.

Firth, John. "Syphilis – Its Early History and Treatment Until Penicillin, and the Debate on Its Origin." *Journal of Military and Veterans Health* 20, no. 4 (November 2012): 49–58.

Giacani, Lorenzo, and Sheila A. Lukehart. "The Endemic Treponematoses." *Clinical Microbiology Reviews* 27, no. 1 (2014). https://doi.org/10.1128/cmr.00070-13.

Harper Kristin, N., Paolo S. Ocampo, Bret M. Steiner, Robert W. George, Michael S. Silverman, Shelly Bolotin, Allan Pillay, Nigel J. Saunders and George J.

Armelagos. "On the Origin of the Treponematoses: A Phylogenetic Approach." *PLoS Neglected Tropical Diseases* 2, no. 1 (2008): e148. https://doi.org/10.1371/journal.pntd.0000148.

Lasègue, Charles. "De la médication hypodermique." *Archives générales de médecine* 7, 6th ser., 7, no. 1 (January 1866): 80–96.

Lewin, Georg. "Ueber Syphilis-Behandlung mit hypodermatischer Sublimat-Injection nebst epikritischen Bemerkungen." *Annalen des Charité-Krankenhauses und der übrigen Königlichen medicinisch-chirurgischen Lehr- und Kranken-Anstalten zu Berlin* 14 (1868): 122–762.

Majander Kerttu, Saskia Pfrengle, Arthus Kocher, Judith Neukamm, Louis du Plessis, Marta Pla-Díaz, Natasha Arora, Gülfirde Akgül, Kat Salo, Rachel Schats, Sarah Inskip, Markku Oinonen, Heiki Valk, Martin Malve, Aivar Kriiska, Päivi Onkamo, Fernando González-Candelas, Denise Kühnert, Johannes Krause and Verena J. Schuenemann. "Ancient Bacterial Genomes Reveal a High Diversity of Treponema Pallidum Strains in Early Modern Europe." *Current Biology* 30, no. 19 (October 2020): 3788–803.

O'Shea, J. G. "Two Minutes with Venus, Two Years with Mercury – Mercury as an Antisyphilitic Chemoterapeutic Agent." *Journal of the Royal Society of Medicine* 83, no. 6 (June 1990): 392–95.

Quétel, Claude. *Le mal de Naples: Histoire de la syphilis*. Paris: Robert Laffont, 1986.

Rabbiosi, Giacomo, and Giovanni Borroni. "Storia della Clinica dermatologica dell'Università di Pavia." In *Storia della dermatologia e della venereologia in Italia*, edited by Gelmetti Carlo, 239–46. Milan: Springer-Verlag Italia, 2015.

Scarenzio, Angelo. "Primi tentativi di cura della sifilide costituzionale mediante la injezione sottocutanea di un preparato mercuriale." *Annali universali di medicina*, 4th ser., 53 (1864): 602–22.

______. "Rivista sifilografica." *Annali universali di medicina*, 4th ser., 56 (1865): 606–84.

Scarenzio, Angelo, and Amilcare Ricordi. "La méthode hypodermique dans la cure de la syphilis." *Journal de Médicine de Chirurgie et de Pharmacologie* 49 (1869): 105–18, 232–39, 360–67, 482–89, 578–85; 50 (1870): 139–46, 224–32, 332–40, 425–30, 530–35.

______. "Il metodo ipodermico nella cura della sifilide." *Annali universali di medicina*, 4th ser., 79 (1871): 19–89, 241–326.

Smirnoff, Georg. *Om behandling af syfilis medelst subkutana Kalomelinjektioner*. Helsingfors: J. C. Frenckell, 1883.

______. *Dévelopment de la méthode de Scarenzio*. Helsingfors: Verlag nicht ermittelbar, 1886.

Sontag, Susan. *Illness as Methaphor*. New York: Ferrar, Straus and Giroux, 1978.

Tognotti, Eugenia. *L'altra faccia di Venere: La sifilide dalla prima età moderna all'avvento dell' AIDS, XV–XX sec.* Milan: FrancoAngeli, 2006.

Truffi, Mario. "Il metodo Scarenzio per la cura della sifilide." In *Ad Angelo Scarenzio in occasione del XL anniversario della prima iniezione di calomelano*, 23–235. Milan: Tipografia degli operai, 1904.

______. "Angelo Scarenzio." In *Annuario della Regia Università di Pavia: Anno accademico, 1904–05*, 266–68. Pavia: Tipografia degli eredi Bizzoni, 1905.

Zeissl, Hermann. *Lehrbuch der constitutionellen Syphilis*. Erlangen: Verlag von Ferdinand Enke, 1864.

Zini, Marco. "Medicamenti mercuriali nella farmacologia risolvente secondo il trattato pratico di farmacoterapia di Giovanni Bufalini dell'Istituto di studi superiori in Firenze (1896)." *Atti e memorie rivista di storia della farmacia* (December 2018): 225–31.

6 The Insufficiency of Science

Skepticism, Polemic and Irony Toward Medicine in Nineteenth- and Twentieth-Century Italian Literature

Federica Massia

Literature and Science in Nineteenth-Century Italy and Europe

In the past few years, the journalistic rhetoric surrounding the COVID-19 pandemic has accustomed us to the representation of doctors and health professionals as heroes of our present day. At the same time, there has never been such widespread distrust of science as in the difficult years we have faced. This is not only because many have felt entitled to their own medical opinions, regardless of guidelines provided by health authorities, but also because beliefs such as the alleged creation of the virus in a laboratory, the inefficacy (if not danger) of vaccines and the economic conspiracy between governments and pharmaceutical companies have been able to spread. In days when the disease was omnipresent, doctors, researchers and science communicators became the positive or negative protagonists of public opinion.

To a certain extent, a similar phenomenon occurred in Italy during the late *Ottocento* (nineteenth century) in the decades following national unification. The emergence of the positivist culture on the one hand and industrial and technological developments on the other increased public interest in scientific discourse. The rise of major epidemics (such as tuberculosis, cholera and malaria), which is a downside of that economic development, drew attention to the role and responsibility of doctors and healthcare workers. It was during those years that they developed a professional class consciousness.

As a result, all major newspapers and publishers moved to respond to new trends and public tastes. Treves successfully launched the periodical *Conversazioni scientifiche* (*Scientific Conversations*, 1856–74) and Sonzogno inaugurated sections dedicated to physiology, anatomy, hygiene, chemistry and physics in the *Biblioteca del Popolo* (*People's Library*). Hoepli and Vallardi published popular science manuals and booklets.[1] There were cases of doctors and scientists becoming successful novelists, such as Paolo Mantegazza (*Un giorno a Madera, A Day in Madera*, 1868). In this context, writers and intellectuals had to engage with the new cultural horizon, in the wake of what critics have recognized a "medicalization of literature" during the period from the unification of Italy to the First World War.[2]

DOI: 10.4324/9781003382805-6

This chapter explores the intricate perception and representation of science in Italian literature of these years. It investigates three periods: the Scapigliatura, Verismo and Crepuscolarismo movements. The intention is not to provide an exhaustive repertoire of occurrences of scientific themes in these literary works. Instead, I highlight how the representation of medicine acquired a specific meaning for these authors, tied to the historical and cultural context of late nineteenth-century Italy. The topic of illness is related to the medical-scientific field and will be taken into consideration throughout, with attention devoted to the representation of contagious diseases.

It is important to first look at the wider European context since the special relationship that developed between science and literature during the *Ottocento* is not limited to the Italian panorama. This phenomenon emerged in Italy relatively late when compared to the rest of Europe. English and German literature demonstrated an early, pronounced interest in morbid and pathological themes, dating back to the eighteenth and nineteenth centuries, coinciding with the onset of the industrial and technological revolution that Italy would experience a century later. Undisputed centrality is given to tuberculosis, which, owing to its long and silent progression, lends itself well to the romantic portrayal of a mysterious inner affliction.[3] In this phase, the disease is not approached so much as a health issue or social matter but rather as a spiritual and distinctive quality of the individual, often an external manifestation of inner distress or destructive passionate love. For this reason, illness can provide writers with a tool for delving into the depths of the human soul.[4]

In Romantic literature, the physical characteristics of tuberculosis (consumption, emaciation, paleness), aptly referred to as the so-called slimming disease, are employed to represent it as what was known at the time as the gentle affliction. The external wasting away of the body – traditionally described in a softened, idealized manner – corresponds to the spiritual and intellectual refinement of the afflicted individual, sometimes revealing a genius or artistic inclination.[5]

However, alongside this idealized portrayal of the disease, tuberculosis came to be seen as a negative consequence of the economic and industrial development, often associated with harsh conditions of the urban proletariat. Following the discovery of the Koch's bacillus in 1882 and the confirmation of the contagious nature of tuberculosis, pulmonary infection came to be recognized as a social problem rather than as a mere expression of an individual condition.[6]

Because of this, realist literature began to adopt illness as a privileged tool for the representation and denunciation of contemporary societal issues. From being a manifestation of spiritual nobility, tuberculosis came to be configured as a sign of the challenging conditions the poorest classes faced, as well as a symbol of vice and moral degradation, mainly affecting women.

France took the lead in moving toward a more raw and realistic representation of illness. As early as the 1830s and 1840s, Auguste Comte's *Cours de philosophie positive* (*Course of Positive Philosophy*) spread the idea that all psychic phenomena, in individuals and societies, were determined by physiological facts. This perspective suggested that human passions and relationships could be studied using the same tools and experimental methods as those employed in the exact sciences. In the 1850s, while Gustave Flaubert was writing *Madame Bovary*, Hippolyte Taine first theorized the principles of naturalism, which were later applied by the Goncourt brothers and Émile Zola, gaining prominence throughout Europe.[7]

In Italy, although with some delay, the Industrial Revolution and economic progress experienced similar developments, with comparable consequences in the cultural and literary realms. However, compared to the rest of Europe, the literary representation of illness and science in Italy took on a distinct connotation, tied to the historical moment the country was undergoing.[8] Scientific advances and positivist thought spread with the completion of national unification. The intellectual class that had played a central role during the Risorgimento found itself marginalized in the new political and cultural system, which promoted the values of utility and economic progress. Consequently, the skepticism expressed by Italian artists and writers toward science and progress should be interpreted as a response to the disappointment both of their expectations and of the ideals of the Risorgimento.[9]

Scapigliatura

Between the 1860s and 1870s, the first and most radical manifestation of this discontent can be attributed to the Scapigliati, a group of intellectuals active in the Piedmont and Lombardy regions, close to the epicenter of cultural and economic development in the country.[10] These writers felt unable to find their place within the new reality to such a degree that it manifested within their literary works and life choices, marked by recklessness, substance abuse and, consequently, in many cases, illness and premature demise.

The need to find a transgressive alternative model – distinct from the new positivist materialism and the political and religious ideology that had characterized Italian literature during the Risorgimento – compelled these authors to look back to European Romanticism. In contrast to a reality dominated by rationality and scientific calculation, the Scapigliati emphasized irrationality, imagination and the fantastic. However, this revival of Romantic motifs should not be interpreted as a retreat and anachronistic rejection of modern times. By asserting art's autonomy and exalting creativity, these writers aimed to defend the literary space of reflection and representation of the world upon which contemporary science sought to intrude.[11]

The theme of illness occupied a central place in Scapigliatura literature, where it is expressed according to the Romantic taste for the deformed, the macabre and the terrifying. In line with the Romantics, the Scapigliati saw illness as a marker of the exceptional nature of the afflicted individual, uncovering an inner condition that medical science could not understand. In the realm of the relationship between mind and body, psychological distress and physical manifestation, Scapigliati writers recognized an unexplored territory that could expose the limitations of contemporary science:

> Science has examined nature; its systems, its laws, its influences are almost all known to us: but it has come to a halt in front of psychological phenomena, and in the face of the relationships that connect these to the others. It has not been able to advance further, and it has retained our beliefs on the threshold of this unexplored realm.[12]

These are the first words of Igino Ugo Tarchetti's *Racconti fantastici* (*Fantastic Tales*, 1869), which investigates mysterious and supernatural phenomena, aiming to instill doubt against the unshakeable certainties of science.[13] In a perspective where health corresponded to normality, rule and order, medicine assumed a socionormative function that expanded outside its traditional dominion, affecting every aspect of human existence with ethical and moral implications.[14] In Scapigliatura literature, medical science is ridiculed, while illness and madness are harnessed to represent an alternative to the order of bourgeois society.[15] In *Fosca*, Tarchetti's most successful work, the doctor is forced to admit his own powerlessness in the face of the neurosis that afflicts the protagonist:

> It is a kind of phenomenon, a wandering collection of all possible evils, where our science falls short in defining them. We can grasp a symptom, an effect, a particular result, but not the totality of its evils, not their overall character, nor their foundation. We can treat it like empirics, not like physicians.[16]

However, Tarchetti's attitude toward science appears ambivalent. Not only does the doctor play a significant role in the narrative but the novel is structured in the form of a genuine medical report. From the first pages, the omniscient narrator declares: "more than the analysis of an emotion, more than the tale of a love passion, here I may be making a diagnosis of an illness."[17] The author used extensive medical-scientific terminology in describing the protagonist's pathology, revealing connections with the theories of Cesare Lombroso, the founder of criminal anthropology.[18]

This provides broader insights into the Scapigliati stance toward science. Between attraction and repulsion, interest and rejection, their relationship with science is shaped by the contradictions and dualisms that underlie their poetic approach.

Carlo Dossi's case is emblematic because he had the opportunity to become acquainted with scientists from an early age (including Lombroso, Mantegazza and Paolo Gorini) and because of his work on *Ritratti umani:*

Dal calamajo di un medico (*Human Portraits: From a Doctor's Inkpot*, 1873). Here, Dr. Ferretti serves as both protagonist and narrator of twelve stories, becoming the alter ego of the author. In the prefatory dedication, Dossi portrays himself as a patient, humorously recounting the medical treatments he has received, and then expresses his intention to assume the role of physician. Balancing the literary trend that medicine took on, where an increasing number of physicians ventured into literature and became writers, Dossi claims his "right to pretend – for a brief artistic whim – the role of the physician."[19] This exchange is justified by the fact that "friendship has always existed between medicine and literature": although one concerns the body and the other the soul, "both lie, the former for the sake of good, the latter for the sake of beauty."[20]

The ambivalent perspective toward science emerges throughout the work, where one can identify nearly all negative and positive topoi of the portrayal of physicians in nineteenth-century literature.[21] In the first chapter, Dossi portrays in caricatural form the social and professional evolution of physicians throughout the *Ottocento*. While in the past the literary scene was dominated by erudite "great-grandfathers doctors," by the end of the century a new breed of "well-dressed and stylishly groomed young doctors" emerged, who were skilled conversationalists and elegant participants in high society salons.[22] Dossi warns that this is a superficial change: "despite exhibiting less erudition and more gracefulness, they scientifically kill nowadays, no more and no less than before."[23] In chapter three, the trope of the "killer doctor" extends to pharmacists, playing on the dual Greek etymology of *pharmakon* (meaning both "medicine" and "poison"). This gives rise to the traditional invective against "lengthy and expensive prescriptions,"[24] written in incomprehensible language and aimed at enriching those who prescribe and sell the medications rather than benefiting those unfortunate enough to take them.

Nevertheless, alongside the negative portrayal of medical practice, Dossi presents an alternative model. In the poignant final chapter, Dr. Ferretti embodies the qualities of a good physician, comforting his young patient and instilling in him the illusion of a potential recovery until the end. However, this caring humanitarian approach, which still aligns with the role of physicians in the early *Ottocento*, is incompatible with the new principles of materialism and scientific positivism.

The utmost ambivalence of the Scapigliati toward science becomes evident in their relationship with death, the ultimate mystery of human life. New techniques of mummification and anatomical studies of the human body held enormous fascination for these authors. An example of the former was Gorini, a scientist and mathematician from Pavia who was close to Dossi. In the eyes of the Scapigliati, Gorini was able to partially overcome death by finding a way to halt the decomposition of dead bodies, preserving the semblance of life and bridging his science with a true art form.[25]

Anatomy represented one of the dearest themes to these writers because it allowed the representation of the macabre and entailed direct confrontation with science and its limitations. Two poems, both titled *Lezione di anatomia* (*Anatomy Lesson*) by Bernardino Zendrini and Arrigo Boito, respectively, focus on the dissection of the heart, the most celebrated organ in literature, traditionally considered the seat of emotions and passions. Zendrini challenges the professor engaged in the operation to:

> Show in what corner
> Or in what nook
> Hatred clings,
> Love oscillates!
> Where do they nestle
> Joys and sorrows?[26]

Science can study the organs, muscles and tissues of the body but is unable to unveil the mystery of the soul. Not every aspect of human life can be explained in materialistic terms as positivist thought claimed, trivializing its complexity and usurping the functions of literature. This contention forms the foundation of Boito's contemporary poem:

> Science, be gone
> With your consolations!
> Give me back the worlds
> Of dreams and soul!
> Let there be peace for the dead
> And the dying.[27]

In the final stanza, the "adorned dreams" to which Boito appeals are unexpectedly contradicted by the discovery of a fetus in the womb of the girl whom he believed to be "pious, sweet, pure," a "virgin without a shroud."[28] Thus, alongside the invective against positivist science, an antisentimental polemic emerges, mercilessly revealing the truth hidden behind the ideal.

Another example of the attraction-repulsion relationship of the Scapigliati toward anatomical studies is the story by Arrigo's brother, Camillo Boito, titled *Un corpo* (*A Body*, 1870). Here the comparison between art and science is embodied in the narrative's two protagonists, a painter and a cold German anatomist named Carlo Gulz. While the former possesses the sensitivity and passion typical of an artist, the latter demonstrates an unwavering materialistic belief: "everything is connected, everything merges. What most people call the soul is one and the same as what everyone refers to as matter." For him, thoughts and feelings are nothing more than "infinite and extremely rapid combinations of infinitely small atoms."[29]

But the true competition between the two unfolds in their attempts, each with their own means, to possess the secret of the extraordinary beauty of the narrative's female character, Carlotta. While the painter protagonist seeks to immortalize his beloved by painting her, the scientist expresses the desire to study her body on his anatomical table, convinced that fate will provide him with this opportunity. The suggestion of this premonition terrifies Carlotta to the point where she is involved in a fatal road accident. The final confrontation between artist and scientist takes place in the presence of her lifeless body lying on the anatomical table. Gulz, who had secretly acquired his rival's artwork, declares that he no longer needs it and returns it to the painter:

> I need the artist to come to my aid, reminding me of the appearance of life from memory. But appearance is merely form: I seek the reasons in substance. The bones, the organs, the tissues of the human being, just as they explain life, also explain beauty.[30]

The story ends with the painter's symbolic decision to cut and burn the portrait. The detail of the destruction of the painting was omitted by Boito in the final version of the text (1895), potentially tempering what remains a triumph of science over art.[31]

Verismo

After the skeptical and hostile reaction of the Scapigliati, a second moment of confrontation between Italian literati and positivism occurred in the 1880s, through the works of Giovanni Verga and Luigi Capuana. While embracing the principles of modern science with renewed interest, Italian verists looked to the French naturalist model's employment of the experimental method, aiming for a representation that was as objective and realistic as possible. However, Verga and Capuana rejected the progressive optimism and utilitarianism of naturalism, which considered literature a tool for addressing societal problems. Like the Scapigliati, Italian verists asserted the specificity and autonomy of art.

The attitude of Verga and Capuana toward science can be examined through the portrayal of doctors and scientists in their works. In the various forms that these characters assume throughout their extensive production, one recognizes a reflection of the evolution of Italian culture in the late *Ottocento*: from the interest in scientific innovations and the experimental method to the cooling of positivist enthusiasms and rejection of the myth of progress. On the threshold of the new century, Capuana interprets the attention directed to the interiority and mystery of the human psyche and to spiritual and occult currents.

Verga's early works, from *Una peccatrice* (*A Sinful Woman*) and *Storia di una capinera* (*A Nun's Story*) to *Eva*, *Tigre reale* (*Royal Tiger*) and *Eros*, employ a representation of illness that still resembles the Romantic and Scapigliatura traditions. It is interpreted at times as the physical manifestation of a destructive passion or a metaphor for the character's moral corruption and social displacement. Even the character of the scientist is mostly portrayed in the traditional guise of a sensitive and compassionate, yet impotent doctor. From a narrative standpoint, the doctor's character may offer a clear objective perspective on the events, contrasting with the delirious vision of the patient overwhelmed by passion.[32]

A similar representation of the scientist is in Capuana's *Povero dottore!* (*Poor Doctor!*, 1882). Despite being a competent physician and sensitive individual, Lorenzo proves incapable of curing his beloved young wife, who has been afflicted by a Romantic rendering of tuberculosis. However, in comparison to Verga, the sincere interest that Capuana demonstrates toward science, as evidenced by his personal studies, often brings his early works closer to enthusiasm for positivist thought.[33]

"Is this man perhaps a God? – He's a scientist; it's almost the same."[34] These words introduce Doctor Cymbalus, the protagonist of the eponymous novella, which was Capuana's first published work (1867). A cultured and competent scientist, Cymbalus successfully performs a surgical operation that prevents the young protagonist, William, from experiencing any emotions and thus dissuading him from committing suicide out of a betrayed love. The intervention seems to demonstrate the omnipotence of science, capable of acting – through the body – even on the inner world of the human being. However, the author's perspective emerges through the doctor's words: Cymbalus tries in every way to dissuade the young lover from undergoing the procedure and acknowledges the inferiority of science in the face of nature, "capable of destroying and not building."[35] In the end, William is unable to bear the inhumane state of apathy he finds himself in and commits suicide, closing the narrative where it had begun. In this way, Capuana warns the reader about a science that operates without moral scruples and is incapable of distinguishing between soul and body. Even Doctor Follini, the protagonist of *Giacinta* (1879), presents himself as the author's alter ego and an embodiment of the positive example of a scientist.[36]

A negative shift in the portrayal of physicians is evident in the works of Verga and Capuana during the transition from the 1870s to the 1880s, coinciding with their renewed attention to Sicily's rural reality. These are the years of Verga's verist masterpieces, ranging from his collections of short stories to the novels of the *Ciclo dei Vinti* (*Cycle of the Defeated*). For Capuana, it includes the novellas gathered in *Paesane* (*Countrywomen*, 1882–92). Illness no longer represented an individual condition or a literary metaphor but rather a social issue belonging to the life of misery and poverty depicted in verist narratives. In the novella where he theorizes his "ideal of the oyster" – an immutable law of human existence – Verga mentions epidemic diseases as one of the many misfortunes that cyclically decimate the population of Aci Trezza: "from time to time, typhoid, cholera, a poor harvest, the storm, come to give a good sweep in that swarming mass."[37]

In *Malaria* (1881), the disease is inherent to the rural reality itself, as inevitable as the air one breathes: "It enters your bones with the bread you eat, and if you open your mouth to speak."[38] The poverty of Sicilian peasants is nothing but the downside of the country's economic progress. Malaria finds optimal conditions to spread in the fertile lands that the poor people cultivate for the wealthy landowners: "Where there is malaria, it is a land blessed by God."[39] In *Malaria*, the juxtaposition of these two distinct and nonintersecting social realities is represented by the train passing through the countryside. The peasants observe the passengers peering out of the train window, as if "a piece of the city were parading right in front of them," images of a bright dazzling world where "malaria simply does not exist."[40] The disease serves to depict the poverty of Sicilian rural life and above all to underline the contrast between that reality and the official representation of the country, highlighting the contradictions and inequalities within the newly unified state.

Significantly for a novella titled *Malaria*, doctors and scientists are absent.[41] In the veristic narratives, the figure of the empathetic benevolent doctor disappears, making way for the cynical professional driven by greed, often portrayed in Italian literature of the late *Ottocento*.[42] In *Nedda* (1874), the doctor visits the dying mother of the unfortunate protagonist only on Sundays, the day he "couldn't dedicate to his own lands,"[43] and prescribes useless medications. Here, the mistrust of the humble characters toward healthcare professionals becomes openly hostile: "More medicine! – mumbled one – after he already prescribed the sacred oil! They're in cahoots with the apothecary, bleeding the poor people dry!"[44]

In parallel with the social and professional rise of the medical class, doctors and scientists were increasingly assimilated in the folk perspective into a political and institutional system perceived as foreign and hostile. An extreme point was reached in the accounts of the cholera epidemic that repeatedly struck the Sicilian population between the 1860s and the 1880s. In *Quelli del colera* (*Cholera's People*, 1884), Verga portrays a disrupted social reality caused by the disease, where neglect of the basic norms of civilized coexistence is accompanied by fear, superstition and ignorance. As a result, a group of wandering actors is assaulted by the local population, who believe them to be government agents tasked with spreading "cholera pills."[45] Upon the arrival of the strangers, the mayor and the pharmacist go to the campsite to inquire about the reason for their presence in town. However, the people have no trust in the reassurances of their representatives:

And that infamous mayor who kept saying, "It's nothing, it's nothing," and showing the blank paper! That was the paper from the Deputy Superintendent instructing them to spread the cholera! Ah! They really wanted to make them die like animals in their den, for heaven's sake![46]

Similar situations occur in *Mastro-don Gesualdo* (1889) and in the stories of Capuana and De Roberto. This was not just a literary invention to again exploit disease as a metaphor but rather the narrative transposition of a historically existing superstition. Evidence can be found Capuana's letters; during the 1887 epidemic, he served as mayor (for the second time) of his hometown, Mineo.[47] In *Il medico dei poveri* (*The Poor People's Doctor*, 1892), Capuana describes the cholera epidemic of 1866:

> Bad news was coming from Palermo, Catania and Messina: people were dying like flies. It was known for certain that the poison-dispensing machine had already reached the magistrate and the carabinieri marshal. Only the parish priest had not yet reached an agreement with the marshal, the magistrate and Dr. La Bella regarding the number of deaths that were supposed to occur in Rammacca. . .. However, it was certain that sooner or later, it had to happen, by order of the government, to reduce the excessive population. And in the meantime, Garibaldi had assured that there would have been no more cholera after the revolution! What could poor Garibaldi do? Vittorio Emanuele wanted it that way because other governments were forcing his hand. Even the Pope was spreading cholera in his own states, and he was a minister of God![48]

Law enforcement, politicians, medical professionals and ecclesiastical figures at all levels are united in representing the new historical and social reality in which the impoverished population felt unrecognized and lacked protection. The illusion that fueled the Risorgimento revolution had quickly crumbled, giving way to a bitter realization that everything had remained unchanged. This interpretation is evident in the novel *I Viceré* (*The Viceroys*, 1894) by the younger Federico De Roberto:

> Most people believed in witchcraft, in poison spread by order of the authorities, and they lashed out against the "Italians," considering them as plague spreaders just like the Bourbons. In 1860, the patriots had implied that there would be no more cholera because Vittorio was not an enemy of the people like Ferdinando; and now, here it was starting all over again! So why had they even had a revolution?[49]

In verist narratives, the theme of political and social discontent, as well as the lack of understanding of Italy's historical evolution, intertwined with the theme of disease. With the unification of Italy, healthcare became the responsibility of the national government for the first time. However, the new authorities proved unprepared to confront the epidemics that struck the country in the late nineteenth century (mainly tuberculosis, which reached its peak between the 1860s and 1880s) and failed to formulate effective reforms and responses to the healthcare emergency.[50] The strongest criticism toward the new unified government comes from authors – such as Verga and Capuana – who operated on the fringes of the Italian state. In the last decades of the *Ottocento*, the widespread presence of Italian regional literature served a dual purpose: to provide material for the construction of the new national society, while contesting the methods and timing of this construction, foregrounding the feelings of exclusion and the identity crisis experienced in the country's peripheries.[51]

Crepuscolarismo

Through the veristic denunciation, the promise and presumption of positivism to dominate reality and change the fate of humankind are revealed as illusory. The awareness of the insufficiency of science in addressing the deeper needs of humanity contributes to the crisis of values that characterizes the fin de siècle. While authors such as Antonio Fogazzaro and Gabriele D'Annunzio sought answers in the direction of metaphysical, spiritualistic and aesthetic sublimation, a decisive embrace of modernity occurred through the works of writers who delved into the shadows of the collective consciousness. Isolated and unheard for a long time, Italo Svevo, Luigi Pirandello and the younger Federigo Tozzi became interpreters of a new introspective realism, an investigation into human reality that proceeds without faith in rational knowledge and without the comfort of a "formula that can open up worlds for you."[52]

In this context, the various facets of mental illness (from madness to psychosis to neurosis) emerged as a privileged tool for investigating a condition of restlessness and uncertainty that was increasingly defined as existential and universal.[53] At the beginning of the twentieth century, illness did not affect artists and exceptional individuals but rather ordinary people, simple company employees, people without qualities. In a now-consolidated political system, illness no longer served the function of contestation typical of Scapigliatura and verist literature but rather continued to highlight the problematic relationship between the modern individual and society, the external world.

Although less prominent compared to the previous century, tuberculosis contributed to this new literary portrayal of illness. While political and health authorities struggled to control the spread of the contagion, tuberculosis continued to affect numerous artists and writers, such as Sergio Corazzini and Guido Gozzano. As with the Scapigliati, the concept of illness occupies a central position in the works and biographies of the Crepuscular poets.

Sergio Corazzini, who would die at age twenty-one from tuberculosis, configured his entire human condition in terms of death and consumption.[54] In a short cycle of poems entitled *Toblack* (1905), the poet recounts life in the eponymous sanatorium in the Val Pusteria: a condition of pervasive and constant melancholy, in the illusion of an impossible cure and awareness of imminent death:

> Gloomy hospital, good penance
> for the merciful brothers
> whom Death has made aware of itself
> in their daily experience,
>
> even if from your sky it rains, relentlessly,
> behind tearful windows
> your livid consumptive patients
> are held by a longing for recovery.

> Always, until the coffin comes,
> quietly, with the crucifix,
> to receive them in the final corridor.[55]

The context of the sanatorium provides an opportunity to depict the sense of a suspended existence, lived on the fringes of reality. For Crepuscular poets, the experience of illness represented the definitive realization of their inability to face life, the ultimate rejection of those who feel excluded from the normal rhythms of everyday existence.

While Corazzini expressed illness as suffering, often still with a polemical attitude, Gozzano explored more original approaches in representing his affliction. Struck by tuberculosis in 1907 at age twenty-four (leading to his premature death in 1916), the writer spent the last period of his life traveling between Liguria, Valle d'Aosta and India in search of relief from his illness. In this state of complete isolation, only letters allowed him to maintain contact with the world. In his correspondence are precious testimonies of his health conditions and his way of dealing with them. While understandably concealing his suffering from his family, Gozzano occasionally opened up to friends Carlo Vallini and Amalia Guglielminetti with more sincere accounts.[56] More often, however, the poet portrays illness in a playful and self-ironic tone. Not only does he regularly use the farewell formula *bacini e bacilli* (kisses and bacilli) in his letters to Vallini but in both sets of correspondence he adds a recurring caricature of himself and his sick body. He describes the inhaler mask as a "contraption" that gives him "the befuddled appearance of a deep-sea diver" and, by taking away "visual symmetry," forces him to "follow the pen with one eye and then with the other, as a hen would do."[57]

In this routine of "dull and peaceful life,"[58] the poet paradoxically found a condition of serenity. The physical separation from the world, commitments and affections offered him the opportunity for that sentimental aridity that is at the core of his poetry. For the Crepuscolari, in addition to being a biographical reality and poetic theme, illness represented a psychological alibi for renouncing life.

Despite the centrality of tuberculosis in his existence, Gozzano addresses the theme of sickness in only two poems. The first, *Alle soglie* (*On the threshold*), later included in the collection *Colloqui* (*Conversations*, 1911), was written shortly after he discovered his condition:

> They knock in their various ways, observing I know not what signs,
> they auscultate me with their instruments, from the front and the back.
>
> And they sense some hidden worms, those knowledgeable elders . . . For what purpose?
> I would almost smile, if it weren't necessary to pay them afterward.
>
> . . .

"Healthy diet . . . no more verses . . . no more sleepless nights . . .
no cigarettes . . . no women . . . experiencing clearer skies:

Nervi . . . Rapallo . . . San Remo . . . chase away melancholy;
and if you allow it, we shall even perform some radioscopies . . .."[59]

In these few verses, the traditional theme of the cost of medical treatment appears, along with the conventional distrust in the usefulness of such treatments and the incompetence of doctors. The true novelty lies in the smile with which Gozzano approaches these topics. Starting from the aseptic description of the medical examination he undergoes, where the radioscope makes internal organs visible, the poet addresses his heart, foregrounding by contrast the theme of the inscrutability of the human soul and emotions. It is an expedient one like the one Boito exploits in *Lezione di anatomia*. However, Gozzano replaces the violent tones of denunciation or polemics with pervasive irony, at times bitter but more often amused, manifested in the catalog of useless behaviors prescribed by doctors and the jarring rhyme between *malinconia* (melancholy) and *radioscopia* (radioscopy) – a typically literary term and a prosaic scientific technicality – which is a distinctive stylistic feature of the Turinese writer. The poet's irony seems to be addressed to medical practices and the noble Italian literary tradition.

A similar motif is found in the only other poem that tackles the scientific theme: *Il commesso farmacista* (*The pharmacist*). Ironically, the pharmacist mourns the death of his young consumptive fiancée, whom his medicines could not save. By restating the example of the scientist who assumes the role of the writer, the pharmacist confesses to writing poetry to alleviate the suffering caused by the loss of his beloved. Gozzano smiles at the "rough rhymes" and "abominations worthy of a melodrama" in his friend's verses, but he warns:

Do not laugh at the solitary sorrow
of that poet; do not laugh, for he is worth
much more than me, than you all,
corroded by the literary consumption.[60]

Irony again permeates literature, becoming more cutting. For the Crepusculars, the attitude of weariness and abandonment represented a physical and literary illness. Even those who had briefly participated in the atmosphere of those years, such as Marino Moretti and Corrado Govoni, who survived long into the twentieth century, recognized it:

At that time, who didn't feel a bit inclined toward consumption and flirt with it? It was a kind of literary ailment, common to all the poets of that era. There had been a too intense orgy of health and roses with D'Annunzio and Carducci, not to feel a certain invincible inclination towards melancholy, paleness, and fever.[61]

In addition to being a physical and existential condition, illness represents a literary choice for the poets of the early twentieth century. For Crepuscolari poets, identifying with suffering and weakness meant asserting the need to distance themselves from the poetic season that preceded them, seeking a new role and a different direction for twentieth-century literature.

Notes

1 Giovanna Rosa, *La narrativa degli Scapigliati* (Rome: Laterza, 1997), 32.
2 Edwige Comoy Fusaro, *La nevrosi tra medicina e letteratura: Approccio epistemologico alle malattie nervose nella narrativa italiana (1865–1922)* (Florence: Edizioni Polistampa, 2007), 69–96.
3 Susan Sontag, *Illness as Metaphor* (New York: Farrar, Straus and Giroux, 1978); and Greta Perletti, *Il mal gentile: La malattia polmonare nell'immaginario moderno* (Bergamo: Sestante Edizioni, 2012).
4 Annamaria Cavalli Pasini, *La scienza del romanzo: Romanzo e cultura scientifica tra Otto e Novecento* (Bologna: Patron, 1982), 29–37; and Gian Paolo Biasin, *Malattie letterarie* (Milan: Bompiani, 1976), 16.
5 Perletti, *Il mal gentile*, 71–76.
6 Eugenia Tognotti, *"Il morbo lento": La tisi nell'Italia dell'Ottocento* (Milan: FrancoAngeli, 2012), 17–18.
7 Cavalli Pasini, *Scienza del romanzo*, 15–16; and Biasin, *Malattie letterarie*, 17–18.
8 Giorgio Cosmacini, *Storia della medicina e della sanità in Italia: Dalla peste europea alla guerra mondiale, 1348–1918* (Bari: Laterza, 1987), 311–422.
9 Gino Tellini, *Il romanzo italiano dell'Otto e Novecento* (Milan: Mondadori, 1998), 113–21.
10 Ibid., 120.
11 Rosa, *Narrativa degli Scapigliati*, 31–35.
12 All translations are the author's. I am grateful to the Laura Bassi Foundation for the linguistic revision of this chapter.
13 Marinella Colummi Camerino, "Ragione e follia, scienza e arte nella narrativa di Tarchetti," in *Igino Ugo Tarchetti e la Scapigliatura* (San Salvatore Monferrato: Comune di San Salvatore Monferrato, 1976), 68–69.
14 Michael Foucault, *Naissance de la clinique* (Paris: Presses Universitaires de France, 1963).
15 Francesco Ruchin, *Iginio Ugo Tarchetti: Anatomia di un'anima* (Prato: Pentalinea, 2011), 156–62.
16 Igino Ugo Tarchetti, *Tutte le opere*, ed. Enrico Ghidetti (Bologna: Cappelli, 1967), vol. 2, 274. In the nineteenth century, the distinction between physical and mental illness was not as clear-cut as today. For the significance of neurosis and the overlap between neurosis and tuberculosis in the nineteenth century, see Comoy Fusaro, *La nevrosi*; for the concept of contagion, see Comoy Fusaro, "Persone vaporose: Sul motivo del contagio nella letteratura scapigliata," *Post-filosofie* 10 (2017): 38–51.
17 Tarchetti, *Tutte le opere*, vol. 2, 243.
18 Elena Coda, "La cultura medica ottocentesca nella *Fosca* di Igino Ugo Tarchetti," *Lettere Italiane* 52, no. 3 (July–September 2000): 438–54.
19 Carlo Dossi, *Ritratti umani: Dal calamajo di un medico*, ed. Marco Berisso (Rome: Bulzoni, 1995), 28.
20 Carlo Dossi, *Note azzurre*, ed. Dante Isella (Milan: Adelphi, 1964), no. 5064; and Maria Gabriella Puglisi, "Un letterato in veste di medico: Medicina e malattia in *Dal calamajo di un medico* di Carlo Dossi," in *Letteratura e Scienze,*

ed. Alberto Casadei, Francesca Fedi, Annalisa Nacinovich, and Andrea Torre (Rome: Adi Editore, 2021), www.italianisti.it/pubblicazioni/atti-di-congresso/letteratura-e-scienze/Intervento%20ADI%20Puglisi%201.8.pdf.

21 Benedetta Montagni, *Angelo consolatore e ammazzapazienti: La figura del medico nella letteratura italiana dell'Ottocento* (Florence: Le Lettere, 1999), 107–70.

22 Dossi, *Ritratti umani*, 32–34.

23 Ibid., 36.

24 Ibid., 46.

25 Numerous of Dossi's *Note azzurre* attest to his friendship and admiration for Gorini, especially the epitaph he composed upon Gorini's death (no. 4849).

26 Roberto Carnero, ed., *La poesia scapigliata* (Milan: Biblioteca Universale Rizzoli, 2007), 296. English translation by author.

27 Ibid., 208.

28 Ibid.

29 Camillo Boito, *Storielle vane: Tutti i racconti*, ed. Roberto Bigazzi (Florence: Vallecchi, 1970), 34.

30 Ibid., 62.

31 Ibid., 59.

32 Mariella Muscariello, *Gli inganni della scienza: Percorsi verghiani* (Naples: Liguori Editore, 2001), 3–40.

33 Valeria Gravina, "Les personnages de médecins et hommes de science dans la littérature narrative de Luigi Capuana: Une approche morale" (PhD diss., Université Côte d'Azur and Università degli Studi di Napoli Federico II, 2018), 104–25.

34 Luigi Capuana, *Racconti*, ed. Enrico Ghidetti (Rome: Salerno Editrice, 1973–74), vol. 1, 236.

35 Ibid., 244.

36 Montagni, *Angelo consolatore*, 229–36.

37 *Fantasticheria* (1879) in Giovanni Verga, *Tutte le novelle*, ed. Carla Riccardi (Milan: Mondadori, 1979), 130–31.

38 Verga, *Tutte le novelle*, 262.

39 Ibid., 264.

40 Ibid., 269–70.

41 Francesca Favaro, "Sulla scienza medica (o sulla sua assenza) nelle novelle di Giovanni Verga," in *Letteratura e Scienze*, ed. Alberto Casadei, Francesca Fedi, Annalisa Nacinovich and Andrea Torre (Rome: Adi Editore, 2021), www.italianisti.it/pubblicazioni/atti-di-congresso/letteratura-e-scienze/Favaro_articolo_ADI.pdf.

42 Montagni, *Angelo consolatore*, 236–70.

43 Ibid., 16.

44 Ibid., 17.

45 Ibid., 596.

46 Ibid.

47 Capuana, *Racconti*, 200–01.

48 Ibid.

49 Federico De Roberto, *Romanzi, novelle e saggi*, ed. Carlo A. Madrignani (Milan: Mondadori, 1984), 813–14.

50 Tognotti, *Morbo lento*, 213–28.

51 Enrico Ghidetti, "Introduzione," in *Capuana, Racconti*, 42; and Tellini, *Romanzo italiano*, 120–21.

52 Tellini, *Romanzo italiano*, 247–53. The quote is from Eugenio Montale's poem *Non chiederci la parola*.

53 Biasin, *Malattie letterarie*, 21–35.

54 Anna Nozzoli and Jole Soldateschi, *I crepuscolari* (Florence: La Nuova Italia, 1978), 32–50.
55 Sergio Corazzini, *Poesie edite e inedite*, ed. Stefano Jacomuzzi (Turin: Einaudi, 1968), 78. English translation by author.
56 See, e.g., Guido Gozzano, *Lettere a Carlo Vallini: Con altri inediti*, ed. Giorgio de Rienzo (Turin: Centro studi piemontesi, 1971), 31.
57 See letters to Guglielminetti and Vallini between December 1907 and January 1908: Gozzano, *Lettere a Vallini*; and Guido Gozzano and Amalia Guglieminetti, *Lettere d'amore*, ed. Franco Contorbia (Macerata: Quodlibet, 2019).
58 Gozzano, *Lettere a Vallini*, 16.
59 Guido Gozzano, *Tutte le poesie*, ed. Andrea Rocca (Milan: Mondadori, 2016), 93. English translation by author.
60 Ibid., 272.
61 Govoni's considerations, published in *Popolo d'Italia* (March 25, 1943), were republished in Filippo Donini, *Vita e poesia di Sergio Corazzini* (Turin: De Silva, 1949), 143; a similar declaration about this "affliction made of paper" is by Moretti (ibid., 242).

References

Biasin, Gian Paolo. *Malattie letterarie*. Milan: Bompiani, 1976.
Boito, Camillo. *Storielle vane: Tutti i racconti*. Edited by Roberto Bigazzi. Florence: Vallecchi, 1970.
Capuana, Luigi. *Racconti*. Edited by Enrico Ghidetti. 3 vols. Rome: Salerno Editrice, 1973–74.
Carnero, Roberto, ed. *La poesia scapigliata*. Milan: Biblioteca Universale Rizzoli, 2007.
Cavalli Pasini, Annamaria. *La scienza del romanzo: Romanzo e cultura scientifica tra Otto e Novecento*. Bologna: Patron, 1982.
Coda, Elena. "La cultura medica ottocentesca nella *Fosca* di Igino Ugo Tarchetti." *Lettere Italiane* 52, no. 3 (July–September 2000): 438–54.
Colummi Camerino, Marinella. "Ragione e follia, scienza e arte nella narrativa di Tarchetti." In *Igino Ugo Tarchetti e la Scapigliatura*, 65–75. San Salvatore Monferrato: Comune di San Salvatore Monferrato, 1976.
Comoy Fusaro, Edwige. *La nevrosi tra medicina e letteratura: Approccio epistemologico alle malattie nervose nella narrativa italiana (1865–1922)*. Florence: Edizioni Polistampa, 2007.
______. "Persone vaporose: Sul motivo del contagio nella letteratura scapigliata." *Post-filosofie* 10 (2017): 38–51.
Corazzini, Sergio. *Poesie edite e inedite*. Edited by Stefano Jacomuzzi. Turin: Einaudi, 1968.
Cosmacini, Giorgio. *Storia della medicina e della sanità in Italia: Dalla peste europea alla guerra mondiale, 1348–1918*. Rome: Laterza, 1987.
De Roberto, Federico. *Romanzi, novelle e saggi*. Edited by Carlo A. Madrignani. Milan: Mondadori, 1984.
Donini, Filippo. *Vita e poesia di Sergio Corazzini*. Turin: De Silva, 1949.
Dossi, Carlo. *Note azzurre*. Edited by Dante Isella. Milan: Adelphi, 1964.
______. *Ritratti umani: Dal calamajo di un medico*. Edited by Marco Berisso. Rome: Bulzoni, 1995.
Favaro, Francesca. "Sulla scienza medica (o sulla sua assenza) nelle novelle di Giovanni Verga." In *Letteratura e Scienze*, edited by Alberto Casadei, Francesca Fedi, Annalisa Nacinovich, and Andrea Torre. Rome: Adi Editore, 2021. www.italianisti.it/pubblicazioni/atti-di-congresso/letteratura-e-scienze/Favaro_articolo_ADI.pdf.

Foucault, Michael. *Naissance de la clinique*. Paris: Presses Universitaires de France, 1963.

Gozzano, Guido. *Lettere a Carlo Vallini: Con altri inediti*. Edited by Giorgio de Rienzo. Turin: Centro studi piemontesi, 1971.

———. *Tutte le poesie*. Edited by Andrea Rocca. Milan: Mondadori, 2016.

———, and Amalia Guglieminetti. *Lettere d'amore*. Edited by Franco Contorbia. Macerata: Quodlibet, 2019.

Gravina, Valeria. "Les personnages de médecins et hommes de science dans la littérature narrative de Luigi Capuana: Une approche morale." PhD diss., Université Côte d'Azur and Università degli Studi di Napoli Federico II, 2018.

Montagni, Benedetta. *Angelo consolatore e ammazzapazienti: La figura del medico nella letteratura italiana dell'Ottocento*. Florence: Le Lettere, 1999.

Muscariello, Mariella. *Gli inganni della scienza: Percorsi verghiani*. Naples: Liguori Editore, 2001.

Nozzoli, Anna, and Jole Soldateschi. *I crepuscolari*. Florence: La Nuova Italia, 1978.

Perletti, Greta. *Il mal gentile: La malattia polmonare nell'immaginario moderno*. Bergamo: Sestante Edizioni, 2012.

Puglisi, Maria Gabriella. "Un letterato in veste di medico: Medicina e malattia in *Dal calamajo di un medico* di Carlo Dossi." In *Letteratura e Scienze*, edited by Alberto Casadei, Francesca Fedi, Annalisa Nacinovich, and Andrea Torre. Rome: Adi Editore, 2021. www.italianisti.it/pubblicazioni/atti-di-congresso/letteratura-e-scienze/ Intervento%20ADI%20Puglisi%201.8.pdf.

Rosa, Giovanna. *La narrativa degli Scapigliati*. Rome: Laterza, 1997.

Ruchin, Francesco. *Iginio Ugo Tarchetti: Anatomia di un'anima*. Prato: Pentalinea, 2011.

Sontag, Susan. *Illness as Metaphor*. New York: Farrar, Straus and Giroux, 1978.

Tarchetti, Igino Ugo. *Tutte le opere*. Edited by Enrico Ghidetti. 2 vols. Bologna: Cappelli, 1967.

Tellini, Gino. *Il romanzo italiano dell'Otto e Novecento*. Milan: Mondadori, 1998.

Tognotti, Eugenia. *"Il morbo lento": La tisi nell'Italia dell'Ottocento*. Milan: FrancoAngeli, 2012.

Verga, Giovanni. *Tutte le novelle*. Edited by Carla Riccardi. Milan: Mondadori, 1979.

7 "Fever Veiled in Mist"
Denying Contagious Diseases in Modern Italian Visual Arts

Sharon Hecker

Introduction

In 1883, critic Luigi Chirtani described the subject of contagious disease in nineteenth-century Italian art as the result of "unhealthy influences,"[1] characterizing the brushstrokes in one such artwork as if infected by "interruptions of a dry cough."[2] Responses to artworks about epidemics included revulsion, expressions of sadness or a pivoting away from the unappealing subject in favor of discussions of artistic form and style. Most of these artworks did not find buyers in Italy: they languished in the artist's studio, were erased or shipped abroad. Their fate has led the subject of contagious disease in Italian art to remain somewhat invisible, or in the words of poet Gabriele D'Annunzio, like a "fever veiled in mist."[3]

This chapter proposes a deep engagement with images of disease and their reception through three case studies.[4] In analyzing these works' visual languages and critical fortunes, I suggest that artistic representations of contagious illnesses involved the personal, public and scientific spheres. In different ways, all three images addressed the horror and fear of epidemics, invisible lethal enemies for which no cure had been found, provoking anxieties ranging from the private to the social to the cultural and political.

Representing Tuberculosis: Giovanni Segantini

A recently rediscovered painting on the theme of tuberculosis is Giovanni Segantini's *Tisi galoppante* (*Galloping Phthisis*, 1881). The work no longer exists – it was scraped down and painted over by the artist. We know about it through exhibition catalogs, press reviews and Segantini's mentions of it in letters to his dealer. The image was found in an X-ray analysis underneath the painting that covers it, and its visual data is known through copies – a charcoal drawing and a watercolor of 1883–84 – by his roommate, the painter Emilio Longoni (Figure 7.1).[5]

Through the X-ray and Longoni's copies, we know that Segantini's erased painting depicted a cropped close-up of the face of a girl lying in bed, with her head resting on a sunken pillow. Her cheeks were flushed, and she wore

DOI: 10.4324/9781003382805-7

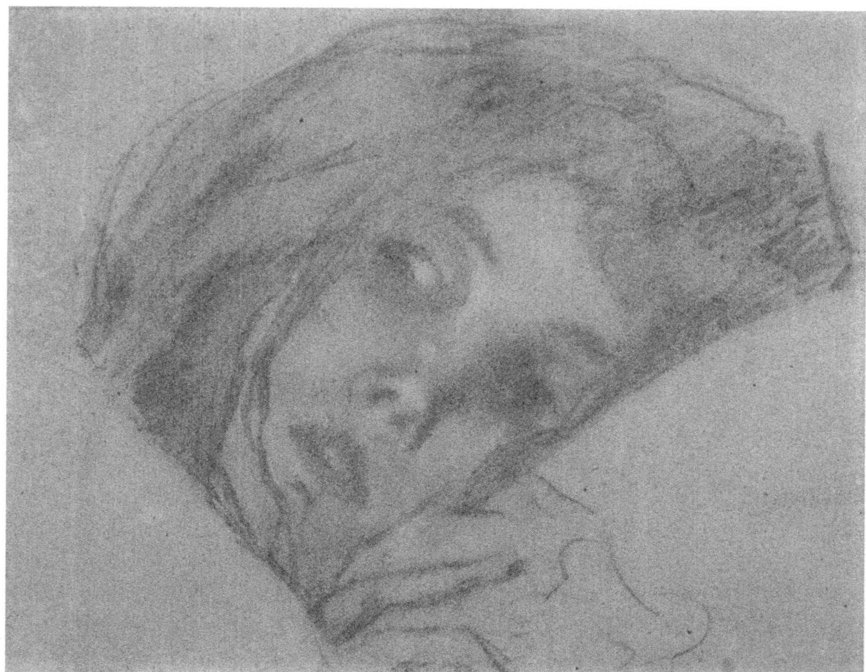

Figure 7.1 Emilio Longoni, *Galloping Phthisis* (1882–84), soft pencil on hazel paper, 24.1 × 30.1 cms.

Source: Barlassina, Banca di Credito Cooperativo.

a dramatic expression of fright, as if responding to some invisible threat coming from outside the painting, perhaps implying that the disease's causes were not understood. A cross hanging on a stoup above her head alluded to her imminent death. The title states that the woman was suffering from tuberculosis.

Segantini's choice of subject deserves contextualization. In her 2012 study of tuberculosis in nineteenth-century Italy, historian of medicine Eugenia Tognotti notes that tuberculosis was the principal cause of death in Italy at the end of the century, generating public worry and private anguish. The disease was little understood in Italy because scientific research on it was delayed in comparison with other European countries. The disease curve rose and the greatest mortality from tuberculosis was in the decades after unification: more than 30,000 deaths per year. The late realization of the problem's enormity was due to political inaction, which resulted in overdue sanitary reforms.[6]

By the 1880s, researchers in Europe and the United States had discovered the role of urban poverty and overcrowding in the spread of tuberculosis's contagion. This was related to industrialization and modern capitalism, which drew people to live and work in crowded, unsanitary quarters. In Italy, this phenomenon was most pronounced in the north. The dramatic conditions seeped into Italian cultural production. In her 1892 poem, Ada Negri referred to "the consumptive blood" of female textile workers in urban Italian factories.[7] The situation was reflected in the different connotations attributed to the disease in the operatic roles of Violetta in Giuseppe Verdi's 1853 *La Traviata*, written before the discovery, whose disease was associated with sensuality, frailty and decadence, and Mimì in Giacomo Puccini's 1893 *La Bohème*, written after the discovery, whose disease derived from poverty and working conditions in the silk industry.[8] In 1882, the German microbiologist Robert Koch discovered the tubercle bacillus and the theory of contagion. Such findings were translated and discussed in Italian newspapers, especially in northern industrialized areas hit hard by tuberculosis. It seems fitting that Segantini, who was working in Northern Italy in the early 1880s, would have familiarity with the topic of tuberculosis and would want to recapture it in his art.

Outside Italy, notably in Britain, tuberculosis gained special appeal for artists. There was a rise in the Romantic and sexual attractiveness of the tubercular aesthetic, for tuberculosis was unique in its ability to replicate the beauty standards of the Victorian woman. This is evident in depictions by British pre-Raphaelite painter and poet Dante Gabriele Rossetti of the pale, beautiful Lizzie Siddal carrying the disease.[9] Some elements in Segantini's paintings also link feminine beauty and frailty with tuberculosis, but unlike Rossetti, Segantini was not depicting the reality of a personal situation. For the model, he used his partner Bice Bugatti, who may have had a fever but was not suffering from tuberculosis. He made her appear younger than she was to intensify the dramatic effect of the subject and perhaps to link the work with earlier Romantic associations of youth and death. While the woman is depicted as attractive, Segantini did not elevate or spiritualize his ill beloved as Rossetti did.

Over the following two years, Segantini showed *Galloping Phthisis* in three Italian venues: refused for the Esposizione Nazionale di Belle Arti, it was shown at the Galleria Grubicy in 1881, then at Rome's Esposizione di Belle Arti and finally at the Esposizione di Belle Arti at Brera in Milan, both in 1883. In an 1881 review, a critic under the pseudonym "Athos" singled it out in the daily *Lombardia*:

[The work] instills a great sadness in the soul and almost gives a sense of creepiness. A woman's head sinks into a pillow. The cheeks are lit with fever, the dumbfounded eyes are lost in the void; the blond tresses fall loose on the forehead and descend on the sheets. A blessed olive branch hangs from the wall.[10]

Evidently, Athos's response reflected a general sense of sorrow and disgust.

Upon seeing the work in Rome in March 1883, Chirtani devoted significant space to reviewing it in *Corriere della Sera*. Surprisingly, he called it "the most pleasant [*simpatico*]"[11] painting by Segantini in the exhibition. However, he noted with exasperation that "literature, painting, sculpture . . . have not yet completely exhausted that period of unhealthy influences that one day prompted art to take an interest in tuberculosis and make it the subject of artistic creations."[12] To prove his point, he described with horror another painting on consumption in the show by the Roman artist Alessandro Morani depicting two "skin and bones" ill women, one with "yellowed ivory pallor" and the other with an "earthy pallor of burial."[13] For Chirtani, it was as if the paintbrush itself was infected by an ill artist:

> It is a scene that is repulsive in pathological truth; the painting is solidly constituted, but it also has an earthy pallor of thin sickness, and the brush feels the effects of that contact by marking the forms in sharp touches, like one straining to speak by accenting words between the interruptions of a dry cough.[14]

In discussing Segantini's work, the critic dissociated from the scene of illness, instead praising its poetic painterly qualities:

> Segantini's *Galloping Phthisis* is completely different. All that can be seen from the sick woman is her head, which stands out against the whiteness of a pillow and a section of the tuck of the sheet, flattened under her chin by loving maternal hands. The pillow standing out against the light ashen damask background of the room's upholstery, the tucking in of the sheet of the finest cloth and of a whiteness different from the whiteness of the pillow and the little blond head sunk in those crisp linens, as in a bed of lilies, form a whole of a moving and singularly poetic original purity.[15]

For Chirtani, the figure's beauty came from Segantini's masterly handling:

> The sick girl is a maiden, almost a child, she has abundant golden hair, an oval face, wispy, but that has not lost all the unconscious festivity of early age, and from the orbits hollowed out by fever with two big blue eyes she stares into the void perhaps [at] a flight of angels who want to kidnap her from her mother. This amplification is my own, but the painting is . . . an ode to candor, a most delicate painting obtained spontaneously with an abundance of impasto, with a masterly glaze and riches of pearl jewel-like mottling that make up for some inexperience in full-body modeling of the genteel forms.[16]

Somewhat similarly, when the Milanese critic for *La Perseveranza*, Filippo Filippi, saw the work at Brera in September 1883, he initially gushed about "a very beautiful head, expressive, and all the intonation is clear, bright, full midday."[17] Yet he had evidently misread the theme, suggesting that nothing in the painting's language clued him in to the subject of disease. After learning the title, Filippi revised his initial response: "that frightened maiden's head by Segantini, beautiful, but impossible to guess, not even to suspect that it is called '*Galloping Phthisis*.' "[18] Chirtani's and Filippi's words suggest that the image was not fully understood as a realistic, convincing depiction of a woman afflicted with tuberculosis and did not resonate with its tragic aspects. The image seemed more like a choreographed performance than a lived reality.

Perhaps because of Segantini's unappealing theme, his tubercular painting did not find a buyer in any of its exhibition venues and returned to the artist's studio, where it remained for almost a decade. The painting's mixed reception and failure to sell may partially explain why nine years later, Segantini decided to paint over the image and change its title. The new painting represented a woman with rosy cheeks, renamed *Petalo di rosa* (Rose Petal, 1890) (Figure 7.2). While her flushed cheeks may still have alluded to symptoms of tuberculosis, the woman's once-frightened expression was softened to give her a dreamy gaze. No longer depicted with clenched fingers desperately holding on to crumpled bed sheets and to life itself, she now sensually played with a golden lock of hair between her fingers. The agitated bed sheets were smoothed, making the work feel more serene. Technical studies show that Segantini scraped the original face away. He made the crucifix smaller, less prominent and no longer hanging from the stoup. He added yellow, white and red gold to render the image brighter and more appealing. Finally, Segantini scattered gold powder overall to give the scene a warm, dreamy feeling.

Today, scholars have hypothesized that these changes could have been due to stylistic developments and Segantini's later embrace of Divisionism. In relation to the movement itself, contagious disease was explicitly mentioned as a rhetorical way *not* to paint – critics denigrated Divisionism as "painted measles,"[19] suggesting that Divisionist works, which were created using spots of pigment, were contaminated and unappealing. Segantini may have felt that the initial subject was not appreciated, convincing or saleable. The change may have been made at the urging of the artist's dealer, Vittore Grubicy, who was known to have a heavy hand in shaping his artists' paintings, a reason why Segantini eventually parted ways with him. The operation was successful: with its reworked subject and innocuous title, the new painting was exhibited in Milan in 1890, the Munich Glaspalast in 1891 and the Esposizione di Torino in 1894. It was bought there by the wealthy Turinese painter Clemente Pugliese Levi for 2,500 lire and remained in the family for two more generations. Until recently, *Rose Petal* has been frequently exhibited without mention of its original title: all traces of tuberculosis were erased from the work, and its original subject was disguised by the new work, remaining buried underneath.

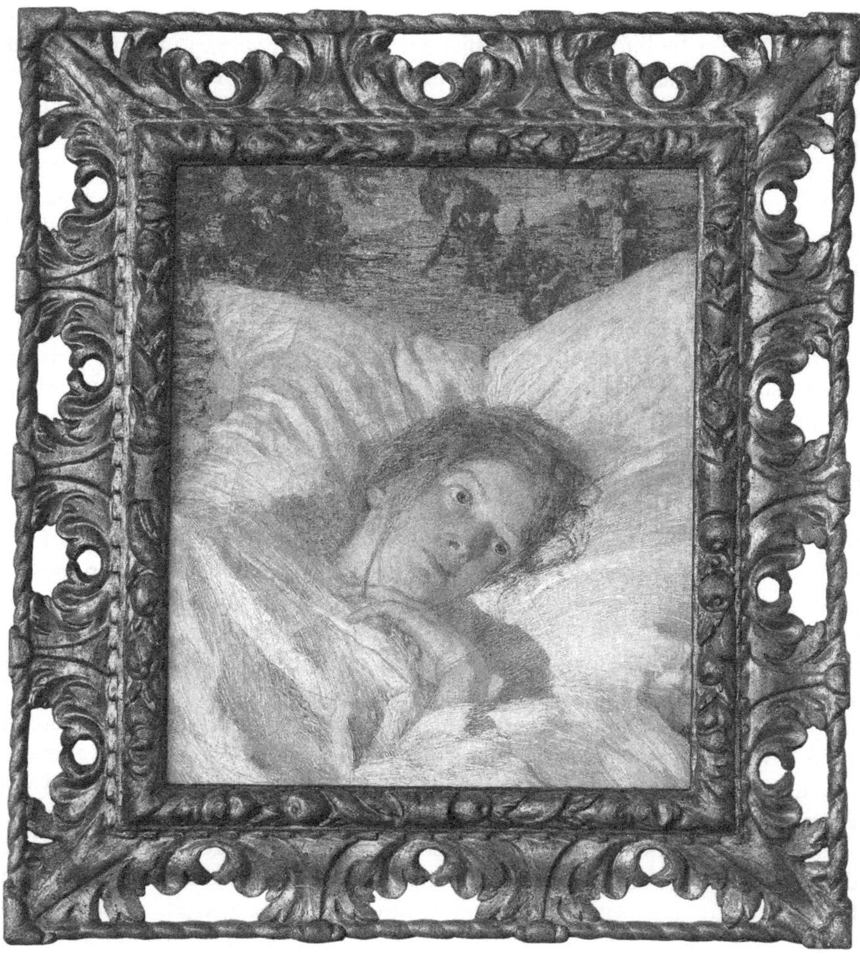

Figure 7.2 Giovanni Segantini, *Rose Petal* (1890), oil on canvas with addition of gold leaf and gold powder, 64 × 50 cms.

Source: Courtesy Gallerie Maspes, Milan.

Imagining Malaria: Giulio Aristide Sartorio

In contrast to Segantini's intimate close-up of a frightened diseased woman's face, Giulio Aristide Sartorio's painting was a direct, politically charged statement about the contemporary problems of another overwhelming contagious epidemic that afflicted Italy: malaria. While Segantini was working in the urban north, Sartorio painted the countryside in the south. The work, dated 1883, depicts a desolate landscape with a woman sitting in the foreground alongside the dead body of a young boy (Figure 7.3). Her hands cover her eyes in grief. The figures are poor: she is clothed in a simple sleeveless dress,

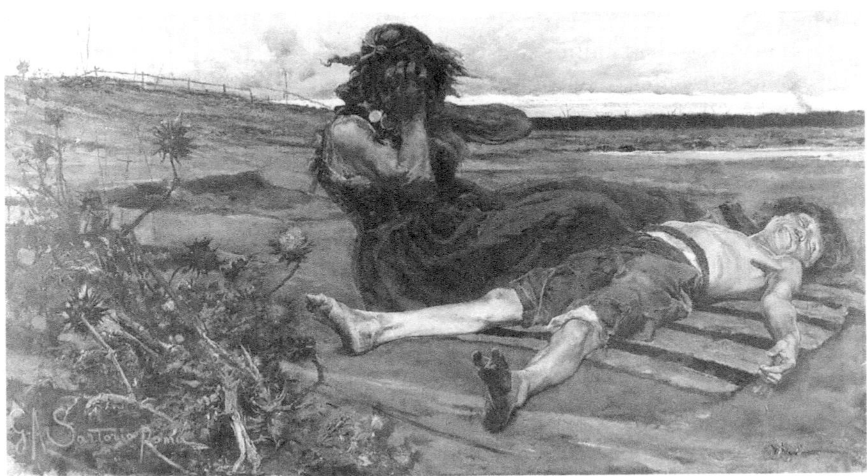

Figure 7.3 Giulio Aristide Sartorio, *Malaria* (1883), originally titled *Dum Romae consulitur, morbus imperat* (While Rome deliberates, the disease rules), oil on canvas, 125 × 223 cms.

Source: Museo Nacional de Bellas Artes, Buenos Aires.

and her hair is wild and unkempt. The boy, presumably her son, is shirtless and shoeless, wearing only pants and a makeshift cord as a belt. Laid out on an improvised mat made of rough wooden slats, his lifeless body is thin, his dirty feet visible to the viewer and his nose seems to have been bleeding. The figures resemble a Christian *Pietà*, with the thistles symbolizing arid land and Christ's Passion. The background includes a grave-like hole in the earth, perhaps for the boy's simple burial. Hovering over the background are large ominous gray clouds that meet the horizon, compressing the scene, with a patch of pink light underneath.

Unlike the small dimensions of Segantini's work, Sartorio's painting was large – 125 by 223 centimeters – a size suitable for a public declaration. Sartorio gave the work a contentious political title: *Dum Romae consulitur, morbus imperat* (While Rome deliberates, the disease rules), rephrasing the Latin locution *Dum Romae consulitur, Saguntum expugnatur* (While Rome deliberates, Sagunto is expunged). This was Livy's bitter commentary on a situation in which the ambassadors of Sagunto needed Rome's help to repel the siege that Carthaginian general Hannibal Barca laid on the city in 219 BC. Rome procrastinated, and after eight months of fighting, the city surrendered and Hannibal razed it to the ground, an attack that occasioned the Second Punic War.

The timeliness of Sartorio's painting merits contextualization. As with tuberculosis, mortality from malaria was at its peak in Italy between 1872 and 1881. According to historian of medicine Gilberto Corbellini's 2022 study, the first results of data were only compiled in 1881, and the first map showing the disease's distribution was published in 1882. By 1887, a nationwide census demonstrated that almost a third of Italy was afflicted with malaria, with two million cases out of a population of 30 million. There were 20,000 deaths per year, more in Southern Italy than in the north.[20]

Today, it is thought that the painting was "of veristic social inspiration,"[21] and that in its time, the work's "crude and violent realism was praised and at the same time provoked debates."[22] This is only somewhat true, for despite Sartorio's confrontational title, the critical responses – like those to Segantini's work – pivoted away from the subject of disease. Critic Ferdinando Fontana's 1883 review ignored the theme, noting only the formal qualities, praising it as: "Most vigorous, painted with an eagerness of a true artist's soul." From Sartorio, "for the personal path he shows to have [taken] and to pursue vigorously, we should expect excellent things."[23] Painter Nino Costa, while recognizing the theme, remained unconvinced by Sartorio's rendering of malaria:

> The young Sartorio in *Malaria* has much nerve, and beneath the skein of color, there is undoubted feeling in the two figures. The landscape of this painting [though] well imagined is, however, dry, poor in form, which is not true to the Roman countryside, and he has not expressed in the air the fat hot humidity of malaria.[24]

Costa's review points to an artistic difficulty with convincingly depicting swampy air, or the *mal-aria* (literally "bad air") that was thought to breed disease.

Only the critic Luigi Bellinzoni fully understood the tragic, frightening subject and the depiction of malaria as an unseen adversary:

> A child lies dead on the ground: a country girl kneeling near him puts her hands in her hair and moans: a line divides the livid sky from the parched earth. Oh! One is quick to realize it: it is a plain scourged by malaria. The intonation of the picture gives one the chills: in that environment, extermination breathes, and we, having come to our senses from such a mournful scene, must tear our hair out, our hands clenched like the poor mother's for not yet having crushed this enemy that decimates us.[25]

At the same time, Bellinzoni expressed concern that the artist had used this subject to gain sympathy with viewers:

> Sartorio, young and inexperienced, has already mastered the secret of flogging our inertia by hiding the blows under the attractive appearances of an original and serious art. I admire in Aristide Sartorio the intrinsic value; I criticize the extrinsic qualities, which need to be

restrained by reflection and study. If he were to continue the path on which his youthful impetus threw him, soon the sympathies of today would fall away from him. This time he has painted a grim subject: that unrestrained form and modeling of his stands its ground: however, one does not always find [a] *malaria* to keep pace with the escapades of a prodigy. And then what?[26]

Others claimed that Italian artists used malaria to galvanize the public and gain notoriety. In an 1885 government survey of malaria in Sardinia, for example, the author warned:

[Malaria] was and is still exaggerated, as well as the intensity of it, and also some of the effects. . .. One writes about it in a novel-esque way in order to make some noise. . .. Malaria lends itself to a gloomy painting; if [an artist] adopt[s] the gloomiest hues, the painting succeeds in being frightening, succeeds as artistically horrifying . . . so that at the mere sight of it, everyone feels the evil fluid of fever running through their veins. The painting often assures the success of the painter. . .. It is well known that in paintings there is more of the fantastic than the real; but I express the painful impression which I always feel when I hear my very first countrymen exaggerate this insalubriousness.[27]

These comments suggest that paintings about epidemics were unwelcome due to political and economic anxieties about projecting a negative public image of the country: people would be afraid to visit if they saw off-putting paintings about the disease, contaminating and destroying the benefits of tourism. Many critics felt that the subject of epidemics in art was better disguised or denied.

As critic Francesco Sapori would later recall, Sartorio's "humanitarian appeal was not heeded."[28] Nor, perhaps due to its controversial title and subject, did Sartorio's depiction of malaria find a buyer, like Segantini's painting on tuberculosis. Sartorio recalled that it "was on the verge of [being bought by] the [national museum, the] Galleria d'Arte Moderna, but ended up in the hands of Sommaruga, who sold it in America."[29] Publisher Angelo Sommaruga took it to Buenos Aires in 1885 and sold it to Susana Rodríguez Viana de Quintana, wife of the president of Argentina Manuel Quintana, who donated it to the Museo Nacional de Bellas Artes in 1910. Today, the work is not on display.[30] Its failure to sell in Italy suggests the risk of representing such a theme at home, given that artists were typically trained in state-sponsored schools, mostly showed their works in government exhibitions and hoped to sell them to public national museums. As a perceived critique of the state's refusal to address epidemics, the painting exposed Italy's lagging acceptance of medical discoveries and the tragic consequences of its delays in implementing cures.

Sartorio's work and its critical response unveil Italy's fragility as a newly united nation, showing how epidemics continued to be politically disguised. The health of the nation depended on the perceived health of its citizens. Contagious disease unsettled social performance, negatively intervening in people's lives. It upset society's self-perception as a strong, well-functioning, unified whole, creating separation between healthy and diseased bodies, as well as pathological tensions and divisions among citizens. Although undiscussed in art-historical analyses of *Ottocento* art, the reluctance to engage with images of fragile, vulnerable, diseased bodies laid the groundwork for the twentieth century during Fascism, when visual arts came directly under the yoke of the Regime and were harnessed to promote and glorify the cult of the strong, healthy Italian body.[31]

Sartorio's mapping of pathological signs of illness onto a male body was unusual. With rare exception, Italian paintings of the malaria-infested Roman Pontine or Maremma swamps did not typically focus on clinical depictions of bodies decaying from disease but rather on the poverty of inhabitants, religious piety or universal themes of death. Maremma artists like Teofilo Patini produced spiritualized images of mortality and bereavement in the 1880 *L'erede* (The Heir), which garnered public success but avoided showing the realities of sickness and contagion. Painter Mario de Maria showed three works in the 1886 Roman exhibition *In arte libertas*, namely, *Sorgente infetta* (Infected Water Source), *La peste di Roma nel 1600* (The Plague in Rome in the 1600s) and *Ospedale degli infetti* (Hospital of the Infected), that may have resonated obliquely with current events. *Peste a Roma* remained rather unknown in Italy but garnered great success abroad: as art historian Anna Mazzanti notes, it won a medal in Munich in 1888, then was exhibited in London and again at the Galleria Schulte in Berlin, where it was bought by William I.[32] Dante Ricci's *Il Mortacino* (The Mortacino Canal, 1927) gestured indirectly to swampy waters, while Amedeo Bocchi's expressionistically colored *Terracina, la malaria* (Terracina, Malaria, 1919) avoided pathological realities.[33] Giuseppe Raggio's empathetic two-meter *La Malaria* (Malaria, 1873) is more direct. Sapori describes the tragic scene:

By the little door of a deserted hut, a man afflicted with malaria lies without strength. Before him, a young woman, accompanied by a young boy, shows that she has no food to feed herself. . .. The clear, indifferent sky looks like a greenish mirror. The unspeakable sadness of those dying of fever, of hunger, spreads across the canvas like an unheard plea for the well-being, the joy they will never know.[34]

For Sapori, Raggio felt pity for those he represented:

creatures condemned to "live by dying" in the Pontine Marshes. . .. [He] had for the workers, forced to die of fever in those moors, boundless pity, which made his colorist's eyes forget the flickering pearl dawns and the peacock-tail-colored orgies of the sunsets, and left traces of real tears in his brushes.[35]

But Raggi never let the painting out of his studio.

In its directness, Sartorio's image seems closer to two celebrated French paintings about Italy and malaria: Eugène Giraud's *Le fiévreux dans la campagne romaine* (The Feverish Man in the Roman Countryside, 1845, Clemont-Ferrand, Musées Bargoin et du Tapis), possibly inspired by an 1835 trip to Italy, and Ernest Hébert's *La Mal'aria* (The Mal'aria, 1848–49, Musée d'Orsay). Both works were praised by French critics, awarded grand prizes and are displayed today in French museums. They led to the writing of poems and engendered public debate in France about infectious diseases.[36]

Sartorio exhibited another version of the subject, titled *Febbre* (Fever), in 1905 at the Esposizione degli Amatori e Cultori.[37] The work's location today is unknown. In 1914, he sent what is assumed to be another version to the Venice Biennale. At 59.5 by 130 centimeters, it was smaller than his bold 1883 manifesto. The earlier polemical title was now gone. He called this work, more poetically, *Alba lunare nelle paludi pontine* (Moonrise in the Pontine Marshes) (Figure 7.4).[38] According to Sapori, at some point Sartorio changed the title to *Trasporto d'una malata* (Transport of an Ill Woman),[39] shifting the focus to the coffin-like boat being used to carry the sick woman. Today, it has been renamed *Malaria*. Here, Sartorio more conventionally projected disease onto a female victim. Sapori commented:

> night compresses, wraps all things in a dreary leaden and turquoise hue . . . the moon rises from the sea: its dull reflection walks meekly over the dead waters of the canals. A hanging hut . . . watches like a dumbfounded eye in the distance. A rope, pulled by an invisible person or horse, leads the sandal [a traditional Venetian rowboat] in which the mother holds the head of a fever-stricken maiden. A nocturnal languor imbues this canvas, from which emanates the sick fascination of incurable malaria.[40]

As with Segantini's woman, frightened by an invisible threat, the boat of death in Sartorio's painting is pulled by an unseen force, symbolizing the disease's unknowable cause and the absence of a cure. Like Sartorio's earlier polemical painting, this one too went unsold, remaining in the artist's studio at his death, as did yet another version titled *Malaria*. It took another century for it to be sold by Sartorio's heirs, in 1983, to the Galleria Nazionale d'Arte Moderna in Rome.[41]

Sartorio's paintings emphasized nature's illness rather than just the ill human suggested by Segantini. The idea that nature might be sick, alluded to by critics' descriptions of unhealthy sky, earth, air and water, contrasted

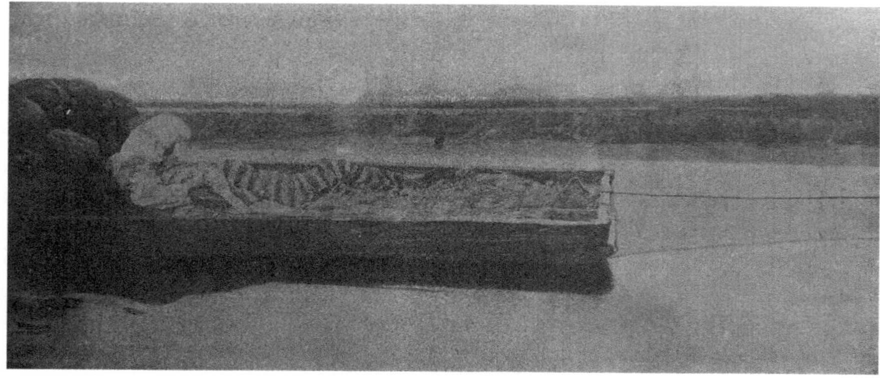

Figure 7.4 1933 photograph of the exhibition catalogue, *Mostra delle pitture di Giulio Aristide Sartorio nella Regia Galleria Borghese, 9 marzo-24 aprile 1933–1* (Rome: Reale Accademia d'Italia, 1933), TAV. XLIII, showing Giulio Aristide Sartorio's, *Malaria* (ca. 1913).

with the enduring Italian identification with the land and nature and the projection onto nature of higher human spiritual values. Such a topos spans modern Italian art from Romanticism to the Tuscan Macchiaioli, to the Lombard Scapigliatura, to Divisionism, Symbolism, Futurism and postwar Arte povera.

Verist art did not focus on nature as unwell. Most *Ottocento* artists created work that showed nature as a retreat into symbolic fantasy spaces or subjects from the past or the natural passage of the seasons, which remained uncontaminated by the unpleasant aspects of contemporary disease. In doing so, they preserved idealized picturesque, nostalgic images of Italy and its landscape, which uplifted natives, fulfilled the expectations of foreigners, raised no political questions and satisfied the market.

Today, historians of the environmental history of modern Italy such as Marco Armiero and Marcus Hall view this narrative critically, arguing that there were "reciprocal relationships between nature and society"[42] that have remained suppressed in Italian culture. They propose a view that takes into account both the enduring picturesque images of Italy's genius loci and the often less-appealing histories of its environment, "coexisting in the same place, neither cursed nor blessed but a hybrid landscape fashioned by history as well as nature."[43]

Vaccinations and Monteverde's *Jenner Inoculates His Son*

Finally, a third case is an artwork that focuses on the role of scientific advances: Giulio Monteverde's 1869–73 *Edward Jenner* (Figure 7.5). The work commemorated British doctor Edward Jenner's 1796 promotion through

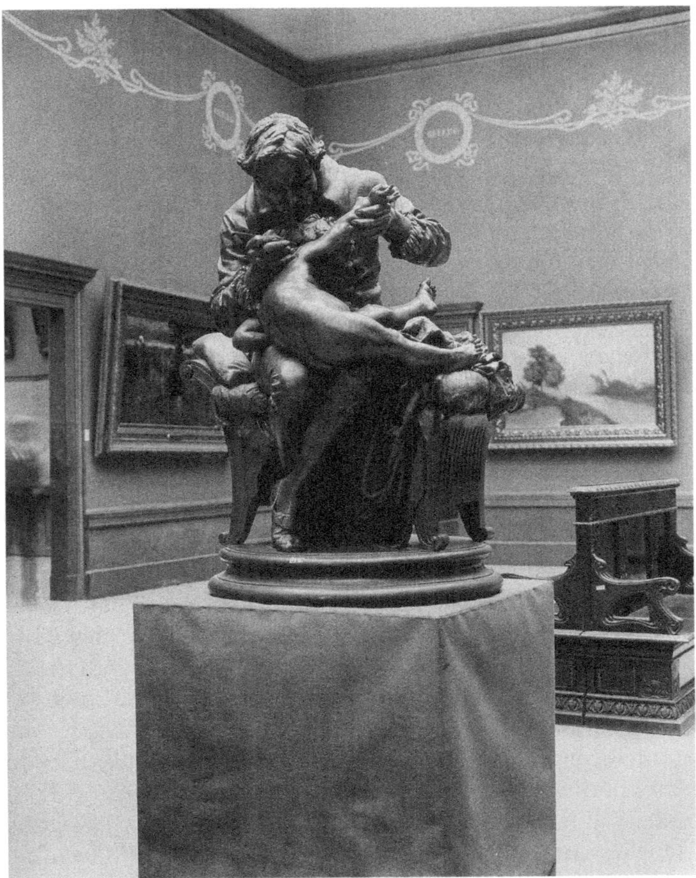

Figure 7.5 Edward Jenner. Photograph of a sculpture by Giulio Monteverde.
Source: Wellcome Collection. Public Domain Mark.

experimentation of the technique of vaccinations to combat smallpox. The sculpture's subject, usually described as Jenner inoculating his son, was somewhat erroneous, given that it was not Jenner's son whom he had vaccinated but rather James Phipps, the son of his gardener. Although Jenner's breakthrough had occurred almost a century earlier and the subject was taken from the past, Monteverde apparently considered its symbolic importance to be valuable for his time. Late in life, he recalled the work's genesis, showing that he read medical history books and became inspired by them:

> [The subject was] an old favorite theme of mine. Stuck in my mind was the phrase of Massimo d'Azeglio, who deplored how Napoleon, hero

of so many human massacres, was so glorified, and so little was known and revered the name of Jenner, who had prevented so many massacres of children with his smallpox vaccine. I had read in a medical history how Jenner had had the revelation of the wonder from the confession of a Peasant Woman. . . . After long research, I got from a German friend of mine who had gone to London a beautiful portrait of Jenner: with my first success I had saved a little money to afford the luxury of a statue; with the fever of singular desire, I modeled this hero of humanism: and I was not satisfied until I had accomplished the work I had long dreamt about.[44]

According to art historian Gianluca Kannès, Monteverde submitted a plaster version to be sent to the Universal Exhibition in Vienna of 1873. It was rejected by the jury of the Accademia di San Luca: according to the rules, all submissions had to be in bronze or marble, given the fragility of plaster. Thanks to the intervention of Stefano Castagnola, a Genoese Minister of Agriculture and Commerce and president of the exhibition committee, the work was accepted belatedly and sent to Vienna. It was awarded a medal and was unanimously praised by critics. Monteverde then sent a marble version, carved at the artist's expense, to the 1878 Exposition Universelle in Paris, where it won Honorable Mention and was favorably reviewed by French critics from Henri Chapu to Anatole de Montaiglon to Paul Mantz.[45] According to Monteverde, the Accademia di San Luca's jury "had not even understood the subject, and when asked by one of them: 'But what could it be?!' The most intelligent of the Commission had replied: 'It must be a doctor!' "[46]

After attempting unsuccessfully to sell the marble to the French state, Monteverde sold it to an Italian residing in France, Maria Brignole Sale de Ferrari, Duchess of Galliera, for half the asking price.[47] According to the duchess's biography, her second son, Andrea, in whom she had placed hopes of passing on her inheritance, died of *malattia esantematica* (measles or scarlet fever) in his adolescence.[48] The positivist subject of vaccinations may have been of personal interest to her.

Although Monteverde's work was bought by a private collector, it continued to circulate, widely reproduced in lithographs and acquiring lasting significance abroad, in contrast to Segantini's and Sartorio's forgotten works. Monteverde cast more copies serially in bronze at the Bastianelli foundry in Rome, selling one to the Galleria Nazionale in Rome in 1913, and other casts have made their way into international collections. The work gained importance when the British pharmaceutical entrepreneur Henry Wellcome acquired a bronze cast for his celebrated collection in 1917, and the sculpture became connected to the role of vaccines in combating contemporary infections.[49] This was again confirmed recently, during COVID-19, when two further bronze casts were commissioned by David B. Agus, MD, one of which was placed at the entrance of the Lawrence J. Ellison Institute for Transformative

Medicine of the University of Southern California in Los Angeles.[50] These casts were made by the Fonderia Artistica Ferdinando Marinelli in Florence from a mold taken from the original plaster in the Galleria d'Arte Moderna in Genoa, housed along with the marble donated to the museum by the Duchess of Galliera through her will of 1884. The work's enduring international success as a statement about the value of medical cures continues to honor Jenner's work through public monuments around the world: in London (in 1862, by William Calder Marshall, RA), Boulogne-sur-Mer (in 1865, by Eugène Paul, to honor Napoleon's 1905 vaccination of his troops) and Tokyo (in 1904, by Yonehara Unkai, sponsored by the Japanese Society of Hygiene).[51] Puzzlingly, in Italy no monument to Jenner was erected, and Monteverde's large sculpture was never contemplated for a public site. Perhaps this had to do with the nineteenth-century suspicion about doctors and medicine in Italy, or with antivaccination movements like the one that emerged after the 1888 Crispi-Pagliano law made vaccination against smallpox obligatory.[52]

Ultimately, the enduring success of Monteverde's sculpture is its representation of faith in human discoveries of medical cures for infectious diseases. This may be why this hopeful image returned to the mind of art historian Maria Flora Giubilei in an essay for a medical journal during the most dramatic and frightening moments of COVID-19: "What artwork is more coherent to present to the public at this time than the portrait that an artist dedicated in the second half of the nineteenth century to the figure of the British doctor, 'father' of the vaccine?"[53] As a productive encounter between art and science, the sculpture continues to remind us of the lasting human capacity to find solutions for epidemics even today.

Acknowledgements

I thank Christopher Calefati, Ughetta Orlando, Arianna Arisi Rota, Judith Hecker, Paolo Mazzarello, Chiara Stefani, Chiara Lanzi, Giovanna Ginex, Elisabetta Staudacher and Maria Flora Giubilei for generously sharing research information. All translations are by the author.

Notes

1 Luigi Chirtani, "L'Esposizione di Belle Arti a Roma/Segantini, il perduto!," in *Corriere della Sera*, March 1883, 4–5.
2 Ibid.
3 Gabriele D'Annunzio, *Laudi del cielo del mare della terra e degli eroi*, vol. 3: *Alcione* (Milan: Treves, 1928), 46.
4 The scope and length of this essay does not permit me to discuss book illustrations, such as painter Gaetano Previati's 1885–87 visionary Symbolist depictions of the 1630 Milan plague for Hoepli's reissue of Alessandro Manzoni's novel *The Betrothed* (1821–27). Nor can I address Italian newspaper illustrations of disease, or art on themes of mental disease or of generic images of death. Italian

art dedicated to social themes does not typically address contagious disease. See Giovanna Ginex, *Staging injustice: Italian Art, 1880–1917* (New York: Center for Italian Modern Art, 2022).

 5 The watercolor was misattributed to Segantini, who later said his dealer Vittore Grubicy had erroneously signed his name on it. See Annie-Paul Quinsac, ed., *Segantini,* Petalo di rosa: *Indagini e scoperte* (Milan: Maspes, 2015), 17. For documentation on Longoni's images and the charcoal's first attribution, see Giovanna Ginex, *Emilio Longoni: Catalogo ragionato delle opere* (Milan: Federico Motta Editore, 1995), 162, 358.

 6 Eugenia Tognotti, *"Il morbo lento": La tisi nell'Italia dell'Ottocento* (Milan: FrancoAngeli 2012), 15–22.

 7 Ada Negri, "Fin ch'io viva e più in là," in *Fatalit*à ed. Negri (Milan: Treves, 1911), 25.

 8 Linda Hutcheon and Michael Hutcheon, *Opera: Desire, Disease, Death* (Lincoln: University of Nebraska Press, 1996), 29–59.

 9 Rhoda F. Lemlein, "Influence of Tuberculosis on the Work of Visual Artists: Several Prominent Examples," *Leonardo* 14, no. 2 (Spring 1981): 114–17. See also Katherine Byrne, *Tuberculosis and the Victorian Literary Imagination* (Cambridge: Cambridge University Press, 2011).

10 Athos [Virgilio Colombo], "Esposizione artistica: Giovanni Segantini," in *La Lombardia,* May 25, 1881.

11 Chirtani, "L'Esposizione di Belle Arti."

12 Ibid.

13 Ibid.

14 Ibid.

15 Ibid.

16 Ibid.

17 Filippo Filippi, "Esposizione di Belle Arti, II," *La Perseveranza* (September 5, 1883), cited in Elisabetta Staudacher, "Segantini e la Permanente, una storia inedita," in Quinsac, *Segantini,* Petalo di rosa, 85.

18 Ibid., 86.

19 Vivien Greene, "Painted Measles: The Contagion of Divisionism in Italy," in *Divisionism/Neo-Impressionism: Arcadia and Anarchy,* ed. Solomon R. Guggenheim Museum (New York: Guggenheim Museum, 2007), 15–27.

20 Gilberto Corbellini, *Storia della malaria in Italia: Scienza, ecologia, società* (Rome: Carocci, 2022), 114–23.

21 Stefano Panci, catalog entry in *Giulio Aristide Sartorio, 1860–1932,* ed. Renato Miracco (Florence: Maschietto, 2006), 230–31.

22 Ibid.

23 Ferdinando Fontana, "Pennelli e scalpelli," in *Esposizione Internazionale di Belle Arti Roma 1883* (Milan: Giuseppe Galli, 1883), 122–23.

24 Giovanni [Nino] Costa, "Prima Esposizione di Belle Arti in Roma, 1883," *Gazzetta d'Italia,* vol. XI, May 21, 1883, cited in Miracco, *Giulio Aristide Sartorio,* 230.

25 Luigi Bellinzoni, *Guida critica della Esposizione Artistica Internazionale di Roma* (Milan: Treves, 1883), 79.

26 Ibid., 79–80.

27 Francesco Salaris, *Atti della Giunta per la Inchiesta Agraria sulle condizioni della classe Agricola,* vol. 14, casc. 1 (Rome: Forzanie C. Tipografi del Senato, 1885), 9–10.

28 Francesco Sapori, "Aristide Sartorio," *Il Circeo* 2 (February 4, 1922).

29 Aristide Sartorio, "Le confessioni e le battaglie di un artista: Note autobiografiche di G. Aristide Sartorio," *Secolo* 20, no. 8 (August 1907): 619–34.

30 I thank Barbara and Claudio Calabi for confirming the work is not on display in the museum.

31 See Sandro Bellassai, "The Masculine Mystique: Antimodernism and Virility in Fascist Italy," *Journal of Modern Italian Studies* 10, no. 3 (February 2007): 314–35, https://doi.org/10.1080/13545710500188338.

32 See Anna Mazzanti, *Simbolismo italiano fra arte e critica. Mario de Maria e Angelo Conti* (Florence: Le Lettere, 2007), 53; Romualdo Pantini, "Mario De Maria," *Emporium* 15, no. 86 (February 1902): 83–107. De Maria also exhibited *La Peste a Venezia* (The Plague in Venice) (Esposizione di Torino, 1898, and Venice Biennale, 1912). See also Flavia Scotton, *Mario de Maria, nell'atelier del pittore delle lune* (Milan: Electa, 1983).

33 See Renato Mammucari and Rigel Langella, *I pittori della mal'aria dalla Campagna romana alle Paludi pontine* (Rome: Newton & Compton, 1999); and Enrico Crispolti, Anna Mazzanti and Luca Quattrocchi, eds., *Arte in Maremma nella prima metà del Novecento* (Cinisello Balsamo: Silvana, 2005).

34 Francesco Sapori, *I maestri di Terracina* (Rome: Romani, 1954), 432.

35 Ibid. Other generic images of illness by Angelo Morbelli, such as *Testa di fanciulla malata* (Head of a Sick Girl, 1897), did not sell and remained in the artist's studio after his death.

36 On Giraud, see Laetitia Levrat, "Eugène Giraud (1806–1881): Un peintre français en Espagne, 1846." *Art et histoire de l'art* (2008), accessed August 19, 2023, https://dumas.ccsd.cnrs.fr/dumas-00385667/file/Eugene_Giraud_un_peintre_francais_en_Espagne_Vol_1.pdf.

37 Giovanni Battista Rossi, "Esposizione di belle arti Roma," *L'Italia industriale artistica* 3, no. 3 (April 15, 1905): 11–12, 14–15.

38 The Italian Ministry's elevated costs for permission to reproduce this image in an academic publication prohibits me from reproducing it. To view it online, see https://catalogo.beniculturali.it/detail/HistoricOrArtisticProperty/1200489567 (accessed October 4, 2023).

39 Sapori, "Aristide Sartorio."

40 Ibid.

41 Stefania Frezzotti, catalog entry in *Galleria Nazionale d'Arte Moderna: Le collezioni; Il XIX secolo*, ed. Elena Di Majo and Matteo Lanfranconi (Milan: Electa, 2006), 339.

42 Marco Armiero and Marcus Hall, *Nature and History in Modern Italy* (Athens: Ohio University Press, 2010), 6. I thank Teresa Kittler for this reference.

43 Ibid. 9.

44 Italo Falbo, "I nostri artisti – Giulio Monteverde," *Il Messaggero*, April 19, 1911, cited in Gianluca Kannès, "Polemica e propaganda attorno alla presentazione in Roma di Edoardo Jenner che inocula il vaccino a suo figlio, scultura di Giulio Monteverde," *Rivista di storia arte archeologia per le province di Alessandria e Asti* 128 (2019): 423.

45 See Matteo Gardonio, "Scultori italiani alle Esposizioni Universali di Parigi (1855–1899): Aspettative, successi e delusioni" (PhD diss., Università degli Studi di Trieste, 2008), 69–71, 76–78, 80, 82, 86, 176.

46 Cited in Kannès, "Polemica e propaganda," 422.

47 Ibid., 423. See Maria Flora Giubilei, ed., *Galleria d'Arte Moderna di Genova* (Florence: Maschietto, 2004), 39.

48 "Maria Brignole Sale de Ferrari Duchessa di Galliera." *Note storiche lette dal gran cancelliere Maurizio Daccà alla cerimonia del Confeugo per il bicentenario della nascita 1811–2011*, https://www.acompagna.org/rivista/2012/1/p04.pdf.

49 Kannès, "Polemica e propaganda," 425n1. Kannès cites three terracotta models: one lost, another at the Accademia di San Luca and another sold at auction. He cites another possible bronze of 1905 in St. Louis and another in Florida.

50 See Galleria Bazzanti, "Il vaccino di Edward Jenner e la scultura di Giulio Monteverde," accessed August 11, 2023, www.galleriabazzanti.it/vaccino-jenner-scultura-monteverde/.

51 John Empson, "Little Honoured in His Own Country: Statues in Recognition of Edward Jenner MD FRS," *Journal of the Royal Society of Medicine* 89 (September 1996): 514–18.

52 See Eugenia Tognotti, *Vaccinare i bambini tra obbligo e persuasione: Tre secoli di controversie* (Milan: FrancoAngeli, 2020). A small pastel by Demetrio Cosola, *La vaccinazione nelle campagne* (Vaccination in the Countryside, 1894, Chivasso, Palazzo Santa Chiara), shows a country doctor vaccinating under the watchful eye of a poster of King Umberto I, implying a connection between vaccines and governmental forces.

53 Maria Flora Giubilei, "Arte e scienza, scalpelli e vaccini: Giulio Monteverde e il suo monumento per Edward Jenner," in *Medicina, cultura ed arte*, ed. E. Baldo, *Orizzonti FC* 17, no. 2 (May–August 2020): 44–45.

References

Armiero, Marco, and Marcus Hall. *Nature and History in Modern Italy*. Athens: Ohio University Press, 2010.

Athos [Virgilio Colombo]. "Esposizione artistica: Giovanni Segantini." *La Lombardia*, May 25, 1881.

Bellassai, Sandro. "The Masculine Mystique: Antimodernism and Virility in Fascist Italy." *Journal of Modern Italian Studies* 10, no. 3 (February 2007): 314–35. https://doi.org/10.1080/13545710500188338.

Bellinzoni, Luigi. *Guida critica della Esposizione Artistica Internazionale di Roma*. Milan: Treves, 1883.

Byrne, Katherine. *Tuberculosis and the Victorian Literary Imagination*. Cambridge: Cambridge University Press, 2011.

Chirtani, Luigi. "L'Esposizione di Belle Arti a Roma/Segantini, il perduto!" *Corriere della Sera*, March 4–5, 1883.

Corbellini, Gilberto. *Storia della malaria in Italia: Scienza, ecologia, società*. Rome: Carocci, 2022.

Costa, Giovanni [Nino]. "Prima Esposizione di Belle Arti in Roma, 1883." Vol. XI. *Gazzetta d'Italia*, May 21, 1883.

Crispolti, Enrico, Anna Mazzanti, and Luca Quattrocchi, eds. *Arte in Maremma nella prima metà del Novecento* (Exhibition catalog). Cinisello Balsamo: Silvana, 2005.

D'Annunzio, Gabriele. *Laudi del cielo, del mare, della terra e degli eroi*. Vol. 3, *Alcione*. Milan: Treves, 1928.

Di Majo, Elena, and Matteo Lanfranconi, eds. *Galleria Nazionale d'Arte Moderna: Le collezioni; Il XIX secolo*. Milan: Electa, 2006.

Empson, John. "Little Honoured in His Own Country: Statues in Recognition of Edward Jenner MD FRS." *Journal of the Royal Society of Medicine* 89 (September 1996): 514–18.

Falbo, Italo. "I nostri artisti–Giulio Monteverde." *Il Messaggero*, April 19, 1911.

Filippi, Filippo. "Esposizione di Belle Arti, II." *La Perseveranza*, September 5, 1883.

Fontana, Ferdinando. "Pennelli e scalpelli." In *Esposizione Internazionale di Belle Arti Roma 1883*. Milan: Giuseppe Galli, 1883.

Gardonio, Matteo. "Scultori italiani alle Esposizioni Universali di Parigi (1855–1899): Aspettative, successi e delusioni." PhD diss., Università degli Studi di Trieste, 2008.

Ginex, Giovanna. *Emilio Longoni: Catalogo ragionato*. Milan: Federico Motta Editore, 1995.

———. *Staging Injustice: Italian Art, 1880–1917* (Exhibition catalog). New York: Center for Italian Modern Art, 2022.

Giubilei, Maria Flora, ed. *Galleria d'Arte Moderna di Genova*. Florence: Maschietto, 2004.

———. "Arte e scienza, scalpelli e vaccini: Giulio Monteverde e il suo monumento per Edward Jenner." *Medicina, cultura ed arte* (*Orizzonti FC*) 17 (May – August 2020): 44–45.

Greene, Vivien, ed. *Divisionism/Neo-Impressionism: Arcadia and Anarchy* (Exhibition catalog), edited by Solomon R. Guggenheim Museum. New York: Guggenheim Museum, 2007.

Hutcheon, Linda, and Michael Hutcheon. *Opera: Desire, Disease, Death*. Lincoln: University of Nebraska Press, 1996.

"Il vaccino di Edward Jenner e la scultura di Giulio Monteverde." *Galleria Bazzanti*. Accessed August 29, 2023. https://www.galleriabazzanti.it/vaccino-jenner-scultura-monteverde/.

Kannès, Gianluca. "Polemica e propaganda attorno alla presentazione in Roma di Edoardo Jenner che inocula il vaccino a suo figlio, scultura di Giulio Monteverde." *Rivista di storia arte archeologia per le province di Alessandria e Asti* 128 (2019): 421–44.

Lemlein, Rhoda F. "Influence of Tuberculosis on the Work of Visual Artists: Several Prominent Examples." *Leonardo* 14, no. 2 (Spring 1981): 114–17.

Levrat, Laetitia. "Eugène Giraud (1806–1881): Un peintre français en Espagne, 1846." *Art et histoire de l'art*, 2008. Accessed August 29, 2023. https://dumas.ccsd.cnrs.fr/dumas-00385667/file/Eugene_Giraud_un_peintre_francais_en_Espagne_Vol_1.pdf.

Mammucari, Renato, and Rigel Langella. *I pittori della mal'aria dalla Campagna romana alle Paludi pontine*. Rome: Newton & Compton, 1999.

"Maria Brignole Sale de Ferrari Duchessa di Galliera." *Note storiche lette dal gran cancelliere Maurizio Daccà alla cerimonia del Confeugo per il bicentenario della nascita 1811–2011*. https://www.acompagna.org/rivista/2012/1/p04.pdf.

Mazzanti, Anna. *Simbolismo italiano fra arte e critica. Mario de Maria e Angelo Conti*. Florence: Le Lettere, 2007.

Miracco, Renato, ed. *Giulio Aristide Sartorio, 1860–1932* (Exhibition catalog). Florence: Maschietto, 2006.

Negri, Ada. *Fatalità*. Milan: Treves, 1911.

Pantini, Romualdo. "Mario De Maria." *Emporium* 15, no. 86 (February 1902): 83–107.

Perciaccante, Antonio, and Alessia Coralli. "The History of Congenital Syphilis Behind *The Inheritance* by Edvard Munch." *JAMA Dermatology* 154, no. 3 (March 2018): 280. https://doi.org/10.1001/jamadermatol.2017.5834.

Quinsac, Annie-Paul, ed. *Segantini, Petalo di rosa: Indagini e scoperte*. Milan: Maspes, 2015.

Rossi, Giovanni Battista. "Esposizione di belle arti Roma." *L'Italia industriale artistica* 3, no. 3 (April 15, 1905): 11–15.

Salaris, Francesco. *Atti della Giunta per la Inchiesta Agraria sulle condizioni della classe Agricola*. Vol. 14, fasc. 1. Rome: Forzanie C. Tipografi del Senato, 1885.

Sapori, Francesco. "Aristide Sartorio." *Il Circeo* 2 (February 4, 1922).

———. *I maestri di Terracina*. Rome: Romani, 1954.

Sartorio, Aristide. "Le confessioni e le battaglie di un artista: Note autobiografiche di G. Aristide Sartorio." *Secolo* 20, no. 8 (August 1907): 619–34.

Scotton, Flavia. *Mario de Maria, nell'atelier del pittore delle lune* (Exhibition catalog). Milan: Electa, 1983.

Tognotti, Eugenia. *"Il morbo lento": La tisi nell'Italia dell'Ottocento*. Milan: Franco Angeli, 2012.

———. *Vaccinare i bambini tra obbligo e persuasione: Tre secoli di controversie*. Milan: FrancoAngeli, 2020.

8 Masking Female Illness in *Tigre Reale*

Tuberculosis from Print to Screen

Catherine Ramsey-Portolano

This chapter analyzes the portrayal and role of tuberculosis in the literary and cinematic versions of *Tigre reale* (*The Royal Tigress*), juxtaposing the 1875 novel by the Italian writer Giovanni Verga to the 1916 film adaptation by the Italian director Giovanni Pastrone in order to identify critical differences between the two genres' portrayal of illness.[1] Both the novel and film hide the true nature of the female protagonist's illness behind a depiction that adheres to socially pervasive perceptions of women as suffering from an overly passionate nature and nervous disorders. While both the novel and the film depict the female protagonist as exhibiting the traditional physical symptoms of tuberculosis, direct references to tuberculosis are avoided, and passion is proposed as the source of her affliction. The ambiguity surrounding the exact nature of the protagonist's illness reflects a portrayal that rejects scientific notions of disease and the depiction of a real sick female body in favor of a version in line with contemporary notions of femininity.[2] The novel's female protagonist Nata is the femme fatale typical of many novels of the period, and illness is explored as part of her alluring yet threatening presence. In the novel, contagious illness ultimately leads to Nata's death and functions as the consequence of her transgressive behavior. The film adaptation of *Tigre reale*, on the other hand, presents her recovery and reserves for her a happy ending. I will examine how the film explores malady as a means for showcasing the figure and character portrayed by the diva but ultimately dissociates her from the role of femme fatale and from the notions and consequences of illness presented in the novel, allotting instead this character a regenerative function within the film.

Literary historian Athena Vrettos notes the seemingly endless "attraction of the 'medical' body, its diseases and diagnoses, as a subject of narrative interest" in the second half of the nineteenth century.[3] Vrettos attributes this literary "desire to talk of diseases" to the endeavor to "answer questions about the material, social, and spiritual nature of human relations."[4] Illness became the lens through which it was possible to understand and portray personal experiences, social classes, genders and much more, as literary historian Barbara Spackman remarks regarding the *"rhetorique obsedante* of the nineteenth century: the rhetoric of sickness and health, decay and degeneration,

DOI: 10.4324/9781003382805-8

pathology and normalcy."[5] A metaphorical portrayal of illness and its causes as a way of communicating certain qualities of a person took precedence within nineteenth-century romantic and decadent literature over a strictly scientific approach to representing disease.[6] It is important to note that this was not due to lack of knowledge regarding the nature of tuberculosis, as exemplified by the doctor's comments regarding the disease in Verga's *Tigre reale* that will be examined below. Susan Sontag argues regarding nineteenth-century romanticization of tuberculosis, for example, that "agony became romantic in a stylized account of the disease's preliminary symptoms (for example debility is transformed into languor) and the agony was simply suppressed."[7]

In numerous novels of the fin de siècle period, illness stood in as a communicator for a variety of conditions: indicator of a refined sensitivity, punishment for transgressive behavior, rebellion against repressive social norms or catalyst for a regenerative convalescence.[8] I will discuss how the portrayal of Nata's tuberculosis, its onset and even her death at the end of the novel is depicted in *Tigre reale* as resulting from an excess of emotion and passion rather than from the unstoppable progression of a disease that was uncurable at that time. This tendency was taken a step further in the film adaptation of *Tigre reale*, which features a different ending from the novel to present the female protagonist's recovery from the disease. I suggest that the elimination of the female protagonist's on-screen death can be attributed to a variety of factors: the influence of the Italian writer Gabriele D'Annunzio on the film adaptation, the primary role of the diva in silent Italian cinema and the desire in the film to mask tuberculosis and its true causes and consequences.

Tuberculosis and Illness in Verga's Novel *Tigre Reale*

The novel *Tigre reale* offers a portrayal of tuberculosis that draws upon scientific conceptions of the illness yet fails to legitimize a medical origin to the female protagonist's condition, thereby enforcing stereotypes of the period regarding women's overly passionate nature. Nata, a Russian countess who spends her winters in Italy for health reasons, is presented as "very sick," "a finished woman" with "that terrible disease" who, the doctor says, has only two years to live.[9] Nata performs the role of femme fatale in the novel through the irresistible yet threatening seduction she exerts on the male protagonist Giorgio La Ferlita, a young Italian aristocrat she meets during her stay in Italy. In presenting Nata, Verga realistically describes the physical symptoms that accompanied tuberculosis: fever, coughing fits, paleness and sunken, feverish eyes with dark circles.[10] However, Nata's illness is romanticized to downplay the unhealthy and accentuate her appeal. She is described as possessing a "sick passion" and her appearance is defined as majestic rather than sickly, reflecting the link in the novel between her illness and her seductive appeal.[11] An aura of sickness reigns over the union of Nata and Giorgio, who are defined "unhealthy products" of modern society, providing another example of the function in the novel, to quote Sontag's work, of illness as metaphor.[12]

Ambiguity surrounds the origin of Nata's illness, as when Giorgio asks what kind of passion has led to her current state. Her condition is only indirectly acknowledged as tuberculosis, when the doctor wryly informs Giorgio that one can only die from passion if it is accompanied by tuberculosis or typhus. Dismissing this scientific approach, Giorgio argues that the doctor does not comprehend the possible effects of authentic passion:

> You speak as a doctor . . . but you completely ignore what a passion is . . . and better for you! Could you overcome death, you who have studied so much? Do you know if there is a remedy for tuberculosis? When one is stricken with that malady, you see . . . it is a misfortune, it is a fatality . . . but it is useless to struggle, and one must suffer it to the end.[13]

Although the doctor indicates the scientific reasons for the cause of contagious illness and death, this perspective is discredited within the novel as the restricted view of a man, limited by his medical training, who fails to understand the true nature of love and passion. The doctor's comments in another encounter with Giorgio further reveal his familiarity with tuberculosis due to what was evidently a common practice in those years, that of Italy serving as a medical refuge for foreign patients afflicted by the disease: "And she went to die in a corner of some hotel, like all these great tubercular ladies. . . . I don't understand why the doctors up there send their sick people here when they are at this extreme."[14] Furthermore, it is interesting to note the doctor's knowledge of the evolution of tuberculosis, again demonstrating his awareness of cases like those of Nata: "we're in the third stage, actually at the end of the third stage; her left lung doesn't have as much left as a child's fist; her right lung is completely gone. . . . All my science will be of use only in delaying death for two weeks or three."[15] Although *Mycobacterium tuberculosis* as the cause of tuberculosis had not yet been discovered at the time Verga wrote *Tigre reale*, the doctor's assertions reveal a medical understanding of the disease that is nonetheless discredited by Giorgio and other characters in favor of the view that Nata's passion is killing her.[16] The novel intentionally masks the scientific causes of tuberculosis, instead portraying it in a way that adheres to socially pervasive perceptions of women as suffering from and paying the price for an overly passionate nature.

The issue of contagion is also presented in a nonscientific fashion in the novel, as the consequence of, or castigation for, excessive passion, rather than resulting from the biological communication of a disease due to close contact. Nata's tuberculosis, for example, is attributed to resulting from an excess of emotions and feeling, as illustrated in the story she tells Giorgio of how her illness began after discovering her previous lover's betrayal:

> I learned that during my time away he had had another affair, and that another woman . . . I don't know who it was, I didn't want to know, had defiled my memory and my love. I set off again without seeing

him, without giving him a reproach; I fell ill on the journey, and when I reached St. Petersburg, they said that I was consumptive.[17]

The link between Nata's overwhelming passion and the onset of her illness is evident, confirming once again the tendency in the novel to attribute the origin of female suffering and illness to women's overly sensual nature.

The novel further explores the theme of contagion and malady through the life-threatening illnesses that afflict Giorgio's wife and son, reinforcing a rhetorical rather than scientific explanation for their conditions. Illness as the physical consequence of excessive passion not only afflicts Nata but risks contaminating Giorgio's family when both his wife and son fall ill, symbolizing the price they must pay for his transgressions with Nata. Giorgio admits to the invincible sway that this female character holds over him and his failure to uphold his duty to his family: "I know I am a wretch! I deceived that poor Erminia, I left my son when it would have been my duty to assist him, I left my home, my happiness . . . my heart was breaking to leave them . . . and I left!"[18] It is not a coincidence that while Giorgio is away visiting Nata, his newborn son falls deathly ill due to the "sudden and threatening onset" of another infectious disease, diphtheria.[19] The young child demonstrates similar symptoms to those associated with Nata's condition, such as fever, difficulty in breathing and a cadaver-like appearance, but the doctor's careful watch and a small surgical intervention save him from death. The sequential link between Giorgio's transgression and his son's illness confirms once again the literary tendency to obscure scientific views of illness and contagion in favor of romantically-contrived notions.

In the course of the novel, Giorgio's wife Erminia is also afflicted by illness, exemplifying another female character in the novel whose illness derives from excessive passion. Although initially portrayed as the epitome of wifely and motherly purity, Erminia becomes distracted with feelings for her cousin Carlo during Giorgio's infatuation with Nata, succumbing to a violent fever after Carlo's forced departure. The novel portrays Erminia as another symbolic victim of Giorgio's deviance, morally contaminated by his wrongdoings to commit those of her own, as well as a victim of the effects of her own overwhelming passion. After her fever breaks, Erminia's first words to Giorgio reveal transgressive emotions as the source of her illness: " 'I loved Carlo! . . . Forgive me.' . . . sobbed the sick woman after a longer silence. 'I need you to forgive me . . . Giorgio!' "[20] The novel explores how Erminia, in straying from the sanctified role of wife and mother, also risks delving into the role of femme fatale. Presenting a symbolic rather than medical perspective of contagion, the novel shows how Erminia, like Nata, suffers the physical consequences of her forbidden and excessive love for a man other than her husband.

The fates of Erminia and Nata differ drastically in the novel, however, due to the different paths they take. After her brief episode of illness, Erminia confesses her error and asks for Giorgio's forgiveness, completely recovering not only her good health but also her role within the family as a beloved and respected wife and mother. Nata, on the other hand, never admits to the error of her adulterous love, asking Giorgio to visit her and declare his love for her until the end. Nata is ultimately punished for her transgressive behavior, first by Giorgio's failure to see her again after his visit during his son's illness and then by the events of the novel's ending. The book's final scene, which takes place at the train station of the town where Nata had awaited Giorgio's arrival, juxtaposes the fates of the two women as leading in separate directions. Erminia, headed toward a summer vacation and a future filled with happiness and fulfilment with her husband and son, encounters the funeral train bearing Nata's coffin departing in the opposite direction. The bright future that awaits Erminia is reflected also in the description of the weather and surrounding countryside at the passing of their train: "gold dust seemed to rain down from the sky, the sea shimmered with silver stripes; the gardens scattered along the train line threw into the carriages the fragrance of orange blossoms."[21] The threatening presence of the femme fatale has been permanently removed with Nata's death, and a happy future awaits the faithful wife and mother. The contrasting fates of the female characters in the novel *Tigre reale* demonstrate once again how medical explanations for illness and contagion are veiled, and even discredited, in the novel in favor of a representation that posits excessive passion as the cause.

Tuberculosis in the Cinematic Adaptation of *Tigre Reale*

The 1916 cinematic version of *Tigre reale* places greater emphasis on the role and character development of the female protagonist Nata, who in the film is renamed Natka, and employs certain plot modifications with respect to Verga's 1875 novel to reflect this change. Notable deviations from the events of the novel, such as the reduction of Erminia to the role of fiancée rather than wife and the happy ending reserved for Natka and Giorgio, serve to elevate the prominence of Natka's character, portrayed in the film by the diva Pina Menichelli. One of the most significant changes to the plot regards Natka's role and the portrayal of her illness, as film historian Fabio Andreazza notes, suggesting the importance of the diva and D'Annunzian influences within Italian cinema of those years as reasons:

> In order to make the plot palatable to an audience sensitive to D'Annunzio's superwomen, precise choices had to be made at the script stage. First, it was necessary to make the Countess the sole object of Giorgio's desire, and then it was necessary to reduce the sense of illness and impending death that pervades the novel. Thus, not only were all the parts that could overshadow the figure of Natka cut out, but the ending was also twisted, precisely because of its funereal atmosphere.[22]

Reflecting the centrality of her character in the film adaptation and the regenerative role assigned to female convalescence in D'Annunzio's literary production, Natka suddenly and rather inexplicably triumphs over her illness in the film's conclusion. It is important to note, however, that up until the end of the film, Natka is associated with images of and references to illness and suffering. I will analyze below the portrayal and function of her illness, as well as the significance of her recovery, in the film adaptation of *Tigre reale*.

Within this context, though, it is important first to understand the figure of the cinematic diva and D'Annunzio's influence on Italian cinema of the silent period. "Diva films," a genre defined by film historian Cristina Jandelli as "entirely constructed around the centrality of the female performer," dominated, together with historical films, the early Italian film industry.[23] The Italian film historian Angela Dalle Vacche provides the following definition of the diva role: "In early Italian cinema, *diva* meant a female star in a feature film that ran at least sixty minutes and included some close-ups for the heroine and a fairly static use of the camera."[24] The three most famous Italian cinematic divas of this period, who all achieved fame in films after beginnings in the theater, were Francesca Bertini (1892–1985), Lyda Borelli (1884–1959) and Pina Menichelli (1890–1984).[25] Demonstrating the diva's significance within the Italian film industry of those early years is the superior number of female stars with respect to male cinematic stars, who furthermore remained subordinate to the diva on screen. The personal lives and professional choices of the divas reflected a more modern and emancipist lifestyle than was typically the case for Italian women of the time. Menichelli, for example, toured with a theater company in South America before returning, as a single mother of two children, to Italy and beginning her film career in 1913. In the two years she collaborated with the cinematic production company Cines, she featured in approximately forty films.[26] In addition to the nontraditional lifestyle she exhibited during the years of her acting career, Menichelli also made nonconventional choices for how she interpreted her roles in film. Dalle Vacche notes, for example, that after starring in the films *Il fuoco* (The Fire) and *Tigre reale*, "Menichelli abandoned her femme fatale roles for a more modern and socially charged character: a single mother obliged to live like a high-class prostitute in Amleto Palermi's *La storia di una donna* (The Story of One Woman, 1920)."[27] Menichelli came to reject acting roles that enforced stereotypical and denigrating models of female behavior upon women of the time. Furthermore, the success of film divas, who were highly compensated and internationally famous, undoubtedly proposed a new professional model for women of the time, offering an example of women who succeeded in breaking away from the restrictive roles of wife and mother. Through their lives, cinematic performances and careers, divas represented a new model to the Italian public of the time – that of a woman renowned not only for her beauty but also for her talent and successful management of her career. Dalle Vacche notes, in fact, that unlike the literary femme fatale, the diva of Italian cinema "was not always and only a projection of male paranoia about the other sex."[28]

The figure of the diva was, however, heavily influenced by literary, artistic and theatrical models from the previous century, as Italian film historian Mario Verdone notes: "the cinema of the Italian 'silent' divas, and all their acting styles, found abundant material for inspiration and imitation in the world and literature of Decadentism, the essential domain of which remains D'Annunzio's *The Pleasure*."[29] His literary fame already solidly established in the 1890s both in Italy and abroad, D'Annunzio became actively involved in the emerging film industry of the 1910s. Italian film historian Gian Piero Brunetta discusses the importance of the writer's engagement in cinema for elevating artistically the new genre, noting that his involvement extended from ceding the rights to certain of his literary works and writing intertitles for films, as in the case of *Cabiria* (1914), to influencing the choice of titles for films, such as *Il fuoco* and *La serpe* (The Serpent), which evoked D'Annunzian titles but were not based on novels by the writer.[30] Given D'Annunzio's international fame and popularity, production companies sought out collaborations with the writer with the goal of attracting audiences for their films.

The female protagonists of D'Annunzio's literary works served as models for many of the characters portrayed by divas in films of the period. Spackman notes that his novels repeatedly featured stories of female illness and subsequent recovery, exploring the eroticization of female convalescence and the creative power for both women and men deriving from that experience. In recognition of the power attributed to D'Annunzian female protagonists, literary historian Mario Praz notes the superwoman quality they exhibit: "woman not only represents the active principle in the distribution of pleasure, but also in ordering the world. The female is aggressive, the male falters."[31] *Tigre reale*'s new plot elements and ending adhere to such a model, positing the erotic suffering diva with power and control, as well as with a regenerating function within the film.

As in the novel *Tigre reale*, the female protagonist's tuberculosis in the film adaptation is hidden behind a metaphorical version of illness, where suffering comes to stand for excessive passion and emotion. Natka's allure is associated with an aura of illness throughout the film. From her initial appearance the film artfully integrates physical malaise into her persona, introducing Natka as a figure suffering from tuberculosis and adept at dissimulation, as Jandelli notes regarding the scene and its goals:

> Its length is not only motivated by the need to present and show the diva, it serves to portray right away Natka's character: Menichelli breathes visibly pained, then as if in apnea, bursts into a smile that marks her entrance into the functional space of the worldly salon, the result of a skillful ploy. In a few seconds, Natka is presented as suffering from tuberculosis and lover of dissimulation.[32]

The film employs vivid imagery and intertitles to accentuate Natka's suffering, with scenes and texts referencing physical ailments (fevers, difficult breathing, fits of coughing, migraine headaches and fainting spells) and attempts at self-treatment, including deliberately overdosing on medication to garner strength for a last meeting with Giorgio. Natka's psychological suffering is also on display through sighs, tears and languid postures. The camera lingers on her afflictions, exemplified in scenes such as her nighttime walk outside that leaves her with a fever the following day, and the diva's dramatic acting style accentuates the gravity of her condition. The film's intertitles further confirm the female protagonist's physical ailments and delicate emotional state, with instances such as "[a]nd the obstinate laugh and convulsive cough shake so much the fragile body that she sways exhausted and falls" and "[y]ou know I have little time left in this life. Goodbye Giorgio! I promise you, I will come to die near you."

Natka's illness serves the additional function of bringing attention to the female character's personal experiences. Exploration of her illness allows for her backstory and suffering to be explored to a further extent in the film than allowed by the novel's cursory reference to the origin of Nata's illness. Dedicating lengthy scenes and narrative detail to Natka's prior romance with Dolski, the film recounts a love that ends in his death by suicide and her tuberculosis. Film historian Vittorio Martinelli notes that the cinematic version of *Tigre reale* presents "an uneven development, as it includes in the story a long flashback – the episode in Russia – which, although beautifully done, appears to stand alone with respect to the dominant context of the story."[33] This narrative arc serves, in fact, to offer insight into Natka's character and justify her seemingly aloof and cold demeanor, which eventually gives way to her acceptance of love and vulnerability, emphasized by exclamations such as "I rejected you and would have wanted to suffocate you in my arms like a jealous tiger. I love you!" Natka's illness not only reinforces her centrality as a character but also justifies her attitudes and actions. Her character evolves in the film from a seemingly superficial and cold figure who takes no interest in her suitors to one with a complex past and a yearning for genuine love. By using illness to develop and expand Natka's story, the film resolves the conflict present in the novel between the female protagonist's transgressive nature and actions and the need to punish her in the eyes of society.

In the film version of *Tigre reale*, illness is not imposed as retribution for transgression as it is in the novel; rather, it serves as a catalyst, propelling the diva into the spotlight, enabling her to act out her own personal narrative. The cinematic approach adopts illness as a conduit, a means to artistically convey the diva's physical allure, while simultaneously presenting the intricacies of her psychology. The diva's performance becomes a channel through which the depths of the female psyche are unveiled – a manifestation of inner feminine experiences communicated through the vocabulary of body language, poses and gestures. The archetype of the woman being punished for her transgressions has given way, replaced by the paradigm of the liberated woman who commands both the screen and the audience's thoughts. Literary historian Michael Subialka notes that the diva films often manage to turn the "femme fatale figure from the cursed harbinger of doom into a vehicle to reject the nihilism of Decadent degeneration."[34] Natka refuses to die or to be punished or cast aside, instead presenting her story and obtaining fulfillment and happiness.

The film's director Pastrone also recognized the necessity to avoid having Natka die from tuberculosis. In his study of the plot changes made to the film version of *Tigre reale*, Andreazza notes the existence in the Museo Nazionale del Cinema di Torino of a production journal for the film containing references to two versions, each with drastically different endings. While the ending of one version faithfully follows the novel's plot, discussed previously in this chapter, the other version presents the ending known to audiences today, in which Natka recovers from her illness, survives the hotel's fire and her husband's rage to find health and happiness with Giorgio as they literally sail away into the sunset. This final scene is accompanied by the intertitle: "In the splendor of a fiery sunset . . . Natka fervently in love with her adored Gorgio feels herself miraculously returning to youth and life." The second version is labeled in the production journal with the heading "Special English Ending Tigre Reale," indicating this version as intended for distribution in the UK, a common practice in the 1910s, as Andreazza notes:

> It is well known that in the 1910s endings underwent transformations depending on the countries to which films were exported. While, for example, a tragic epilogue was packaged for Russia if the original was a happy ending, the opposite was done for England.[35]

Verga himself confirms as much in a letter to a friend dated October 31, 1916, where he explains why the different ending was adopted for audiences abroad:

> Itala-Film, since the censorship of certain foreign countries, as you say, would perhaps not tolerate the death of the protagonist of *Tigre reale* from tuberculosis on the movie screen, could suppress this last scene or adapt to it that variant you will think best. I do not object and you can give the assurance on my behalf.[36]

According to Verga, Natka's death from tuberculosis was deemed unacceptable for certain foreign audiences in 1916 and recognized explicitly as the reason for the production company's changes to the film's ending. However, the fact that this version is the one that is known today by audiences everywhere indicates that ultimately it was chosen for circulation also in Italy, over the version faithful to Verga's novel.

One might question what had changed in the forty-one years since the novel's publication in 1875 that would lead the production company to reject the on-screen portrayal of Natka's death from tuberculosis even for Italian audiences, who were obviously familiar with the original ending of Verga's novel. Contemporary reviews of the film help answer this question. Italian film critic Pio Fasanelli writes in *Cine-Fono* in November 1916 that Menichelli's "performance was not too faithful to the protagonist painted for us by Giovanni Verga" because she offered the viewer a version of Countess Natka as "a normal woman, profoundly in love with her lover."[37] This observation, striking in its simplicity, suggests that audiences had tired of witnessing women objectified as nervous and overly passionate creatures, forced to choose between wife and mother or femme fatale. Furthermore, Fasanelli recognized the diva's role in representing this new sensibility when he wrote that "in *Tigre reale* they had in mind to rest all the work on the prima donna."[38] The film adaptation employs illness as a tool to relay Natka's personal story, complicating her character and transforming her into the "normal woman" noted by Fasanelli. She does not endure her illness, like the novel's Nata, but rather embodies it as a means toward self-fulfillment. The film and its new ending resolutely challenge established conventions, portraying Natka as an empowered woman who shapes her own narrative. It is the diva, exhibiting both D'Annunzian influences and a modern sensibility, who accomplishes the evolution of *Tigre reale*'s female protagonist from the literary to the cinematic context.

The diva reflected fin de siècle artistic and cultural models for women of the time while also projecting new forms of behavior. As film historian Mary P. Wood writes: "divas encapsulated a combination of feminine models from the previous century and the energetic impulses of the new one."[39] Brunetta notes regarding the revolutionary function of the diva within Italian cinema and society of the time:

> The Diva, with her behavior, affirms new rights, overturns century-old values and models, reveals new dimensions of the human soul, but more than anything revitalizes the romantic imagination put into crisis by positivist culture and reaffirms its relevance in an age that witnesses the triumph of heroic, vitalistic models and a virility that finds in the Great War the highest manifestation of itself.[40]

The context of Italy's participation in World War I precisely during the years that witnessed the triumph of the diva films should, in fact, be noted as subtext for the making of *Tigre reale*. Perhaps it is the experience of the Great War, as Brunetta suggests, that also influenced the decision to allow *Tigre reale*'s female protagonist to live. Natka's story, exemplified through the diva's performance, portrays a journey of self-determination for audiences of the time that provided a look toward a future where women could realize aspirations other than those traditionally allowed. Dalle Vacche points out, in fact, the liminal role of the diva, recognizing her as a figure who "grew out of the struggle for change in Italian culture."[41] *Tigre reale*'s cinematic format showcases the empowerment of women through the performance of the diva's embodiment of illness, allowing for the challenging of the period's gendered stereotypes that associated women with nervous disorders and an overabundance of emotions. This new woman, exemplified by the figure of the diva, stands as a definitive signifier of shifting eras and customs, indicating women's quest for new societal roles, as Jandelli suggests when referring to the diva as "an accurate indication of changing times and customs, a symptom of women's search for a new social role."[42]

Notes

1 Giovanni Pastrone worked under the pseudonym Piero Fosco, given to him by the Italian writer and poet Gabriele D'Annunzio. Pastrone and D'Annunzio collaborated on the films *Cabiria* (1914), *Il fuoco* (1915) and *Tigre reale*. Pastrone was a pioneer in the Italian film industry; during his leadership of Itala film company, he invented and patented the *carrello* (carriage), the mobile camera stand that would become a standard in the industry, and conceived of the first colossal film (*Cabiria*) that would revolutionize filmmaking.
2 For an overview of the nineteenth-century scientific and cultural debate in Italy on women's physical and mental inferiority and tendency toward nervous disorders, see Catherine Ramsey-Portolano, "Denigrated Femininity in Fin de Siècle Italy," in *Performing Bodies: Female Illness in Italian Literature and Cinema (1860–1920)*, ed. Ramsey-Portolano, 7–36. (Madison, NJ: Fairleigh Dickinson University Press, 2018).
3 Athena Vrettos, *Somatic Fictions: Imagining Illness in Victorian Culture* (Stanford: Stanford University Press, 1995), 1.
4 Ibid.
5 Barbara Spackman, *Decadent Genealogies: The Rhetoric of Sickness from Baudelaire to D'Annunzio* (Ithaca, NY: Cornell University Press, 1989), vii.
6 Consider the role of disease in general, and tuberculosis in particular, in the works of nineteenth-century European writers such as John Keats, Percy Bysshe Shelley, Stendhal and Novalis.
7 Susan Sontag, *Illness as a Metaphor and Aids and Its Metaphors* (New York: Anchor, Doubleday, 1989), 32.
8 For the role of illness in Italian literature, see, e.g., Spackman, *Decadent Genealogies*; and Ramsey-Portolano, *Performing Bodies*.
9 Giovanni Verga, *Tigre reale*, in *I romanzi brevi e tutto il teatro*, ed. Verga (Rome: Newton, 1996), 317, 319, 325.
10 Ibid., 317, 318, 322 and 325.
11 Ibid., 318.
12 Ibid.
13 Ibid., 350.
14 Ibid., 342.
15 Ibid.
16 The German physician Johann Schonlein coined the term "tuberculosis" in 1834, naming a disease that has existed for thousands of years. On March 24, 1882, the German physician Robert Koch announced his discovery of the bacteria that causes tuberculosis, *Mycobacterium tuberculosis*; however, a cure for the disease was not found until 1943, when American scientists Selman Waksman, Elizabeth

Bugie and Albert Schatz developed streptomycin, a compound that acted against *Mycobacterium tuberculosis*. See Centers for Disease Control and Prevention, "History of World TB Day," accessed September 3, 2023, www.cdc.gov/tb/worldtbday/history.htm.

17 Verga, *Tigre reale*, 333.
18 Ibid., 352.
19 Ibid., 356.
20 Ibid., 371.
21 Ibid., 373.
22 Fabio Andreazza, "*Tigre reale*, uno e due: Aspetti D'Annunziani in un film degli anni Dieci," *Italianist* 32, no. 2 (2012): 275–76.
23 Cristina Jandelli, *Breve storia del divismo cinematografico* (Venice: Marsilio, 2007), 39.
24 Angela Dalle Vacche, *Diva: Defiance and Passion in Early Italian Cinema* (Austin: University of Texas Press, 2008), 1.
25 Pina Menichelli (Giuseppina Menichelli), the daughter of Sicilian actors, started her film career in 1913 with the Italian production company Cines. Her filmography includes approximately 60 films, although less than one-third have survived. She retired from working in cinema in 1923.
26 Dalle Vacche, *Diva*, 263.
27 Ibid.
28 Ibid., 15.
29 Mario Verdone, "La recitazione 'Liberty,'" in *Lyda Borelli*, ed. José Pantieri (Rome: Museo Internazionale del Cinema e dello Spettacolo, 1993), 20.
30 See Gian Piero Brunetta, *Storia del cinema italiano: Il cinema muto, 1895–1929* (Rome: Riuniti, 1993), 97–103.
31 Mario Praz, *La carne, la morte e il diavolo nella letteratura romantica* (Segrate: Biblioteca Universale Rizzoli, 2012): 239.
32 Cristina Jandelli, *Le dive italiane del cinema muto* (Palermo: L'Epos, 2006), 198.
33 Vittorio Martinelli, ed., *Pina Menichelli: Le sfumature del fascino* (Rome: Bulzoni, 2009), 94.
34 Michael Subialka, "Diva Decadence: Conflicted Modernity from Death to Regeneration," in *The Poetics of Decadence in Fin-De-Siècle Italy: Degeneration and Regeneration in Literature and the Arts*, ed. Stefano Evangelista, Valeria Giannantonio, and Elisabetta Selmi (Oxford: Peter Lang, 2018), 287.
35 Andreazza, "*Tigre reale*, uno e due," 278.
36 Ibid., 277.
37 Pio Fasanelli, "*Tigre reale*," in *Verga e il Cinema*, ed. Nino Genovese and Sebastiano Gesù (Catania: Giuseppe Maimone Editore, 1996), 260.
38 Ibid.
39 Mary P. Wood, *Italian Cinema* (Oxford: Berg, 2005), 156.
40 Gian Piero Brunetta, "Il corpo glorioso delle dive," in Martinelli, *Pina Menichelli*, 17.
41 Dalle Vacche, *Diva*, 3.
42 Jandelli, *Breve storia del divismo cinematografico*, 38.

References

Andreazza, Fabio. "*Tigre reale*, uno e due: Aspetti D'Annunziani in un film degli anni Dieci." *Italianist* 32, no. 2 (2012): 273–84.
Brunetta, Gian Piero. *Storia del cinema italiano: Il cinema muto, 1895–1929*. Rome: Riuniti, 1993.

______. "Il corpo glorioso delle dive." In *Pina Menichelli: Le sfumature del fascino*, edited by Vittorio Martinelli, 11–17. Rome: Bulzoni, 2009.

Centers for Disease Control and Prevention. "History of World TB Day." Accessed September 3, 2023. www.cdc.gov/tb/worldtbday/history.htm.

Dalle Vacche, Angela. *Diva: Defiance and Passion in Early Italian Cinema*. Austin: University of Texas Press, 2008.

Fasanelli, Pio. "*Tigre reale*." In *Verga e il Cinema*, edited by Nino Genovese and Sebastiano Gesù, 259–60. Catania: Giuseppe Maimone Editore, 1996.

Jandelli, Cristina. *Le dive italiane del cinema muto*. Palermo: L'Epos, 2006.

______. *Breve storia del divismo cinematografico*. Venice: Marsilio, 2007.

Martinelli, Vittorio, ed. *Pina Menichelli: Le sfumature del fascino*. Rome: Bulzoni, 2009.

Praz, Mario. *La carne, la morte e il diavolo nella letteratura romantica*. Segrate: Biblioteca Universale Rizzoli, 2012.

Ramsey-Portolano, Catherine. *Performing Bodies: Female Illness in Italian Literature and Cinema (1860–1920)*. Madison, NJ: Fairleigh Dickinson University Press, 2018.

Sontag, Susan. *Illness as a Metaphor and AIDS and Its Metaphors*. New York: Anchor, Doubleday, 1989.

Spackman, Barbara. *Decadent Genealogies: The Rhetoric of Sickness from Baudelaire to D'Annunzio*. Ithaca, NY: Cornell University Press, 1989.

Subialka, Michael. "Diva Decadence: Conflicted Modernity from Death to Regeneration." In *The Poetics of Decadence in Fin-De-Siècle Italy: Degeneration and Regeneration in Literature and the Arts*, edited by Stefano Evangelista, Valeria Giannantonio, and Elisabetta Selmi, 273–98. Oxford: Peter Lang, 2018.

Verdone, Mario. "La recitazione 'Liberty.'" In *Lyda Borelli*, edited by José Pantieri, 15–25. Rome: Museo Internazionale del Cinema e dello Spettacolo, 1993.

Verga, Giovanni. *Tigre reale*. In *I romanzi brevi e tutto il teatro*, edited by Verga, 313–73. Rome: Newton, 1996.

Vrettos, Athena. *Somatic Fictions: Imagining Illness in Victorian Culture*. Stanford: Stanford University Press, 1995.

Wood, Mary P. *Italian Cinema*. Oxford: Berg, 2005.

9 The Old, the Frail and the Misinformed

Cholera and Aging in Visconti's *Death in Venice* (1971)

Brendan Hennessey

In Thomas Mann's *Death in Venice* (1912), cholera slowly spreads through the city, eventually infecting and killing the book's protagonist, Gustav Von Aschenbach. While a cholera outbreak in Venice also structures Luchino Visconti's film adaptation, the director once claimed that in his film, Aschenbach died of other causes. As actor Dirk Bogarde recounted:

> Visconti of course had been working on this for a long time, and once in his house, I asked him, "But when is the precise moment he catches the plague?" Luchino looked at me with those great, gray eyes and said, "Never. He dies of grief. If you must have a reason, it's a heart attack."[1]

On its face, changing Aschenbach's death appears as just one of the many liberal transformations that were signatures of Visconti's irreverent approach to literary sources. In *Morte a Venezia* (*Death in Venice*, Visconti, 1971), Visconti famously musicalized Mann's novella, exchanging Aschenbach's occupation from writer to composer, then organizing his characterization around episodes from the life of Austrian composer Gustav Mahler. Mahler's presence was amplified by the repetition of the adagietto from his Fifth Symphony, which – together with the overall lack of dialogue – helped Visconti compose "virtually a silent film."[2] A second cardinal alteration to Mann's original regards the young character Tadzio. Expanding on the theme of same-sex desire that was present but restrained in the novella, Visconti remodeled Tadzio from the passive, unaware boy to a flirtatious young man who reciprocates the older man's gaze in the film. These major modifications are key interpretative coordinates guiding more than fifty years of scholarship on *Death in Venice*, making it a paragon of auteur adaptation in postwar European cinema (Figure 9.1).

Far less critical attention has been paid to the decision to ambiguate Aschenbach's cause of death. Perhaps, as some have suggested, Visconti was only transmitting an ambiguity already present in the original text.[3] In what follows, I will explore the transmission of cholera from Mann's novella to Visconti's film. Visconti was first associated with his cinematic portrayals

DOI: 10.4324/9781003382805-9

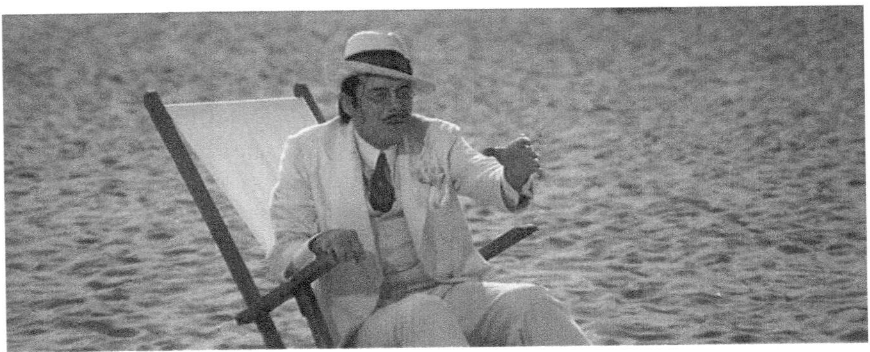

Figure 9.1 Aschenbach dying on the beach. *Death in Venice*, Luchino Visconti, 1971.

of exploited proletarians in films like *La terra trema* (*The Earth Trembles*, Visconti, 1948) and *Rocco e i suoi fratelli* (*Rocco and His Brothers*, Visconti, 1960). In *Death in Venice*, he continued to imagine the marginalized through a focus on another disregarded casualty of post-unification Italy: old people. Equating old age with disease, Visconti highlighted the plight of this neglected group, whom he portrayed as victims of Italy's ambitions for modern statehood in the early twentieth century. At the center of both the book and the film is an infamous chapter of disease cover-up in which Italian prime minister Giovanni Giolitti personally silenced any news of a cholera outbreak through the summer of 1911. To appreciate how Mann's subtle rendering of this historical episode becomes a critique of the elderly as an acceptable loss in Visconti's film, we must begin with the cholera outbreak of 1911 as seen from the perspective of Mann.

Fact and Fiction: Mann, Giolitti and Visconti's Historical Films

In Mann's novella, Aschenbach is a celebrated German author whose trip to Venice is inspired by a need for creative renewal. Once there, he finds himself compelled by a beautiful ephebe named Tadzio, whom he stalks along the seashore and through the city's streets and canals. The intoxicating pleasures Aschenbach derives from this undertaking have deadly consequences. The writer ignores rumors that cholera has arrived in Venice, then eats tainted strawberries that infect him with the deadly pestilence. Contrasting youth with senility, erotic genesis and denouement, Mann accentuates the power of physical decline to magnify aesthetic sensibilities, asking, is the artist doomed by his attempts to recreate a magnificent form from the real world? About Tadzio, Mann writes, "lovelier he was than words could say, and as often the thought visited Aschenbach, and brought its own pang, that language could extol, but not reproduce, the beauties of the senses."[4]

Such a literary representation of a European port beset by an exotic disease harkens back to the age of European expansion in the nineteenth century, an era when Europeans regarded cholera as a strange and sinister foreign import. Early chronicles underscored cholera's origins in the Indian subcontinent and the Ganges Delta, ferried to Europe across new routes of economic and political exchange. "Venice," writes literary historian Amrita Ghosh, "in Mann's text becomes a liminal space that opens up to a 'contact' with the East – within this space two binaries are set up – the sanitized trope of the West against the source of unclean bodies in the East."[5] In Mann's *Death in Venice*, this historical context was accompanied by a biographical one. Mann was on a family trip to Venice from May 19 until June 2 of 1911, then left prematurely after learning that cholera was spreading through the city.[6] The author reflected his personal itinerary that summer in his fictional characters; Aschenbach departs from Munich "on a day between the middle and the end of May,"[7] heading first by train to Trieste, then like the author, on to Pola and the island of Brioni by boat. When he finally arrives in Venice, Aschenbach struggles to learn of the disease's spread from his secretive Italian hosts who were presumably also those of his author. What Mann learned later was that he had played witness to one of the most ignominious cover-ups in the history of the young Italian republic. Motivated by political, economic and social concerns, Prime Minister Giolitti had directed sanitary institutions and media outlets to keep quiet as cholera circulated through Italian ports in 1911, managing to successfully hide the outbreak until August. Mann's trip and his later *Death in Venice* were set in the midst of what is now known as the sixth cholera pandemic (1899–1927), when between 1910 and 1912, an estimated 18,000 Italian lives were lost, most of them in 1911.[8]

What motivated Giolitti to such an egregious breach of international relations (Italy signed onto the Paris Convention in 1903, an international pact to inform of any outbreaks and collaborate on quarantines) reveals the unsteady state of Italy on the eve of the 50th anniversary of unification. In the early twentieth century (not unlike today), cholera outbreaks signaled a weak state whose failure to control a familiar disease indicated a substandard, unmodernized country. Nineteenth-century outbreaks in Italy were associated with social disorder, panic and uprisings against police, foreigners and soldiers or, as author Edmondo De Amicis once commented, anyone deemed to be "poisoners" by the volatile crowds.[9] Unlike previous cholera outbreaks, however, the timing of the 1911 one presented a new set of circumstances. Plans were in place to celebrate the Italian sesquicentennial, promising the arrival of foreign and domestic tourists to Turin and Rome to visit international exhibitions and see the unveiling of the monument to Vittorio Emmanuele II during the summer months.[10] Beyond the hit to tourism that news of an outbreak might cause, there were further implications for the anemic Italian economy. An outbreak would delay the delivery of Italian produce to international markets, and quarantines would thwart the departures of immigrants to North America, delaying the remittances they sent home and a crucial source of foreign capital. For a prime minister who had touted his record on social welfare, placing his citizens at risk to celebrate Italian unification demonstrates the limits of neoliberal reforms during the Giolittian Age (1901–14).[11]

Mann was well aware of the cover-up when he composed *Death in Venice*. The death of Anton Franzky, an Austrian who had contracted cholera in Venice during the last week of May, was a major headline in the German press throughout the summer of 1911. Mann certainly followed what became "The Franzky Affair" when he returned to Germany, and historian Thomas Rütten suggests the running story may even have prompted Mann to leave Venice early.[12] Mann references the case directly in *Death in Venice*:

> A man from the Austrian provinces, who had visited Venice for pleasure for a few days, died, once back in his home town, of unambiguous symptoms, and so the first rumours of the visitation upon the city made their way into the German newspapers.[13]

When he later describes Aschenbach combing the foreign press for any news on cholera in Venice, he continues the delicate highlighting of officialdom begun previously, as in references to the arrival of the sanitation inspector also seen in the film (Figure 9.2).

As I will discuss below, the film transmits this lack of faith in innovative ways. For Visconti, adapting such historical episodes associated with Italian unification would be nothing new. His first historical film, *Senso* (Visconti, 1954), was an adaptation of Camillo Boito's 1883 novella set during the last war of independence between Italy and Austria in 1866. The film interprets this chapter in the independence saga from the viewpoint of Livia Serpieri (played

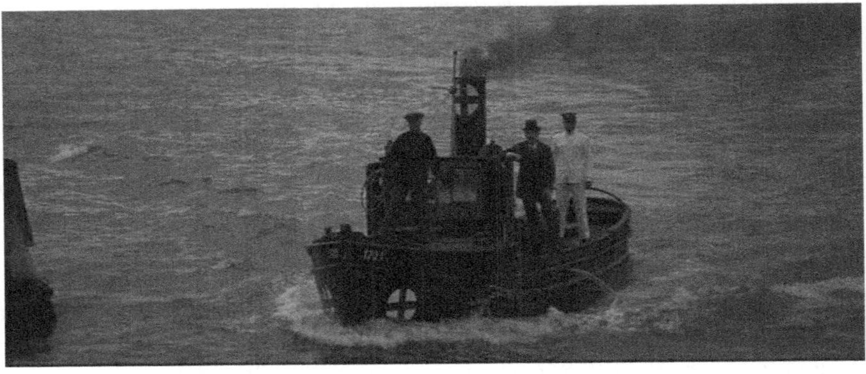

Figure 9.2 The arrival of the sanitation inspector at the beginning of the film. *Death in Venice*, Luchino Visconti, 1971.

by Alida Valli), a Venetian noblewoman who betrays the nationalist cause by diverting funds destined for Italian soldiers to her lover, the Austrian officer Franz (played by Farley Granger). His next historical feature, *Il Gattopardo* (*The Leopard*, Visconti, 1963), observes Garibaldi's landing in Sicily in 1860 from the point of view of the Prince of Salina (portrayed by Burt Lancaster), the main character from author Giuseppe Tomasi di Lampedusa's homonymous novel that the film adapts. Over the ensuing months, the prince witnesses the alignment of Italian elites old and new, who exploit the rhetoric of a nationalist cause to strengthen their position on the newly unified peninsula. By focusing on the consolidation of power in Northern Italy in *Senso*, then the incorporation of the South into a northern-led state-building process in *The Leopard*, Visconti composed a powerful diptych crystallizing Marxist philosopher Antonio Gramsci's analysis of the Italian Risorgimento as a passive revolution.[14] For Gramsci, Italian unification occurred without any real revolution, perpetuating social and political structures that were previously in place.

Despite its historical setting in Italy on the eve of unification's sesquicentennial celebrations, *Death in Venice* is rarely – if ever – regarded alongside these Risorgimento films. It is often not even considered a historical film at all, lacking the specificity of these previous films and purportedly using a background in the chronicled past "only for setting."[15] When asked why he seemingly abandoned history for this film, making no explicit mention of Giolitti or Italy's disastrous military foray into Libya, Visconti replied:

> I'll tell you that in an early stage I expected something of the sort . . . an allusion to the war in Libya overheard in discussions in the hallway of the hotel or on the beach. But I immediately decided against it. . .. A certain pseudo-historical didacticism in these cases doesn't work and is instead counterproductive.[16]

Aschenbach, not history, was apparently the director's central focus.

This apparent curtailment of recorded history is curious given that *Death in Venice* was made at a moment in the director's filmography dominated by historical films. It is the middle chapter of what critics call Visconti's "German Trilogy" – *Götterdamerung: La caduta degli dei* (*The Damned*, Visconti, 1969), *Death in Venice* and *Ludwig* (Visconti, 1973) – a trio of films featuring German protagonists. *The Damned* examines a family of German industrialists during the rise of Nazism in Munich in the early 1930s. *Ludwig* is a biopic of "The Mad King" Ludwig II of Bavaria, set from 1864 to 1886. Like *Senso* and *The Leopard*, *The Damned* and *Ludwig* meticulously recreate historical events and feature notable figures from history. *The Damned*, for example, references the burning of the Reichstag, while *Ludwig* uses the Austro-Prussian War of 1866 as a narrative context. Interacting with historical characters, episodes and discourses, these films exude "historiphoty," the term used by historian Hayden White to denote "the representation of history and our thought about it in visual images and filmic discourse"[17] that is now somewhat of a prerequisite for defining historical films. Given Visconti's established interest in how historical films dramatize and problematize the relationship with history, why might he diminish the historical in *Death in Venice*?

Disease and Old Age in Art and Autobiography

The choice to dissociate Aschenbach's cause of death from cholera may have been a practical one. In general, cholera's cinematic footprint has been limited by its physical manifestations. "The nature of its symptoms," writes historian Richard J. Evans, is

> massive vomiting and diarrhea, in which a quarter of the body's fluids along with essential body salts may be lost within a few hours, reducing the victim to a comatose, apathetic state, with sunken eyes and blue-grey skin . . . might almost have been designed to achieve the maximum shock effect on a society that, perhaps more than any other, was concerned to conceal bodily functions from public view.[18]

In literature, the physical wasting caused by massive fluid loss would align cholera with other diseases, such as smallpox and polio, portrayed as "indecent" in the works of Flaubert and Tolstoy.[19] Cholera was unlike more Romantic illnesses in literature, such as tuberculosis, which as Susan Sontag notes, features symptoms that were "nothing but a disguised manifestation of the power of love; and all disease is only love transformed."[20] Cholera did appear with relative frequency in the literary imagination in France, beginning with Eugène Sue's *The Wandering Jew* (1844), and Italy with Francesco Mastriani's *The Children of Luxury* (1866), then occasionally in cinema.[21] Given the kind of literary acrobatics used in describing the disease and its symptoms in classic works such as *Death in Venice* and W. Somerset Maugham's *The Painted Veil* (1925), cholera would prove largely difficult to represent.

In the late part of Visconti's career, portraying an illness like cholera would not have been out of the ordinary. *Death in Venice* was made during a period critics refer to as Visconti's "decadent phase" that lasted from around the making of *The Leopard* in 1963 through the end of the director's life in 1976. Old people, a social group often overlooked by critics in Italy and elsewhere, were at the forefront of these late films.[22] Recent Italian film scholarship has taken a greater interest in how cinema represents older people. Films about the societal plight of elderly men in isolation, those that address the beauty and repulsiveness of senior citizen desire and comedic works that satirize the dilemmas faced by this growing population have all been richly analyzed in the past few years.[23] Visconti's interest in the dilemmas of the old was also very much a look in the mirror. Born in 1906, his late works were frequently associated with his own perspective as an aging artist. "As Visconti grew older," writes film historian Henry Bacon, "his artistic work acquired a tone of resignation. An almost oversensitive feeling for time and place eventually led him to concentrate on the questions of old age and decay."[24] In the critical establishment, he was part of Italian cinema's old guard, who in interviews often lamented the "inauthentic" and "squalid" filmmaking in Italy in the years that followed the student uprisings of 1968.[25] In the news and celebrity press, his position as an older man was often emphasized through his relationship with actor Helmut Berger, who was 38 years his junior.

Visconti infused this public identity as an aging artist into his main characters, an autobiographical development that can be observed in two works starring American actor Burt Lancaster. In *The Leopard*, Visconti's personal background as a count helped adapt Giuseppe Tomasi di Lampedusa's aristocratic worldview as seen through the eyes of the Prince of Salina, played by Lancaster. Lancaster's next role in a Visconti film was as the professor from *Gruppo di famiglia in un interno* (*Conversation Piece*, Visconti, 1974). This character's encounter with a young American family demonstrates another figure out of step with the times, while his attraction to a young German radical, played by Helmut Berger, clearly references Visconti himself. *Conversation Piece*'s frank representation of homosexual men demonstrates a mainstay of Visconti's filmmaking beginning with *Death in Venice*, further establishing his central position as a gay figure in Italian culture. In this transition from young(ish) to old in these Visconti films, Lancaster provides something of a more nuanced, intellectually challenging "hero of aging" that has cinematic examples elsewhere.[26]

Themes of physical decay, disease, madness and the inevitable desuetude of the older generation also appeared in some of Visconti's other films of the period. The demolition and recreation of female image is central to "The Witch Burned Alive," his episode of the portmanteau film *Le streghe* (*The Witches*, De Sica, Fellini, Monicelli and Visconti, 1968). A famous film actress (Silvana Mangano) passes out at a party and is subjected to crude scrutiny by those who regard the physical signs of growing old as symptoms to be cured through interventionist techniques and products. This stripping away is reversed at the conclusion of the film, when her image is reconstituted via cosmetics and clothing, a kind of recapture of the diva's symbolic capital within a consumer culture.[27] The fabrication of sublime imagery will transition from the physical in *The Witches* to the architectonic in *Ludwig*, where the king is punished for his ruinous investments in his castles, ornately decorated in a maximalist style of imaginative decor. When added to Lancaster's aged professor from *Conversation Piece* and the diminishing sexual potency of the character from the posthumous *L'innocente* (Visconti, 1976), one can trace a persistent interest in the failing faculties associated with old age. And although the casting of Dirk Bogarde, fifty years old when he played Aschenbach, may resist interpretations of an entirely geriatric death in *Death in Venice*, one might recognize how his performance echoes the stock character of the old "curmudgeon who likes no one"[28] that is typical in Hollywood cinema.

Adapting Aschenbach, Victim of History

Where the intersection of old age and disease becomes most explicit is with Aschenbach's physical transformation and demise that occur at the end of the film. This is the culmination of a slow adaptational build that features Visconti's own creative interventions together with elements borrowed directly from Mann's text. Aschenbach's death concludes a process that portrays him as a victim of an Italian cover-up, in which local characters conspire to keep him from the information that might motivate him to flee. A weak man, exposed by a city that colludes to suppress news of a lethal illness, Aschenbach becomes an aged embodiment of the most unifying theme tying all of Visconti films together: defeat. As esteemed Visconti scholar Lino Micciché once opined, "his are all, systematically, stories of definitive, absolute, irredeemable, and almost all historical defeats, even in those films that do not aim to be, and are not, *historical* [Micciché's emphasis]."[29] Whether the penniless wanderer from his first film or the rich but degraded aristocrat from his last, Visconti characters inevitably fail to match their stated goals with the harsh realities they encounter. "I always prefer to narrate defeats, describe the victims, the destinies ruined by reality,"[30] Visconti once commented.

Aschenbach's specific isolation and eventual vanquishment are assembled through a series of nine flashbacks that were based on sources outside of Mann's *Death in Venice*. Three were taken from the biography of Gustav Mahler, suffusing Aschenbach's past with questions of disease and death from the Austrian composer's life (one refers to Mahler's daughter who died from scarlet fever; another displays the composer strewn upon a couch, diagnosed with a weak heart). It is notable that Mahler was also a model for Mann, who gave his protagonist Mahler's first name and facial features. During the early screenwriting phase, Visconti was fascinated by an anecdote Mann told him in which the writer claimed to have met Mahler on a train from Venice, looking ill and with dyed hair. According to Mann, Mahler commented, "I've just come from Venice, and I've fallen in love with a boy of thirteen."[31]

Other flashbacks in *Death in Venice* that likewise accentuate physical decline and contagion are adapted from Mann's 1947 novel, *Doktor Faustus*, a rekindling of the Faust myth set in Germany in the early twentieth century. In early shots, we notice that the ship transporting Aschenbach to Venice is called the "Esmeralda": the name given to the prostitute from *Doktor Faustus* who infects the main character Adrian Leverkühn with syphilis. Visconti ties this infected prostitute directly to Tadzio when a scene of the boy playing Beethoven's *Für Elise* on the piano in the hotel lobby cuts to a flashback of the prostitute playing the same song in a brothel. Given the prominence of Esmeralda's syphilis in *Doktor Faustus*, it is through her that Visconti connects a diabolical, potentially deadly element to Tadzio. The linkage to Mann's prostitute serves to further sexualize the young boy, what, as one reviewer noted, "made Tadzio a bit prostitute and the prostitute a bit Tadzio."[32] While iconic in the history of LGBTQ representation on screen,

Death in Venice has come under scrutiny since the release of the documentary *The Most Beautiful Boy in the World* (Lindström and Petri, 2021), where the nonprofessional actor who played Tadzio, Björn Andrèson, claimed he was mistreated by Visconti and his crew during the promotion of the film.

With these extratextual insertions in mind, Visconti also hews closely to the Mann original in bringing out the theme of contagion. To buttress the idea of Aschenbach's susceptibility to contagion, Visconti scrupulously conveyed Mann's portrayal of Venice's peculiar climate that enabled the spread of illness and disease. In the early part of the book, Mann makes abundant reference to humidity ("the wind was humid"), the condition of the air ("Flakes of sodden, clammy soot fell upon the still undried deck"), weather ("Before the boat was an hour out a canvas had to be spread as a shelter from the rain") and, generally, "the stagnant odour of the lagoon."[33] The author pays particular attention to the wind, which has a disconcerting effect on Aschenbach: "[the wind] had been so bad as to force him to flee from the city like a fugitive. And now it seemed beginning again – the same feverish distaste, the pressure on his temples, the heavy eyelids."[34]

It is worth noting how Mann's fixation on connecting the city's climate with disease reverberates with a certain nineteenth-century understanding of cholera. Now established as a waterborne sickness, caused by the ingesting *vibrio cholerae* bacteria, cholera arrived in Europe during a moment in epidemiological history when miasma theory had yet to be supplanted by modern germ theory. Miasma theory, dominant throughout Europe from the classical age to the nineteenth century, was the belief that disease originated in the earth and was transmitted through the air in the form of vapors wafting up from the soil or foul-smelling, stagnant water. Germ theory had been established in the scientific community since the 1850s, but uprooting the deeply ingrained "humoral-miasmatic paradigm"[35] would take decades. Mann would certainly have been aware of this shift in the science of disease. His scientific knowledge was sophisticated and based on his extensive research on cholera for *Death in Venice* and other diseases, such as tuberculosis in preparation for *The Magic Mountain*.[36]

Visconti teased this folk concept of environmental factors through the repetitive mention of the sirocco wind as a potentially deadly climatic condition. Sirocco, which appears briefly in the novella, refers to a hot, humid wind that periodically sweeps across Southern Europe from North Africa. In Victorian-era medical literature about Mediterranean health resorts, for example, it was one of the winds deemed to be particularly lethal, draining the life out of the sick: "the Sirocco, Liebeccio, and Leste depleted the vitality with blasts followed by copious dews."[37] In the film, we first hear of the sirocco from the hotel manager (Romolo Valli), who provides a rather unscientific formula for understanding the timing of this meteorological phenomenon. When asked when the foul weather would dissipate, the manager responds that it all depends on the sirocco: if it starts on Tuesday, it will be followed by three days of bad weather; if it starts on Friday, nine days will follow; if a tenth day comes to pass, the sirocco will blow for twenty more Mondays. The evasiveness evinced by this absurd calculus indicates the layered conspiracy to hide cholera's spread that will soon emerge. When Aschenbach later asks him directly if cholera is in Venice, he takes issue with media coverage of epidemics, stating that foreign newspapers take advantage of rumor to discourage tourism to Italy. Other marginal characters repeatedly parrot official-sounding justifications, explaining visible sanitation efforts (government signs warning of consuming shellfish, pouring of disinfectant on the city walls and walkways) as a mere formality.

It is not until Aschenbach inquires with the English money exchanger that he receives the news that cholera has arrived in Venice. That this foreign source is the only one to provide any clarity on the situation solidifies the overall depiction of Italians as smooth-speaking dissemblers, complicit in the national whitewash campaign. Instead of the scientific understanding of illness as spread through germs, commonplace by 1911, Italian characters nefariously voice the archaic notion of miasma as a way to divert attention away from evidence of disease. This continues from Mann's portrayal, where Venice is a metonym for Byzantine Italy and the tropical East, a strange borderland separating Northerners (Germans, of course, but also English, Polish and Russian) from Southerners, who are represented by the crass, even demonic characters from Italy.[38] Visconti augments Mann's characterization of Italians as swindlers taking advantage of an old man. Italian characters like the hotel manager collude with the official storyline on cholera or like the barber deceive the aging man with rhetorical tropes of vivacity, youth, beauty and health. We first see a victim of the disease in the train station when Aschenbach's early attempt to leave is thwarted by a mistake with his luggage. The man, shown pale-faced and sweating (classic symptoms of cholera), crumples to the floor to the horror of the bystanders. Tones that mark poor Italians as a disease threat are spotlighted when the band of street musicians arrives at the Hotel des Baines. After Aschenbach receives the same platitudes doubting the alleged spread of cholera from the lead bandmember, there is a marked interruption in the film's otherwise meticulously organized soundtrack. In the place of Mahler's mellifluous compositions, the band's popular songs irritate both characters and audience in a kind of sonic infection of the hotel. This musical contamination is later accompanied by an olfactory one, when Aschenbach comments on the malodors of disinfection, then cringes from the noxious smoke of burning fires throughout Venice's streets.

The transformation of the city, which empties out as the film proceeds, increases the focus on Aschenbach's isolation but also on his appearance. As in the book, the character's fight with old age reaches its apogee with the trip to the barber, where the hair styling, dye and makeup are procedures designed to cheat time through interventions that erase signs of aging.

Beauty treatments have long been associated with a Foucauldian control of women and constitute a problematic space of containment (and potential liberation) of older women.[39] One might observe a similar operation here when deployed on an older man. The dialogue from the barber, who spouts clichés of renewing youth and repossessing natural beauty, underscores the sense of the aesthetic treatments as another ruse from one of Aschenbach's Italian hosts (Figure 9.3).

These attempts to look younger are themselves transgressions that highlight the social difference of the aged body, subject to its own age-appropriate norms, rituals and customs.[40] This difference increases as Aschenbach moves out to the beach, where the dripping hair dye and smudged makeup create a clown-like impression that abases his former appearance of upper-class propriety. If the reaction of the horrified beachgoers who discover his body is any indication, it is, as Simone de Beauvoir suggests, that "in the old person that we must become, we refuse to recognize ourselves."[41]

Despite the final image of this destitute man, alone and humiliated on the Venetian beach, Aschenbach's death actually reflects an empathetic representation of old age for Visconti. In his first published work on cinema, the caustic 1941 *Cadaveri* (*Cadavers*), he used ridiculous old men to symbolize the state of the Italian film industry under Fascism. Written in the first person, Visconti envisioned two aged creators and afficionados of Italian cinema: "An old man hopping about the room in a frenzy, gripped by an inspiring fury while under the gaze of his contemporary with the wattle of an aged turkey and sits motionless . . . watching his companion while munching urotropine pills."[42] Seen in light of postwar Italian cinema, Visconti was calling for an end of Italian Fascist cinema, haunted by zombies "in the process of decomposition . . . already long dead, but with body intact, conserved by a mighty magnetic will."[43] In its place, he suggested something new and vital: something young. Inspired by *Obsession*, Visconti's and Neorealism's first work, a new generation of director, actors and film professionals would assert Italian

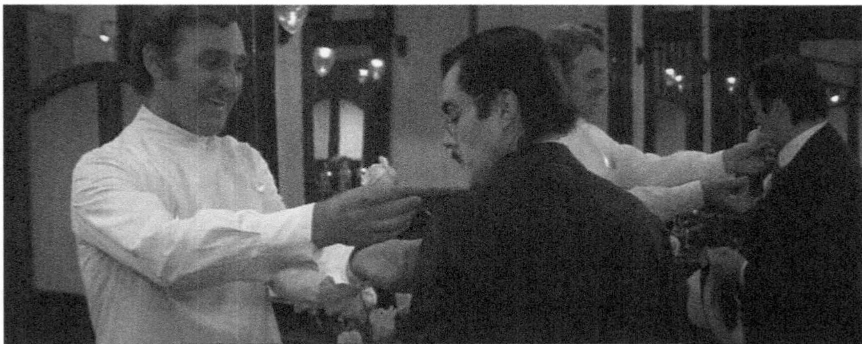

Figure 9.3 Aschenbach receiving beauty treatments at the barber's.

cinema's position at the forefront of world cinema, famous internationally for its compassionate representations of the economically marginalized.

Some 30 years later, Visconti would be celebrated again for this effort to renew Italian cinema, this time in the form of eulogy in 1976 on the occasion of his death at the age of 69. Sadly, *Death in Venice*'s fictional representation of disease, physical decline and death would become all too real in the years that followed the film's release. In 1972 after completing the filming of *Ludwig*, Visconti suffered a debilitating stroke that paralyzed the left side of his body. Alongside other Italian auteurs of the era who died during the 1970s (Vittorio De Sica, Roberto Rossellini, Pier Paolo Pasolini), his death would mark the end of a certain era of Italian cinema, when Italy became synonymous with politically charged films that sought to reconstitute the image society in the years following the Second World War.

In *Death in Venice*'s final flashback, when Aschenbach is publicly jeered following a disastrous performance, his interlocutor Alfred comments: "And in the whole world there is no impurity as impure as old age." Combining the lethality of Venice's environment with the Italian machinations to keep word of a disease outbreak under wraps ultimately creates the natural and human conditions for the character's demise. "In the context of a late capitalist culture," writes scholar Martine Beugnet, "old age is a disease, equivalent to the categories of low consumer value and low productivity; a social stigma that is acutely reflected in its status in terms of representation."[44] Through Aschenbach's decline and death, Visconti folded back upon the predicament of the marginalized individual, staying true to his concept of Neorealism's mission, laid out in 1943, when he published *Cinema antropomorfico* (*Anthropomorphic Cinema*), one of Neorealism's foundational manifestos. There, he implored his fellow directors to abandon the artificiality of Fascist cinema and make "an affectionate and objective examination of human cases" that would aid humanity's understanding of "a suffered experience."[45] Unlike that of the economically marginalized from Visconti's early films, Aschenbach's experience in *Death in Venice* was grounded in the twilight of the director's life.[46] With age, Visconti was finally able to address the suffering from the standpoint of the sufferer, the old from the perspective of an old man.

Notes

1 Hollis Alpert, "Visconti in Venice," *Saturday Review*, August 8, 1970, 16–18, www.unz.com/print/SaturdayRev-1970aug08-00016/.
2 Will Aitken, *Death in Venice: A Queer Film Classic* (Vancouver: Arsenal, 2011), 113.
3 Philip Kitcher, *Death in Venice: The Cases of Gustav Von Aschenbach* (New York: Columbia University Press, 2013), 129.
4 Thomas Mann, *Death in Venice and Seven Other Stories*, trans. H. T. Lowe-Porter (New York: Vintage Books, 1954), 51.
5 Amrita Ghosh, "The Horror of Contact: Understanding Cholera in Mann's *Death in Venice*," *Transte(x)ts Transcultures* 12 (2017): 1.

6 Thomas Rütten, "Cholera in Thomas Mann's *Death in Venice*," *Gesnerus* 66, no. 2 (2009): 259.

7 Mann, *Death in Venice*, 15.

8 Joseph Patrick Byrne and J. N. Hays, *Epidemics and Pandemics: From Ancient Plagues to Modern-Day Threats*, vol. 2 (Santa Barbara: ABC-CLIO, 2021), 248.

9 Tullio Seppilli, "Presentazione: Il colera, il Mezzogiorno e il nuovo stato italiano; Una testimonianza di Edmondo De Amicis," *AM: Rivista della società italiana di antropologia medica* 9–10 (October 2000): 152.

10 Frank M. Snowden, *Naples in the Time of Cholera, 1884–1911* (Cambridge: Cambridge University Press, 1995), 302.

11 Maria Sophia Quine, *Italy's Social Revolution: Charity and Welfare from Liberalism to Fascism* (Basingstoke: Palgrave, 2002), 67–95.

12 Rütten, "Cholera in Thomas Mann's *Death in Venice*," 259.

13 Mann, *Death in Venice*, 53.

14 Brendan Hennessey, *Luchino Visconti and the Alchemy of Adaptation* (Albany: State University of New York Press, 2021), 120.

15 Lino Micciché, *Visconti: Un profilo critico* (Venezia: MarsilioEditore, 2002), 78.

16 Giuliana Callegari and Nuccio Lodato, eds., *Leggere Visconti: Scritti, interviste, testimonianze e documenti di e su Luchino Visconti; Con una bibliografia critica generale* (Pieve del Cairo: Arti grafiche La Cittadella, 1977), 142.

17 Hayden White, "Historiography and Historiophoty," *American Historical Review* 93, no. 5 (December 1988): 1193.

18 Richard J. Evans, "Epidemics and Revolutions: Cholera in Nineteenth-Century Europe," *Past & Present* 120 (August 1988): 127.

19 Philippe Ariès, *The Hour of Death* (New York: Oxford University Press, 1991), 568.

20 Susan Sontag, *Illness as Metaphor* (New York: Farrar, Straus and Giroux, 1978), 21.

21 Roberta Pelagalli, *Le choléra dans la littérature européenne: Les multiples visages de la Némésis (1829–1923)* (Canterano: Aracne Editrice, 2018).

22 William Hope, "Introduzione: Marginalizzazione, esclusione sociale e disagio ambientale nel cinema italiano del Ventunesimo secolo," in *Un Nuovo Cinema Politico Italiano?*, vol. 2, ed. Silvana Serra Hope and Luciana D'Arcangeli (Leicester: Troubadour, 2014), 176–77.

23 Roberta Di Carmine, *Cultural Metamorphoses in Contemporary Italian Cinema* (New York: Peter Lang, 2018); Guglielmo Giumelli, *Vecchi, vecchie e vecchiaie nella letteratura e nel cinema* (Genova: Il Nuovo Melangolo, 2018); and Lisa Dolasinski, "Old Age and Italian (Film) Comedy: Why Cry When You Can Laugh?," *Italianist* 41, no. 2 (2021): 284–307.

24 Henry Bacon, *Visconti: Explorations of Beauty and Decay* (Cambridge: Cambridge University Press, 1998), 3.

25 Callegari and Lodato, *Leggere Visconti*, 134.

26 Mike Featherstone, "Post-Bodies Aging and Virtual Reality," in *Images of Aging: Cultural Representations of Later Life*, ed. Featherstone and Andy Wernick (New York: Routledge), 227.

27 Deborah Chambers, "Sexist Aging Consumerism and Emergent Modes of Resistance," in *Aging, Performance, and Stardom: Doing Age on the Stage of Consumerist Culture*, ed. Aagje Swinnen and John A. Stotesbury (Zurich: LIT, 2012), 162.

28 Timothy Shary and Nancy McVittie, *Fade to Gray: Aging in American Cinema* (Austin: University of Texas Press, 2016), 5.

29 Micciché, *Luchino Visconti*, 79.

30 Callegari and Lodato, *Leggere Visconti*, 142.

31 Mauro Giori, *Scandalo e banalità: Rappresentazioni dell'eros in Luchino Visconti (1963–1976)* (Milano: Lettere Economia Diritto, 2012), 244.

32 Callegari and Lodato, *Leggere Visconti*, 141.
33 Mann, *Death in Venice*, 28.
34 Ibid.
35 Carlo Cipolla, *Miasmas and Disease: Public Health and the Environment*, trans. Elizabeth Potter (New Haven, CT: Yale University Press, 1992), 5.
36 Valerie D. Greenberg, "Literature and the Discourse of Science: The Paradigm of Thomas Mann's *The Magic Mountain*," *South Atlantic Review* 50, no. 1 (1985): 59–73.
37 Vladimir Jankovic, "Gruff Boreas, Deadly Calms: A Medical Perspective on Winds and the Victorians," *Journal of the Royal Anthropological Institute* 13, no. 1 (2007): S151.
38 Carlo Testa, *Masters of Two Arts: Re-Creation of European Literatures in Italian Cinema* (Toronto: University of Toronto Press, 2002), 184.
39 Angela King, "The Prisoner of Gender: Foucault and the Disciplining of the Female Body," *Journal of International Women's Studies* 5, no. 2 (2004): 29–39; and Terryl Bacon and Kate Brooks, "Pleasures, Pains, and Paradoxes: Approaching the Beauty Salon in Feminist Research," in *Aging Femininities: Troubling Representations*, ed. Josephine Dolan and Estalla Tincknell (Newcastle upon Tyne: Cambridge Scholars Publishing, 2012), 87–89.
40 Pamela H. Gravagne, *The Becoming of Age: Cinematic Visions of Mind, Body and Identity in Later Life* (Jefferson, NC: McFarland, 2013), 43–45.
41 Simone de Beauvoir, *Old Age*, trans. Patrick O'Brian (London: Andre Deutsch, 1972), 4.
42 Micciché, *Luchino Visconti*, 98.
43 Ibid.
44 Sally Chivers, *The Silvering Screen: Old Age and Disability in Cinema* (Toronto: University of Toronto Press, 2011), 14.
45 Micciché, *Luchino Visconti*, 100.
46 Cipolla, *Miasmas and Disease*, 5.

References

Aitken, Will. *Death in Venice: A Queer Film Classic*. Vancouver: Arsenal, 2011.
Alpert, Hollis. "Visconti in Venice." *Saturday Review* (August 8, 1970): 16–18. www.unz.com/print/SaturdayRev-1970aug08-00016/.
Ariès, Philippe. *The Hour of Death*. New York: Oxford University Press, 1991.
Bacon, Henry. *Visconti: Explorations of Beauty and Decay*. Cambridge: Cambridge University Press, 1998.
Bacon, Terryl, and Kate Brooks. "Pleasures, Pains, and Paradoxes: Approaching the Beauty Salon in Feminist Research." In *Aging Femininities: Troubling Representations*, edited by Josephine Dolan and Estalla Tincknell, 83–96. Newcastle upon Tyne: Cambridge Scholars Publishing, 2012.
Byrne, Joseph Patrick, and J. N. Hays. *Epidemics and Pandemics: From Ancient Plagues to Modern-Day Threats*. Vol. 2. Santa Barbara: ABC-CLIO, 2021.
Callegari, Giuliana, and Nuccio Lodato, eds. *Leggere Visconti: Scritti, interviste, testimonianze e documenti di e su Luchino Visconti; Con una bibliografia critica generale*. Pieve del Cairo: Arti grafiche La Cittadella, 1977.
Chambers, Deborah. "Sexist Aging Consumerism and Emergent Modes of Resistance." In *Aging, Performance, and Stardom: Doing Age on the Stage of Consumerist Culture*, edited by Aagje Swinnen and John A. Stotesbury, 161–76. Zurich: LIT, 2012.
Chivers, Sally. *The Silvering Screen: Old Age and Disability in Cinema*. Toronto: University of Toronto Press, 2011.

Cipolla, Carlo M. *Miasmas and Disease: Public Health and the Environment*. Translated by Elizabeth Potter. New Haven, CT: Yale University Press, 1992.

de Beauvoir, Simone. *Old Age*. Translated by Patrick O'Brian. London: Andre Deutsch, 1972.

De Sica, Vittorio, Federico Fellini, Mario Monicelli, and Luchino Visconti, dirs. *Le streghe*. Film. Dino De Laurentiis Cinematografica (Italy), Les Productions Artistes Associés (France), 1961.

Di Carmine, Roberta. *Cultural Metamorphoses in Contemporary Italian Cinema*. New York: Peter Lang, 2018.

Dolasinski, Lisa. "Old Age and Italian (Film) Comedy: Why Cry When You Can Laugh?" *Italianist* 41, no. 2 (2021): 284–307.

Evans, Richard J. "Epidemics and Revolutions: Cholera in Nineteenth-Century Europe." *Past & Present* 120 (August 1988): 123–46.

Featherstone, Mike. "Post-Bodies Aging and Virtual Reality." In *Images of Aging: Cultural Representations of Later Life*, edited by Featherstone and Andy Wernick, 227–44. New York: Routledge, 1995.

Ghosh, Amrita. "The Horror of Contact: Understanding Cholera in Mann's *Death in Venice*." *Transte(x)ts Transcultures* 12 (2017): 1–10.

Giori, Mauro. *Scandalo e banalità: Rappresentazioni dell'eros in Luchino Visconti (1963–1976)*. Milan: Lettere Economia Diritto, 2012.

Giumelli, Guglielmo. *Vecchi, vecchie e vecchiaie nella letteratura e nel cinema*. Genoa: Il Nuovo Melangolo, 2018.

Gravagne, Pamela H. *The Becoming of Age: Cinematic Visions of Mind, Body and Identity in Later Life*. Jefferson, NC: McFarland, 2013.

Greenberg, Valerie D. "Literature and the Discourse of Science: The Paradigm of Thomas Mann's *The Magic Mountain*." *South Atlantic Review* 50, no. 1 (1985): 59–73.

Hennessey, Brendan. *Luchino Visconti and the Alchemy of Adaptation*. Albany: State University of New York Press, 2021.

Hope, William. "Introduzione: Marginalizzazione, esclusione sociale e disagio ambientale nel cinema italiano del Ventunesimo secolo." In *Un Nuovo Cinema Politico Italiano?*, vol. 2, edited by William Hope, Silvana Serra, and Luciana D'Arcangeli, 159–86. Leicester: Troubadour, 2014.

Jankovic, Vladimir. "Gruff Boreas, Deadly Calms: A Medical Perspective on Winds and the Victorians." *Journal of the Royal Anthropological Institute* 13, no. 1 (2007): S147–64.

King, Angela. "The Prisoner of Gender: Foucault and the Disciplining of the Female Body." *Journal of International Women's Studies* 5, no. 2 (2004): 29–39.

Kitcher, Philip. *Death in Venice: The Cases of Gustav Von Aschenbach*. New York: Columbia University Press, 2013.

Lindström, Kristina, and Kristian Petri, dirs. *The Most Beautiful Boy in the World*. Film. Mantaray Film (Sweden), 2021.

Mann, Thomas. *Death in Venice and Seven Other Stories*. Translated by H. T. Lowe-Porter. New York: Vintage Books, 1954.

Micciché, Lino. *Visconti: Un profilo critico*. Venice: Marsilio Editore, 2002.

Pelagalli, Roberta. *Le choléra dans la littérature européenne: Les multiples visages de la Némésis (1829–1923)*. Canterano: Aracne Editrice, 2018.

Quine, Maria Sophia. *Italy's Social Revolution: Charity and Welfare from Liberalism to Fascism*. Basingstoke: Palgrave, 2002.

Rütten, Thomas. "Cholera in Thomas Mann's Death in Venice." *Gesnerus* 66, no. 2 (2009): 256–87.

Seppilli, Tullio. "Presentazione: Il colera, il Mezzogiorno e il nuovo stato italiano; Una testimonianza di Edmondo De Amicis." *AM: Rivista della società italiana di antropologia medica* 9–10 (October 2000): 151–207.

Shary, Timothy, and Nancy McVittie. *Fade to Gray: Aging in American Cinema.* Austin: University of Texas Press, 2016.

Snowden, Frank M. *Naples in the Time of Cholera, 1884–1911.* Cambridge: Cambridge University Press, 1995.

Sontag, Susan. *Illness as Metaphor.* New York: Farrar, Straus and Giroux, 1978.

Testa, Carlo. *Masters of Two Arts: Re-Creation of European Literatures in Italian Cinema.* Toronto: University of Toronto Press, 2002.

Visconti, Luchino, dir. *La terra trema.* Film. AR.TE.AS. Universalia (Italy), 1948.

______, dir. *Senso.* Film. Lux Film (Italy), 1954.

______, dir. *Rocco e i suoi fratelli.* Film. Titanus (Italy), Les Filmes Marceau (France), 1960.

______, dir. *Il Gattopardo.* Film. Titanus (Italy), S. N. Pathé (France), SGC (France), 1963.

______, dir. *Götterdämerung: La caduta degli dei.* Film. Italnoleggio (Italy), Praesidens (Italy), Pegaso (Italy), Eichberg Film (Germany), 1969.

______, dir. *Morte a Venezia.* Film. Alfa Cinematografica (Italy), Warner Bros (USA), PECF (France), 1971.

______, dir. *Ludwig.* Film. Mega Film (Italy), Cinétel (France), Dieter Geissler Film Produktion (Germany), 1972.

______, dir. *Gruppo di famiglia in un interno.* Film. Rusconi Film (Italy), Gaumont International (France), 1974.

______, dir. *L'innocente.* Film. Rizzoli Film (Italy), Les Films Jacques Leitienne (France), Imp.Ex.Ci (France), Fracoriz Production (France), 1976.

White, Hayden. "Historiography and Historiophoty." *American Historical Review* 93, no. 5 (December 1988): 1193–99.

10 Tuberculosis, Queerness and Luxury Guests
The Hidden Stories of Capri's Hotel Quisisana

Ewa Kawamura

The Origin of the Name "Quisisana"

Today, the Grand Hotel Quisisana, one of the most luxurious hotels in the world and an icon of the Island of Capri, remains a symbol of exclusive and relaxed life for those on a Mediterranean summer holiday (Figure 10.1). However, when it was founded in the mid-nineteenth century, it was a facility for consumptive patients. It soon began to accept mainly healthy guests, including those seeking to keep private their homosexual affairs. This chapter seeks to uncover this origin by critically examining how the facility became a renowned resort hotel and how the story of its early founding was disguised.

The name Quisisana originated from the Italian phrase *qui si sana*, or "here one becomes healthy," which means recovery through the good quality of the air in a favorable climatic location. Before the foundation of the Capriote Grand Hotel Quisisana, Quisisana was already known as the name of a royal villa in Castellammare di Stabia in the Campania region. The villa, built by the will of King Robert I of Anjou in 1310, became the Bourbon palace (Figure 10.2). An eighteenth-century scholar, Lorenzo Giustiniani, explained that before calling itself Quisisana, the locality had been known as Casasana (healthy house). He described the place as a "district of the Royal city of Castellammare di Stabia, known today as Quisisana. It is located on a mountain, where you can breathe perfect air and enjoy a horizon that is as extensive as it is delightful."[1] After the unification of Italy, the Stabiese royal villa was transformed into Quisisana, the best hotel in Castellammare di Stabia. In 1876, the Stabiese composer Luigi Denza wrote a cheerful serenade "Souvenir de Quisisana" before penning "Funiculì funiculà" (in Neapolitan dialect: the funicular) his best-known song.[2] Around 1860, a villa called Quisisana was also built in Capri. It was founded by a physician named George Sidney Smith Clark, who spoke "pure Italian with an Edinburgh accent."[3] The villa functioned as a therapeutic facility "for invalids, especially those suffering from rheumatism and chest infections."[4]

The second (1855) and third (1858) editions of Murray's *Handbook for Travellers in Southern Italy* finally included the list of hotels on Capri but left out Villa Quisisana. In the fourth (1862) and fifth (1865) editions, Quisisana

DOI: 10.4324/9781003382805-10

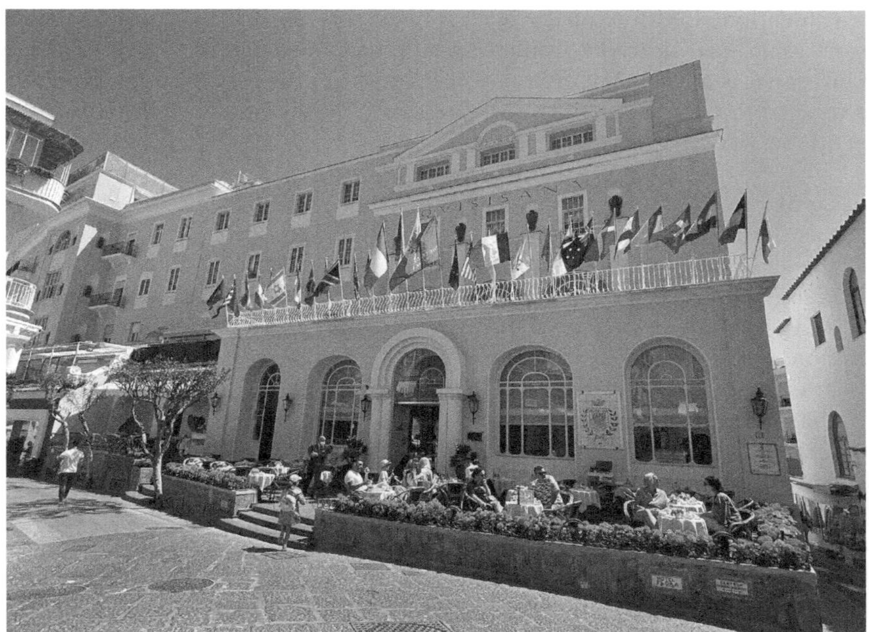

Figure 10.1 Grand Hotel Quisisana in Capri.

Source: Photo by the author taken in May 2022.

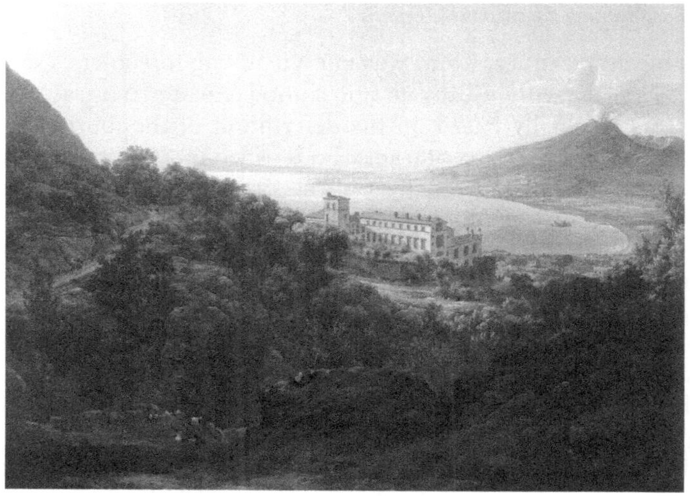

Figure 10.2 Johan Christian Dahl (1788–1857), view of Quisisana in Castellammare
di Stabia with the Bay of Naples, 1825, oil on canvas, private collection.

Source: Public domain, via Wikimedia Commons.

was mentioned but on a page separate from the hotel list: "On the S. of the town of Capri, near the Camerelle, now occupied by Dr. Clark's Villa of Quisisana, is a long row of arches, which were probably the foundations of a road from the Castiglione to the Tragara."[5] In the fourth edition, its therapeutic service was described in detail:

> Until lately the want of medical attendance and of a suitable residence has deterred invalids from resorting to this island in search of health; this drawback now no longer exists, since Dr. Clark, an English physician, has settled here in search of health, and constructed a large villa at Quisisana, in one of the most agreeable of its picturesque situation, where English comforts will be found in connection with medical attendance on the spot. Dr. Clark's house is at a short distance from the village of Capri; it is surrounded by open colonnades, and with a large garden, where at all seasons the invalid can move about, whilst inside each room has a good English chimney. Terms, including, board, medical attendance, and servants, 18 paul (6 s.) a day; less for families during a lengthened stay.[6]

Villa Quisisana offered food and lodging like a hotel, with "Breakfast, Dinner, Tea, or Supper, wine and service" at the rate of "18 carlins" per person (or "six shillings" in British currency).[7] It was a very reasonable and honest price because the Neapolitan first-class hotel of that time cost 8–12 carlins, excluding board.[8]

Villa Quisisana as a Therapeutic Facility

In the eighteenth century, Capri was known among foreigners, especially the English, as a place with healthy air and a good climate.[9] Murray's guidebook on Italy was originally based on the description of the journey written by the British traveler Mariana Starke, who testified in 1797 to the presence of doctors and the good curative effect of the air on the Island of Capri: "Here are three physicians appointed by the king to attend to the people gratis; nevertheless, their practice is very inconsiderable, the air being so particularly salubrious that scarcely any maladies visit this island."[10]

This quality of Capri appears in numerous guidebooks, such as the one by archaeologist Rosario Mangoni, which reports in 1834 that "[t]he climate of the island is generally temperate and sweet; and since there is no stagnant water, the air is pure and healthy."[11] Similarly, the 1832–37 editions of Vallardi's guide to Italy explain that its "healthy air invites the sick and the curious to dwell there."[12] The English doctor James Henry Bennet, who himself suffered from consumption, settled in Menton in 1860, where he recovered. He mentioned Capri as a recommendable place in his book about the Mediterranean climatic resort: "The Naples physicians are in the habit of sending convalescents there, and with the best results."[13]

Advertisements further confirmed this association. The first one for the Villa Quisisana, which depicted its building and pleasant landscape, was printed around 1860 by the Neapolitan typographer Gatti and Dura and designed by engraver Gaetano Dura (Figure 10.3). The piece was accompanied by a detailed description:

> In building this Hotel the goal of the Proprietor has been to meet all the requirements and comforts of Travellers or Invalids . . . so well calculated at all seasons to promote health or returning health where climate is available. . .. The peculiar effect of the Scirocco so distressing throughout Southern Italy is never experienced here, nor will the sufferer from pulmonary consumption (the disease of all others most benefitted by this climate) be exposed to those rapid vicissitudes from heat to cold.[14]

Similar information appeared in the 1862–68 editions of Murray's guide to Southern Italy, omitting Dr. Clark's name: "From some years' observations an English medical gentleman, settled at Capri, informs us that the lowest temperature he had observed in the house was 55 degree and the highest 75

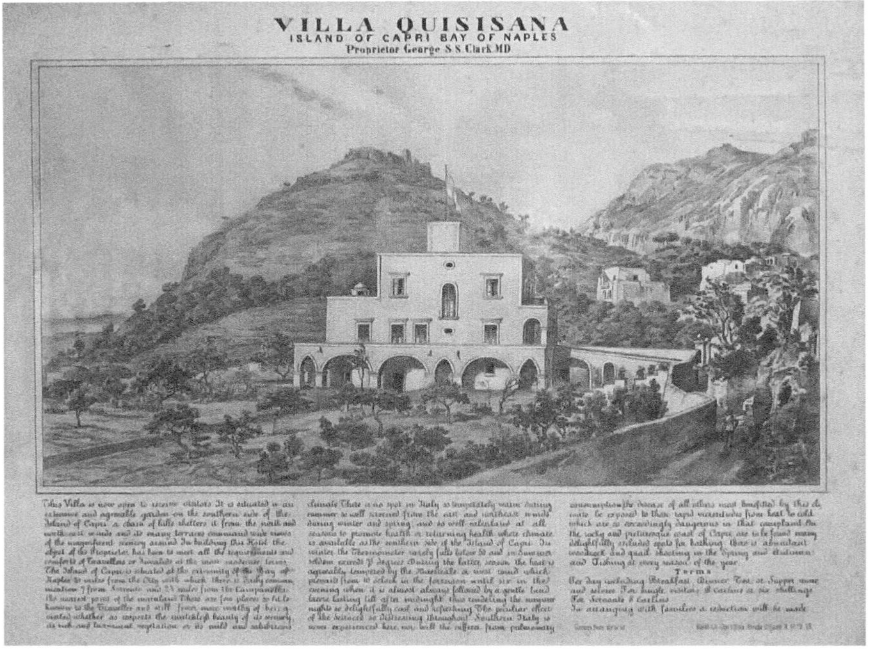

Figure 10.3 Advertisement of the Villa Quisisana in Capri in the form of an engraving printed in Naples by Gatti e Dura, around 1860 (Gianfranco Campione collection).

degree during the summer, the periodical breezes moderating the extreme heat."[15]

Various editions of Murray's guidebooks on Italy and other countries with an advertising appendix specialized for the year 1862 announced the opening of Villa Quisisana through text that resembled Dura's engraving, but with some additional information, such as: "he [Clark] begs to observe that the use of a library of books, newspapers, a good pianoforte, and medical attendance, are advantages for which no extra charge will be made."[16] An 1855 article documents that Dr. Clark did hydrotherapy at the villa.[17] He died at the age of 49 in 1868, and a marble plaque was installed on the Town Hall of Capri's wall in 1908 to commemorate his generous contributions 40 years after his death. The award was meant to emphasize only his medical services to poor people without mentioning the foundation of the Hotel Quisisana.

Hotel Quisisana for Consumptive Guests

Dr. Clark's death created the conditions for the transformation of the resort, now managed by his Capriote wife Anna Lembo, into a hotel that was open to healthy people, as well.[18] The second edition (1869) of Baedeker's guidebook to Southern Italy presented the former Villa Quisisana, renamed "Hotel Quisisana" and managed by an "English landlady, pension 7 1.[lire], well-spoken of."[19] In the German Gsell Fels's 1873 travel guidebook, the Quisisana is represented as an English pension.[20] The seventh (1873) and subsequent (1878–83) editions of Murray's Southern Italy guidebooks reported the following: "Hotel Quisisana, kept by Mrs. Clark, the widow of an English physician, a very well situated house, clean and comfortable; charges moderate; pension 7 to 8 frs. a day."[21]

From the 1870s until his death in 1913, the young and capable Capriote Federico Serena managed the Hotel Quisisana. Serena had experience working in hotels in England.[22] In fact, Baedeker's travel guide of 1876 mentioned Serena as the new hotelier of the Quisisana.[23] Giambattista De Curtis, poet of the famous Neapolitan song "Torna a Surriento" (in Neapolitan dialect: Come back to Sorrento), composed a duet entitled "Custantina" (in Neapolitan dialect: the female name Costantina), which contains the following verses: "If you are sick, come to Quisisana; Serena keeps everything good and God."[24] Even though it was labeled as a hotel, its main target guests were patients with mild symptoms hoping to recover from disease; the verses of the song confirm that the reputation gained by the hotel had grown wider and more famous.

From the winter of 1872 to the spring of 1873, the British historian John Richard Green stayed there and commented: *"Here-you-get-well Hotel,* which is cheering and instructive."[25] He wrote to fellow novelist Mary Augusta Humphry Ward on March 4, 1873: "Not that I long as yet for my winter has passed very happily, in spite of the 'inevitables' of an invalid hotel;

and I love Capri more than ever."[26] Green reported on Quisisana: "Its rough inns, its wants of English doctors, the difficulties of communication with the mainland from which its residents are utterly cut off in bad weather, make Capri an unsuitable resort for invalids."[27] Yet Green returned to Capri in winter in 1878 and 1880 to receive treatment at Quisisana.

At the time, like many other health resorts, Capri's high season was winter and spring, while summer was its low season as the popularity of summer bathing only began in the 1920s. The guidebook *Hygienic-Medical Hand-Book for Travellers in Italy* (1878) commented on summer stays in Capri: "its climate is healthy. . ... As a place, of residence it is not very attractive; although anybody who is fond of solitude may like to spend the summer there. The air is pure but during summer it is very warm, therefore it is not adapted to a long sojourn."[28]

In 1880, the German writer Konrad Telmann, who was transferred to Italy for treatment of consumption, testified that Hotel Quisisana was frequented only by the English and the wealthy.[29] In 1886, the English landscape painter Adrian Stokes, who sojourned in Capri, similarly wrote, "The Quisisana is patronized principally by English visitors."[30]

According to the observation of the German painter Christian Wilhelm Allers, who lived on Capri:

> So far, the English have not been very present on the island, probably because there aren't enough comfortable hotels. In the stiff, quiet Quisisana, it is indeed clean and the waiters are well washed, but the level of comfort naturally does not reach that of the comfortable grandiose hotel palaces of the mainland and that of the English and American hotels of the first rank.[31]

Only the Quisisana Hotel served as a place of gathering for the British and Americans.[32]

Local doctor Vincenzo Cuomo, who received patients every morning at his office in Hotel Quisisana, analyzed in his book the possibility of the winter Capri climate curing consumption.[33] He saw 60 cases of foreign patients in Capri, among whom the majority were German, while only five cases were British and Americans.[34]

Baedeker's 1903 travel guidebook still presented Capri as a favorable location for treating lung disease: "Naples is often trying for persons with weak lungs. . ... Capri is generally much more congenial to patients of this class."[35] An article in a 1905 English travel journal reported the same about Capri:

> The climate, owing to the absence of dust and of sudden variations of temperature, is suited to those in early stages of consumption. The best months in Capri are October, November, April, and May. There are numerous hotels on the island the Quisisana being the best.[36]

On October 2, 1906, hoping for recovery from consumption, the Russian writer Maxim Gorky landed in Capri with his partner, the actress Maria Andreyeva, and his son.[37] They stayed at Hotel Quisisana as guests until November 22nd.[38] Another Russian writer, Ivan Bunin, winner of the 1933 Nobel Prize, had stayed at the Quisisana several times between winter and spring in the years 1909 and 1913. His novel *The Gentleman from San Francisco* (1915) is set in the best hotel on Capri, undoubtedly modeled on the Quisisana. The protagonist is a 58-year-old wealthy American gentleman from San Francisco who was traveling in Europe with his wife and daughter to cure her disease, perhaps consumption. However, the American gentleman suddenly died in the hotel's reading room during dinner time. The manager of the hotel, inspired by the actual Serena, decided that the body could not be moved back to its suite because no one would want to sleep there if they knew a dead body had occupied it. Thus, the body was brought momentarily into a small room of "No. 43, the smallest, wretchedest, dampest, and coldest room at the end of the bottom corridor."[39] The following day, the body was promptly removed from the hotel to be transported back to its homeland.

In 1887, the American writer William Chauncy Langdon documented another case of the death of a compatriot gentleman at the Hotel Quisisana. In the magazine *The Atlantic Monthly*, he recounted his trip to Capri to meet his friend who died at the Quisisana. The widow of Dr. Clark had graciously agreed to preserve the body of his friend in the hotel without charging additional fees.[40] For infirm clients who sojourned on Capri, dying in the hotel was not uncommon. Several foreign guests of the Quisisana are buried in the non-Catholic cemetery of Capri, including its British founder George Hayward, who also stayed at the Quisisana.[41] Langdon's visit to Capri was probably before the non-Catholic cemetery was founded in 1878 because he documented the difficulty of transporting the body to Catholic churches, even if it was only to be held there temporarily. This event shows that the Quisisana still had some ill guests, but it was also beginning to dislike their presence in the hotel.

From Patients to Clients: Spielhagen's Novel *Quisisana*

A key shift in the perception of Hotel Quisisana from tuberculosis sanatorium to *locus amoenus* occurred with the publication of a novel written by a German guest which produced an immediate and successful branding for the Quisisana. Even though the hotel had ill clients, death was concealed. Its image could now shift to that of a hotel for relaxation through the novel *Quisisana* by Friedrich Spielhagen, who wrote it there in 1876.[42] His first stay there dates back to as early as 1873, documented in a chapter in his collection of travel descriptions published in 1874, titled *Quisisana*, in which he recalls the young Federico Serena as a skilled hotelier. The chapter begins by linking the name "Quisisana" to health: "Quisisana! Here one recovers!

That is the name of our inn on Capri, and it is not just called that, not just by me, who needed the friendly help of a mild, clear climate and good, clean lodging."[43] Spielhagen often underlined the meaning of the hotel's name in his memory of Capri:

> Here one recovers, one must recover, here in this white two-story house, with its simple, white-painted rooms equipped with simple furniture, which from their windows, verandas, and balconies in front of the windows facing south, north, east and west, and all sides, points of the compass rose, mastering the most delicious parts of the delicious whole that is called Capri.[44]

Spielhagen repeats the healthiness of the Quisisana: "Here, one must be healthy! The world is far too beautiful to be ill within, and melancholy itself should only come about as contraband."[45]

Spielhagen was enchanted by the name Quisisana. In 1876, he wrote a comedy *Der lustige Rath* (The Merry Council), where the character Trechow talks assiduously about his beautiful memory of his stay at the Quisisana in Capri: "Quisisana: here you heal! I tried it long ago! At a critical time in my life. . ... It is very beautiful and sweet to breathe in the orange garden of Quisisana!"[46] Finally, Spielhagen published the volume entitled *Quisisana: Novelle* (1880) (Figure 10.4), which was a great success. It was translated in 1881 into English and in 1883 into Italian. The second edition was already printed in 1880, and the 21st edition came out in 1919.

While the Quisisana is referred to by the two protagonists several times in conversations in Spielhagen's novel, the story is not set in Capri. Both have experienced staying at the Hotel Quisisana at different times; one is the wise

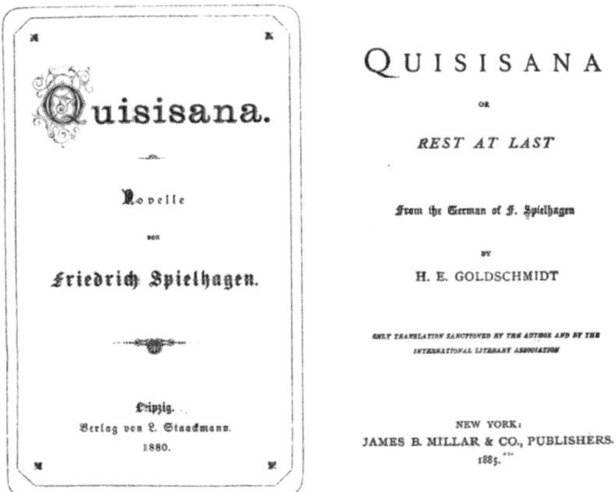

Figure 10.4 Frontispiece of *Quisisana: Novelle* by Friedrich Spielhagen from the 1880 edition (left) and from the 1885 English translation (right).

50-year-old Betram, and the other is his 18-year-old niece Erna, who loves her uncle. In the first part of the novel, Bertram talks to Erna about Hotel Quisisana:

> In Capri there stands amidst orange groves, with sublimest view of the blue infinity of the ocean, a fair white hostelry, embowered in roses, Quisisana. Years ago, I was there, and I have longed ever since to be back again: Qui si sana! What a sound of comfort, of promise! Qui si sana! Here one gets well! Even those who are fairly well physically, have something to recover from. Why, life itself – what is it but a long disease, and death its only cure?"[47]

Hotel Quisisana was again mentioned in the final part. Bertram, who had rejected his niece Erna's courtship, received an affectionate letter from her while she was honeymooning on Capri, written on the balcony of the Quisisana. Erna remembers Uncle Betram's story about Quisisana, explaining, "I wanted first to see the house which had, since then, remained in your fond remembrance, where you 'ever since longed to be back again,' and the very name of which was always to you 'a sound of comfort, of promise: Qui si sana!'"[48] Echoing this sentiment from his niece, Bertram takes his diary to check the date of his arrival in Capri, which coincidentally falls on Erna's birthday: "May 1. Arrived in Capri, and put up at a house which I found it hard to climb up to; the name had an irresistible attraction for me: Quisisana – Sit omen Qui si sana!"[49] Bertram then sends a telegram so that it arrives in time for Erna's birthday. In it, he emphasizes the name of the hotel and wishes her a happy celebration: "All hail – happiness and blessing – to-day and forever – For my darling child in Quisisana."[50] To conclude the novel, Spielhagen repeats the name: "Qui si sana!"[51] The English translation of the novel has a slightly modified title, *Quisisana; Or, Rest at Last*. In fact, the last scene depicts two types of rest: the sudden death of Bertram, who could not recover from his sickness, and the relaxing stay of his niece at the Quisisana. This novel also describes the guests of the Quisisana as changing from patients to clients.

With the success of Spielhagen's novel, Hotel Quisisana became better known.[52] Later, several German literary works were published with titles containing the name Quisisana. Novelist Reinhold Ortmann wrote *Quisisana: Ein görbersdorfer Roman*[53], set in the luxury hotel-like, mountain air treatment tubercular sanatorium in Görbersdorf, earlier than Thomas Mann's *The Magic Mountain*. Playwright Heinrich Ilgenstein composed a three-act comedy titled *Quisisana* (1914), while Liesbet Dill named her novel *Pension Quisisana: Ein heiterer Roman* (The Quisisana Boarding House: A Cheerful Novel, 1944). In this way, by adding the term "Quisisana" to the title, the writers were trying to increase the value of their literary works by associating with a place whose brand had by this point achieved international renown.

Internationalization of the Name "Quisisana"

After the publication of Spielghagen's novel, from the 1880s onward and in the interwar period, the name "Quisisana" acquired the power of a well-known brand. Other than the original Quisisana in Castellammare di Stabia, the Quisisana on Capri became so influential that its name was used for other hotels and pensions around the world until the 1920s (Figure 10.5). In Italy, pensions named Quisisana existed in Naples, Ischia, Castel di Sangro, Rome, Florence, Levico, Bordighera, Milano Marittima and Fasano, while Montecatini Alto had the Grande Albergo Ristorante Quisisana. To accommodate those seeking wellness, some spa towns, such as Chianciano and Abano Terme, had their own Hotel Quisisanas. Lodgings named Villa Quisisana existed in San Remo, Nervi, Lido di Venezia and Arco. An elegant Croatian Hotel Quisisana stood in Opatija (Abazzia) when it was a part of Italy. Many resort hotels built in mild climates were often named Quisisana. Santa Cruz de Tenerife in Spain had a Hotel Quisisana, which was frequently discussed in tourist postcards during the early twentieth century. Green Cove Springs, Florida, in the United States, and Poços de Caldas Minas, in Brazil, also had Hotel Quisisanas.

With the success of Spielhagen's *Quisisana*, the number of hotels, pensions, villas and sanatoriums called Quisisana in Germany increased, especially in

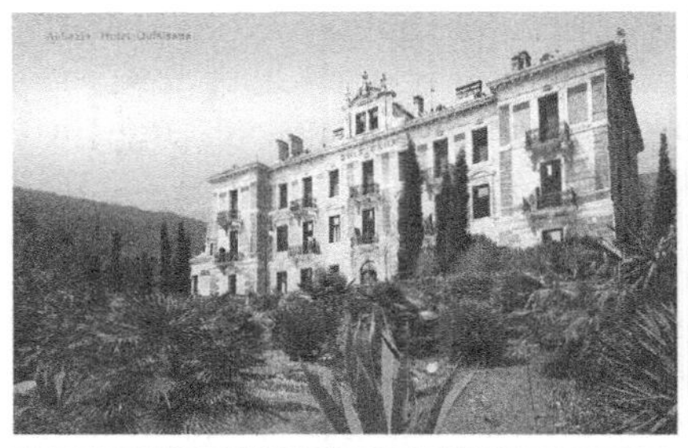
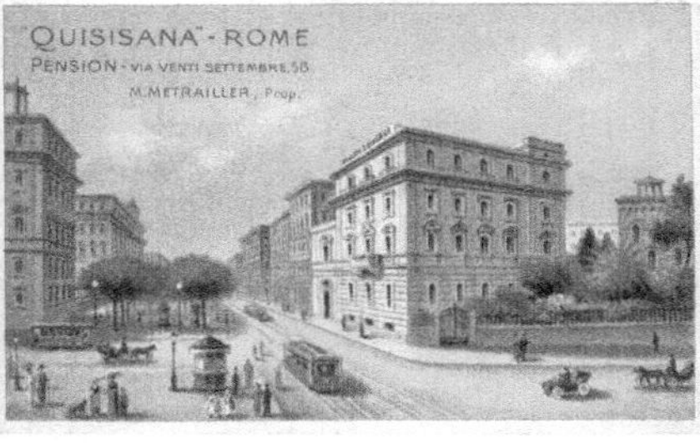
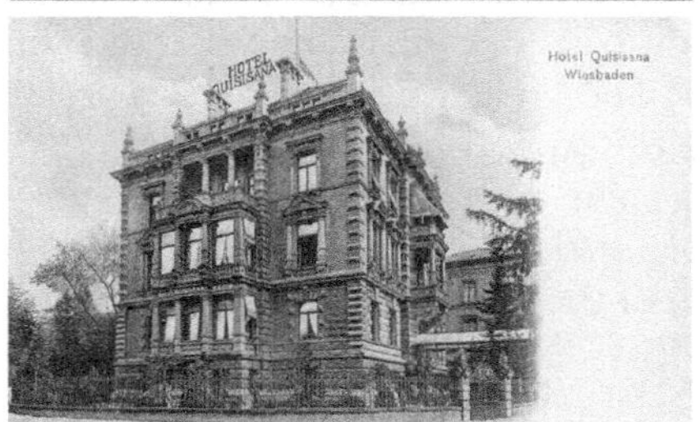
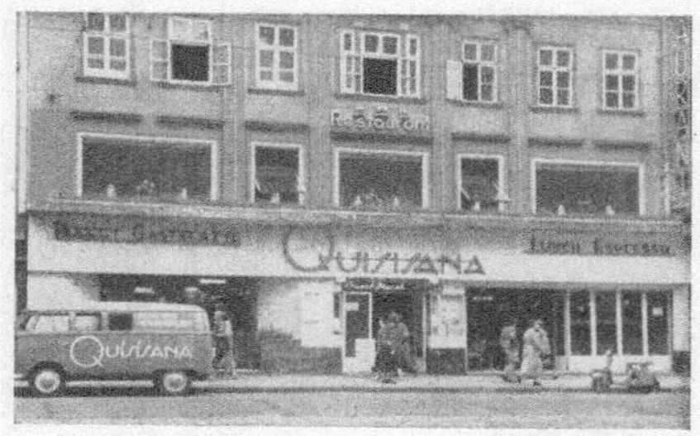

Figure 10.5 Postcards from the early twentieth century depicting the Hotel Quisisana in Abazzia (above left), the Pension Quisisana in Rome (above right), the Hotel Quisisana in Wiesbanden (below left) and the Restaurant Quisisana in Vienna (below right).

spa towns.[54] Wiesbaden, Bad Schandau, Bad Liebenstein, Bad Wildungen and Bad Salzhausen had Hotel Quisisanas. In Baden Baden, Bad Schwalbach, Bad Orb, Bad Königsborn, Ebenhausen and Neckargemünd, there was a Pension Quisisana. Pension Quisisanas also existed in Munich, Westerland and Göhren on the Island of Rügen and Norderney, as well as in Switzerland in Locarno, Zurich and Bern. Hotels named Villa Quisisana were in Bad Elster, Bad Ems, Bad Pyrmont, Bad Reichenhall, Finsterbergen, Halstenbek and Königstein im Taunus. In addition, there were restaurants called Quisisana in Berlin, Vienna, Budapest and Saint Petersburg, and a Café Quisisana in Gera and Malmo in Sweden. For restaurants and cafés, the name Quisisana was used to capture the pleasant and relaxed vibe of the place.

The Triumph of the Quisisana and Its Eccentric Guests

Between the Nineteenth and Twentieth Centuries

During the time that Federico Serena managed it, Hotel Quisisana became the first and only grand hotel on the island. A guidebook to Capri of 1898 praised the state of the hotel under his management:

> There is one large, most excellent, and in every sense first-rate Hotel, called the Quisisana. . ... Beneath Mr. Serena's hospitable roof, many crowned heads and other transient celebrities have satisfactorily slumbered. It faces south and has accommodation for about 120 people; the cooking is excellent, the rooms most comfortably furnished, and the garden which surrounds it beautifully kept.[55]

The garden of Hotel Quisisana offered natural landscaped vegetation in the English style (Figure 10.6), which Baedeker's 1912 guidebook called an "English Garden."[56] The American writer Henry James Forman described the Quisisana's garden in his travel impressions: "There is a beautiful garden at the hotel, with orange and lemon trees and many flowers, and thus a delightful place in which to linger."[57] The French writer Roger Peyrefitte in his novel *L'exilé de Capri* (The Exile of Capri, 1959) quotes Serena: "the mayor and owner, a handsome smiling man, contemplated the triumph of Quisisana and Capri."[58] The importance of the hotel is mentioned again in another part of the novel: "The triumph of the Quisisana was always that of Capri."[59]

This literary work of Peyrefitte deals with the exiled life of the French-Swedish count Jacques d'Adeswärd Fersen in Capri. He was a descendant of the Swedish nobleman Hans Axel von Fersen, the lover of Queen Marie Antoinette. The young Fersen first arrived in Capri in 1897 in the company of his friend, the viscount Robert de Tournel, an amateur poet 18 years his senior. During their stay at the Quisisana, they witnessed the hotel's rejection of the great English poet Oscar Wilde, who was on Capri

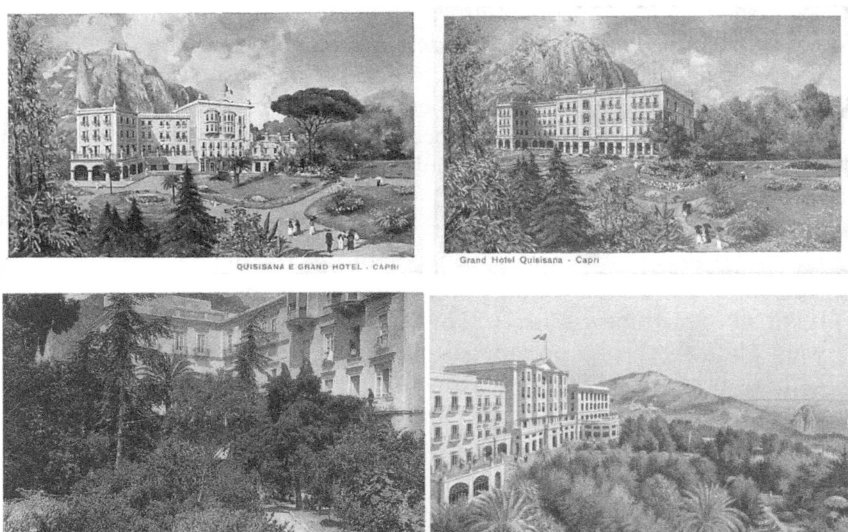

Figure 10.6 Postcards of the Hotel Quisisana seen from the garden in the early twentieth-century illustration (above left), around 1910 (above right), photo from the 1920s (below left) and a 1920s illustration (below right).

in 1897 with his lover Lord Alfred Douglas after his detention in Reading prison for homosexuality.[60] The two lovers had appeared in the dining room but were not allowed in as guests. Fellow hotel guests refused to sit at a table in the same room as Wilde and Douglas, who were asked to leave the hotel by Serena.[61]

Fersen settled in Capri in 1904 after having had to flee Paris, where his scandalous sexual relationship with boys during a satanic mass had been exposed. In the next year, Fersen built a house on Capri, where he would live with his beloved Italian boyfriend Nino Cesarini. The house, named the Villa Lysis, was where he died at 43 from a cocaine overdose. While waiting for its construction, Fersen stayed at the Quisisana. This fact is documented in Scot writer Compton Mackenzie's novel *Vestal Fire* (1927), which recounts the eccentric life of high society on Capri: "Marsac [i.e., Fersen] decided not to take another villa, but to live at the Hotel Augusto [i.e., Quisisana] until his house was finished."[62]

Fersen also authored an autobiographical novel *Messes noires: Lord Lyllian* (Satanic Masses: Lord Lyllian, 1905), in which he wrote about a well-known homosexual guest at the Quisisana, a German industrial entrepreneur who preferred Capri.[63] While the name was not revealed in the novel, Fersen was referring to Friedrich Alfred Krupp, the descendant of a famous family engaged in the steel supply industry. Krupp was a magnate and great arms manufacturer in Essen. Peyrefitte described Krupp's contribution to the hotel in the novel: "He had enlarged and embellished the Hotel Quisisana where he lived; he had the owner Federico Serena elected mayor."[64]

Krupp arrived in Capri in 1898, officially for reasons concerning consumption treatment, and returned there every winter to relax and have fun while hiding his homosexuality. He occupied a series of rooms on the ground floor of the Hotel Quisisana, at an unbelievably high price.[65] He even called the musicians to his hotel room:

> He paid bands to play every evening on the Piazza and the Piazetta [*sic*]. The bandmaster and his musicians being out at the elbows, Krupp set them all up with new suits. . ... The musicians habited in fantastic suits, went about with him on land, or gave concerts for which invitations had not been issued, in his apartments in the Hotel Quisisana. He had there an isolated wing, with a separate entrance, and a wide terrace that looked down on the sea.[66]

In 1902, Krupp bought a *dépendance* of the Hotel Quisisana in Marina Grande, the Hotel Schweizerhof, with a refined French restaurant called "Quisisana."[67] During the same year, Krupp was forced to leave Capri due to a scandal over his alleged homosexuality with Capriote boys. He died shortly after from a suspected suicide. In 1913, Serena died. The First World War broke out, and Hotel Quisisana served as a kind of hospital for convalescent soldiers on leave.[68] Immediately after the war, in 1918, the widow of Serena, Maria Quinton, sold the Quisisana. These changes in the management brought a new spirit of freedom in the hotel.

The Free Atmosphere of Capri and the Quisisana Between the Two Wars

In the interwar decades, the island ceased to be a place for patients, expanding its target clientele to all vacationers, including homosexuals.[69] People felt that tuberculosis was not cured here, and lesbians were treated like normal clients with a tacit form of understanding. The novel *Extraordinary Woman* (1928) by Mackenzie about the lesbian community on Capri told the story of two guests who had occupied the rooms at the Quisisana where Krupp once stayed. The protagonists' names in the novel are Aurora Freemantle and Rosalba Donsante, who are fictional stand-ins for the real-life wealthy Australian Francis Lloyd and his lover Mimì Franchetti, daughter of opera composer Alberto Franchetti. Rosalba (Mimì) was faced with the new atmosphere of the Quisisana, when it was under new management by a Milanese company: "The new manager came forward to assure the Signorina she would find the August [i.e., Quisisana] as anxious to serve her under his direction as in the day of the lamented Don Cesare [i.e., Serena]."[70] In other words, the manager valued this lesbian client.

The new owner changed the name to "Quisisana & Grand Hotel."[71] In 1928, the magazine of the Touring Club Italiano praised the hotel "above all for a livelier showiness and for a tone of modernity and elegance that is particularly felt in the 'Quisisana,' which is the main hotel, the summit of the island."[72]

From July 1, 1936, management of the Quisisana was entrusted to Giorgio Campione, son of a well-known family of hoteliers, who managed two important Neapolitan hotels: Hôtel de Londres and Hotel Santa Lucia.[73] His father, Alfredo Campione, was the CEO of the Compagnia Italiana dei Grandi Alberghi (CIGA), the first luxury hotel chain in Italy. At this time, the high season of Capri had shifted from the winter to care for consumption to the summer for bathing. The English newspaper *Daily Mail* reported on October 18, 1938, the significant increase in the number of summer guests and the construction of the swimming pool for summer bathers:

> The brilliant summer quite capped previous records in the number and quality of visitors. Those who remained have been amply rewarded by the beauty and interest of the island this smiling October, and new visitors are making Capri autumn crowds quite normal again. . .. The Quisisana Hotel, Capri, will double the area of its garden during the winter and will install a modern swimming pool in readiness for the next summer season.[74]

The collection of periodical articles and advertisements on the "Quisisana & Grand Hotel" compiled by Giorgio Campione conveys the shift in the hospitality mindset in Capri (Figure 10.7). For example, the advertisement for the tourism magazine *Giornale della CIT* dated September 1938 included the following catchphrase: "The island that frees you from the bonds of the world."[75] The text was accompanied by a photo of two smiling island girls almost touching each other, which could suggest freedom for lesbian tendencies. The January 1939 issue of *Harper's Bazaar* reported the sojourn of the stylist Coco Chanel, with her companion Misia Sert showcasing their ways of dressing in the Capri style, which was inspired by primitiveness:

> It is gay now. And the most attractive people in the world come there in the summer. Chanel roams about on a donkey. Mme. Sert shops for armloads of stick coral. . .. No one ever wears an evening dress. No one wears anything but the flattest of primitive sandals – it is impossible to get about on the rocky paths without them. All day long, slacks and shorts and jerseys splash their colors among the cypresses. . . . At night, dancing at the Quisisana, you still wear them. But because it's evening, you plaster yourself with pearls and coral and fresh flowers, with great bracelets and necklaces of gold.[76]

Freedom on the island did not only concern lesbians but also people of different skin colors. An advertisement about the Quisisana in the tourism journal *Giornale della CIT* dated June 1939 used the photo of an African boy against a background of the Faraglioni rocks symbol of Capriote nature, who holds the announcement panel of the film festival from June 8 to September 15 at the Quisisana, with the following catchphrase: "A stay in Capri makes you experience the delight of life."[77] Another advertisement in the *Giornale della CIT* from August of the same year took advantage of physicist Marie Curie's visit in 1918, expressing how the island could tone one's body: "Mrs Curie was surprised by the radioactivity of Capri in 1913 [*sic*] . . . to tone up your physique there is only one choice, Capri."[78]

In 1939, the new space for the Quisisana night club appeared and was called "Qui sì", the positive term of the answer *qui sì* ("here, yes"). It was renovated in the style of the island by the skillful manager Giorgio Campione.[79] At this point, the Quisisana had become a symbol of the *dolce vita* (sweet life) in Capri, where clients could relax and did not have to worry about their medical issues or hidden sexual proclivities. The hotel became free from the concept of being a healthy place or of offering recovery from illness: its enduring reputation is still today that of a summer luxury resort where celebrity guests come from all over the world just to enjoy relaxing in a *locus amoenus*.

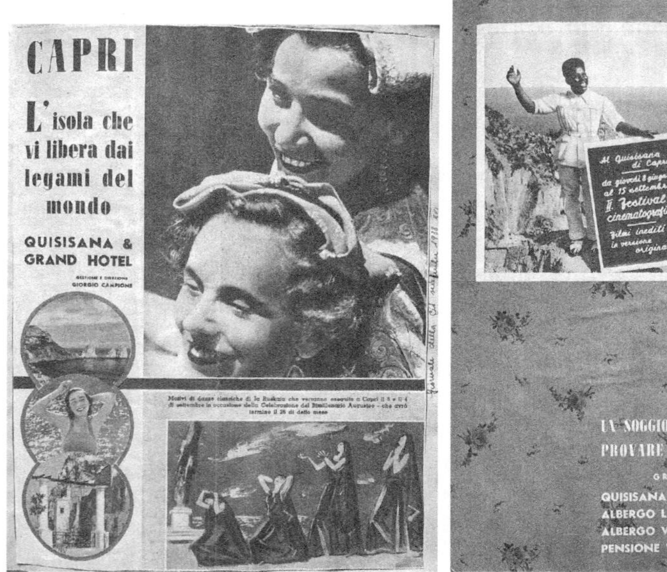

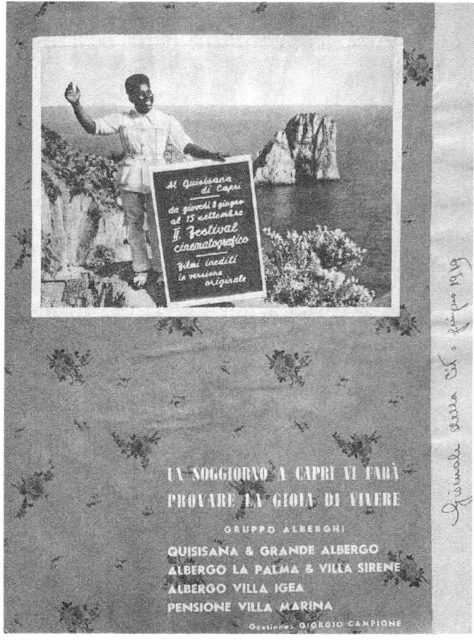

Figure 10.7 Advertisement for the contemporary Quisisana & Grand managed by Giorgio Campione appeared in the *Giornale della CIT* of September 1938 (left); the *Giornale della CIT* of June 1939 (right).

Source: Collection of Giorgio Campione.

Notes

1 Special thanks to Gianfranco Campione (Siena, Italy) and the Atomi University (Tokyo, Japan) for the support with a Special Research Grant for the 2024 academic year.
   Lorenzo Giustiniani, *Dizionario geografico ragionato del Regno di Napoli*, vol. 3 (Naples: Vincenzo Manfredi, 1797), 232.

2 The Stabiese Quisisana remained a hotel until the mid-twentieth century, after which it was abandoned for many years. Now, it has been transformed into an archaeological museum.

3 M. O. W. O. [pseud.], "Life in an Island," *Blackwood's Edinburgh Magazine* 97 (January–June 1865), 88.

4 James Money, *Capri: La storia e i suoi protagonisti*, trans. M. Buzzi (Milan: Rusconi, 1993), 56.

5 John Murray, *A Handbook for Travellers in Southern Italy*, 4th ed. (London: John Murray, 1862), 265; Murray, *A Handbook for Travellers in Southern Italy*, 5th ed. (London: John Murray, 1865), 277; and Murray, *A Handbook for Travellers in Southern Italy*, 6th ed. (London: John Murray, 1868), 288.

6 Murray, *A Handbook for Travellers*, 269.

7 Ewa Kawamura, *The Quisisana: A Biography of the Grand Hotel of Capri* (Capri: Edizioni La Conchiglia, 2011), 20.

8 Murray, *Handbook for Travellers*, 4th ed., 70.

9 Ibid., 17.

10 Mariana Starke, *Letters from Italy between the Years 1792 and 1798*, 2 vols. (London: T. Gillet for R. Phillips, 1800), 2, 165.

11 Rosario Mangoni, *Ricerche topografiche ed archeologiche sull'isola di Capri* (Naples: Torchi di Gennaro Palma, 1834), 2.

12 Giuseppe Vallardi, *Itinerario d'Italia*, 20th ed. (Milan: Pietro e Giuseppe Vallardi, 1832), 293; and Vallardi, *Itinerario d'Italia*, 22nd ed. (Milan: Pietro e Giuseppe Vallardi, 1835), 303.

13 James Henry Bennet, *Winter and Spring on the Shore of the Mediterranean*, 4th ed. (New York: D. Appleton, 1870), 246; and Bennet, *Winter and Spring on the Shores of the Mediterranean*, 5th ed. (London: J. and A. Churchill, 1875), 224.

14 Private Collection, Gianfranco Campione, Siena Italy. The advertisement has been published in Kawamura, *Quisisana*, 21.

15 Murray, *Handbook*, 4th ed., 268; Murray, *Handbook*, 5th ed., 280; and Murray, *Handbook*, 6th ed., 292.

16 Quoted in Kawamura, *Quisisana*, 20.

17 W. P. Bayley, "Visits to the Paradise of Artists. IV," *Art-Journal* 28 (May 1866): 132.

18 Kawamura, *Quisisana*, 21.

19 Karl Baedeker, *Italy: Handbook for Travellers, pt. 3, Southern Italy* (Koblenz: Karl Baedeker, 1869) 142.

20 Theodor Gsell Fels, *Unter-Italien* (Hildburghausen: Bibliographisches Institut, 1873), 471.

21 Murray, *A Handbook for Travellers in Southern Italy*, 7th ed. (London: John Murray, 1873), 271; and Murray, *A Handbook for Travellers in Southern Italy*, 8th ed. (London: John Murray, 1878), 271.

22 Kawamura, *Quisisana*, 33–37.

23 Karl Baedeker, *Unter-Italien*. 5th ed. (Leipzig: Karl Baedeker, 1876), 159.

24 Manfredi Fasulo, *L'isola di Capri* (Sorrento: T. d'Onofrio, 1906), 106.

25 John Richard Green, *Letters of John Richard Green*, ed. Leslie Stephen (London: Macmillan, 1901), 339.

26 Ibid., 350.

27 John Richard Green, *Stray Studies from England and Italy* (London: Macmillan, 1876), 392.
28 Camillo Liberali, *Hygienic-Medical Hand-Book for Travellers in Italy* (Rome: Luigi Piale, 1878), 86.
29 Conrad Telmann, *Auf der Sireneninsel Capri* (Cologne: Tonger, 1880), 30.
30 Adrian Stokes, "Capri," *Art Journal* 48 (1886): 166.
31 Christian Willhelm Allers, *La bella Napoli* (Berlin: Union Deutsche Verlagsgesellschaft, 1893).
32 Christian Willhelm Allers, *Capri* (Naples: Grimaldi and Cicerano, 1892).
33 Harold E. Trower, *The Book of Capri* (Naples: Emil Prass, 1906).
34 Vincenzo Cuomo, *L'isola di Capri come stazione climatica* (Naples: A. Trani, 1894).
35 Baedeker, *Handbook for Travellers*, pt. 3, *Southern Italy*, 14th ed., xxvii.
36 Travel Editor, *The "Queen" Newspaper: Book of Travel* (London: Horace Cox, 1905), 83.
37 Tito Fiorani, *Le case raccontano: Storie e passioni delle dimore del mito a Capri* (Capri: Edizioni La Conchiglia, 2002), 43.
38 Aleksej Kara-Murza, *Napoli russa* (Rome: Teti, 2005), 137.
39 Ibid., 43.
40 William Chauncy Langdon, "An Experience on the Island of Capri," *Atlantic Monthly* 59, no. 352 (February 1887): 241–42.
41 Dieter Richter, *Il giardino della memoria: Il cimitero acattolico di Capri* (Capri: Edizioni La Conchiglia, 1996), 124–35.
42 Friedrich Furchheim, *Bibliografia della isola di Capri e della penisola sorrentina* (Naples: Ditta F. Furchheim di Emilio Prass, 1899), 29.
43 Friedrich Spielhagen, *Aus meinem Skizzenbuche* (Leipzig: L. Staackmann, 1874), 183. The same description was published in other travel writings by Spielhagen about Southern Italy; see *Von Neapel bis Syrakus: Reiseskizzen* (Leipzig: L. Staackmann, 1878), 101.
44 Spielhagen, *Aus meinem Skizzenbuche*, 188–89.
45 Ibid., 191.
46 Friedrich Spielhagen, *Der lustige Rath: Lustspiel in 4 Acten* (Leipzig: Der Verfasser, 1876), 92.
47 Friedrich Spielhagen, *Quisisana; Or, Rest at Last* (New York: James B. Millar, 1885), 16.
48 Ibid., 308–09.
49 Ibid., 311.
50 Ibid., 316.
51 Ibid.
52 Reinhold Schoener, *Capri: Natur, Volkstum, Geschichte und Altertümer der Insel* (Vienna: A. Hartleben's Verlag, 1892), 111.
53 Reinhold Ortmann, *Quisisana: Ein görbersdorfer Roman* (Leipzig: C. Reissner, 1889).
54 Johannes Proelss, *Deutsch Capri in kunst, dichtung, leben* (Oldenburg: Schulzesche hof-buchhandlung und hof-buchdrudkerei, 1901), 29.
55 Harold E. Trower, *Guide to Capri* (Naples: R. Tipografia Francesco Giannini and Figli, 1898), 6.
56 Karl Baedeker, *Southern Italy and Sicily*, 16th ed. (Leipzig: Karl Baedeker, 1912), 182.
57 Henry James Forman, *The Ideal Italian Tour* (Boston, MA: Houghton Mifflin, 1911), 62.
58 Roger Peyrefitte, *L'esule di Capri* (Capri: Edizioni La Conchiglia, 2003), 58. Serena was the mayor of Capri between 1895 and 1909.

59 Ibid., 127.
60 Ibid., 20.
61 Ibid., 21–24.
62 Compton Mackenzie, *Vestal Fire* (London: Chatto and Windus, 1951), 175. He lived in Capri from 1913 to 1920.
63 Jacques d'Adelswärd-Fersen, *Messes noires: Lord Lyllian* (Paris: Librairie Leon Vanier, 1905), 49.
64 Peyrefitte, *L'esule di Capri*, 52–53.
65 Carlo Knight, *Krupp a Capri: Uno scandalo d'altri tempi (e uno dei tempi nostri)* (Naples: S. Civita, 1989), 39; and Norman Douglas, *Biglietti da visita: Un viaggio autobiografico*, 2nd ed. (Milan: Adelphi, 1983), 174.
66 "Notes from Paris: The German Steel King," *Truth* 52, no. 1353 (December 4, 1902), 1395.
67 Ewa Kawamura, *Alberghi storici dell'isola di Capri: Una storia dell'ospitalità tra Ottocento e Novecento* (Capri: Edizioni La Conchiglia, 2005), 238–40.
68 Francesco Caravita di Sirignano, *Capri: Immagini e personagg* (Naples: Società Editrice Napoletana, 1985), 90.
69 A pioneer of the nude and naturalist commune, the German painter Karl Willhelm Diefenbach moved to Capri in 1899 after setbacks. As shown in Italian director Mario Martone's film *Capri-Revolution* (2018), inspired by Diefenbach's life in Capri, it was already considered a place amenable to sexual freedom by 1900.
70 Compton Mackenzie, *Extraordinary Women* (London: Hogarth Press, 1986), 53.
71 Karl Baedeker, *Italien von den Alpen bis Neapel* (Leipzig: Karl Baedeker, 1926), 429.
72 Ulderico Tegani, "Per l'avvenire di Capri," *Le vie d'Italia* 10 (October 1928): 800.
73 Kawamura, *Quisisana*, 81.
74 From the scrapbook made by Giorgio Campione in Gianfranco Campione' private collection.
75 Ibid.
76 Ibid.; and "On the Isle of Capri." *Harper's Bazaar* 73 (January 1939): 71.
77 Giorgio Campione scrapbook, Gianfranco Campione collection.
78 Ibid.
79 M. Balma, "Un rinnovamento ben riuscito: Il 'Qui si' del Grande Albergo 'Quisisana' di Capri," *L'Albergo in Italia* 5 (September–October 1939), 300.

References

Allers, Christian Wilhelm. *Capri*. Naples: Grimaldi and Cicerano, 1892.
______. *La bella Napoli*. Berlin: Union Deutsche Verlagsgesellschaft, 1893.
Baedeker, Karl. *Italy: Handbook for Travellers*. Pt. 3, *Southern Italy*. 2nd ed. Koblenz: Karl Baedeker, 1869.
______. *Unter-Italien*. 5th ed. Leipzig: Karl Baedeker, 1876.
______. *Italy: Handbook for Travellers*. Pt. 3, *Southern Italy*. 14th ed. Koblenz: Karl Baedeker, 1903.
______. *Southern Italy and Sicily*. 16th ed. Leipzig: Karl Baedeker, 1912.
______. *Italien von den Alpen bis Neapel*. Leipzig: Karl Baedeker, 1926.
Balma, M. "Un rinnovamento ben riuscito: Il 'Qui si' del Grande Albergo 'Quisisana' di Capri." *L'Albergo in Italia* 5 (September–October 1939): 300–02.
Bayley, W. P. "Visits to the Paradise of Artists. IV." *Art-Journal* 28 (May 1866): 129–32.
Bennet, James Henry. *Winter and Spring on the Shore of the Mediterranean*. 4th ed. New York: D. Appleton, 1870.

______. *Winter and Spring on the Shores of the Mediterranean.* 5th ed. London: J. and A. Churchill, 1875.

Blewitt, Octavian. *Handbook for Travellers in Southern Italy and Sicily.* London: John Murray, 1853.

______. *A Handbook for Travellers in Southern Italy and Sicily.* 2nd ed. London: John Murray, 1855.

______. *A Handbook for Travellers in Southern Italy and Sicily.* 3rd ed. London: John Murray, 1858.

Bunin, Ivan. *The Gentleman from San Francisco.* Translated by D. H. Lawrence and S. S. Koteliansky. New York: Leonard and Virginia Woolf at Hogarth Press, 1934.

Caravita di Sirignano, Francesco. *Capri: Immagini e personaggi.* Naples: Società Editrice Napoletana, 1985.

Cuomo, Vincenzo. *L'legami di Capri come stazione climatica.* Naples: A. Trani, 1894.

d'Adelswärd-Fersen, Jacques. *Messes noires: Lord Lyllian.* Paris: Librairie Leon Vanier, 1905.

Douglas, Norman. *Biglietti da visita: Un viaggio autobiografico.* 2nd ed. Milan: Adelphi, 1983.

Fasulo, Manfredi. *L'isola di Capri.* Sorrento: T. d'Onofrio, 1906.

Fiorani, Tito. *Le case raccontano: Storie e passioni delle dimore del mito a Capri.* Capri: Edizioni La Conchiglia, 2002.

Forman, Henry James. *The Ideal Italian Tour.* Boston: Houghton Mifflin, 1911.

Furchheim, Friedrich. *Bibliografia della isola di Capri e della penisola sorrentina.* Naples: Ditta F. Furchheim di Emilio Prass, 1899.

Giustiniani, Lorenzo. *Dizionario geografico ragionato del Regno di Napoli.* Vol. 3. Naples: Vincenzo Manfredi, 1797.

Green, John Richard. *Stray Studies from England and Italy.* London: Macmillan, 1876.

______. *Letters of John Richard Green.* Edited by Leslie Stephen. London: Macmillan, 1901.

Gsell Fels, Theodor. *Unter-Italien.* Hildburghausen: Bibliographisches Institut, 1873.

Kara-Murza, Aleksej. *Napoli russa.* Rome: Sandro Teti, 2005.

Kawamura, Ewa. *Alberghi storici dell'isola di Capri: Una storia dell'ospitalità tra Ottocento e Novecento.* Capri: Edizioni La Conchiglia, 2005.

______. *The Quisisana: A Biography of the Grand Hotel of Capri.* Capri: Edizioni La Conchiglia, 2011.

Knight, Carlo. *Krupp a Capri: Uno scandalo d'altri tempi (e uno dei tempi nostri).* Naples: S. Civita, 1989.

Langdon, William Chauncy. "An Experience on the Island of Capri." *Atlantic Monthly* 59, no. 352 (February 1887): 241–46.

Liberali, Camillo. *Hygienic-Medical Hand-Book for Travellers in Italy.* Rome: Luigi Piale, 1878.

Mackenzie, Compton. *Vestal Fire.* London: Chatto and Windus, 1951.

______. *Extraordinary Women.* London: Hogarth Press, 1986.

Mangoni, Rosario. *Ricerche topografiche ed archeologiche sull'isola di Capri.* Naples: Torchi di Gennaro Palma, 1834.

Money, James. *Capri: La storia e i suoi protagonisti.* Translated by M. Buzzi. Milan: Rusconi, 1993.

M. O. W. O. [pseud.]. "Life in an Island." *Blackwood's Edinburgh Magazine* 97 (January–June 1865): 72–91.

Murray, John. *A Handbook for Travellers in Southern Italy.* 4th ed. London: John Murray, 1862.

______. *A Handbook for Travellers in Southern Italy.* 5th ed. London: John Murray, 1865.

______. *A Handbook for Travellers in Southern Italy*. 6th ed. London: John Murray, 1868.

______. *A Handbook for Travellers in Southern Italy*. 7th ed. London: John Murray, 1873.

______. *A Handbook for Travellers in Southern Italy*. 8th ed. London: John Murray, 1878.

______. *A Handbook for Travellers in Southern Italy*. 9th ed. London: John Murray, 1890.

"Notes from Paris: The German Steel King." *Truth* 52, no. 1353 (December 4, 1902): 1394–95.

"On the Isle of Capri." *Harper's Bazaar* 73 (January 1939): 71.

Peyrefitte, Roger. *L'esule di Capri*. Capri: Edizioni La Conchiglia, 2003.

Proelss, Johannes. *Deutsch Capri in Kunst, Dichtung, Leben*. Oldenburg: Schulzesche hof-buchhandlung und hof-buchdrudkerei, 1901.

Richter, Dieter. *Il giardino della memoria: Il cimitero acattolico di Capri*. Capri: Edizioni La Conchiglia, 1996.

Schoener, Reinhold. *Capri: Natur, Volkstum, Geschichte und Altertümer der Insel*. Vienna: A. Hartleben's Verlag, 1892.

Spielhagen, Friedrich. *Aus meinem Skizzenbuche*. Leipzig: L. Staackmann, 1874.

______. *Der lustige Rath: Lustspiel in 4 Acten*. Leipzig: Der Verfasser, 1876.

______. *Von Neapel bis Syrakus: Reiseskizzen*. Leipzig: L. Staackmann, 1878.

______. *Quisisana; Or, Rest at Last*. New York: James B. Millar, 1885.

Starke, Mariana. *Letters from Italy between the Years 1792 and 1798*. 2 vols. London: T. Gillet for R. Phillips, 1800.

Stokes, Adrian. "Capri." *Art Journal* 48 (1886): 165–69.

Tegani, Ulderico. "Per l'avvenire di Capri." *Le vie d'Italia* 10 (October 1928): 793–803.

Telmann, Conrad. *Auf der Sireneninsel Capri*. Cologne: Tonger, 1880.

Travel Editor. *The "Queen" Newspaper: Book of Travel*. London: Horace Cox, 1905.

Trower, Harold E. *Guide to Capri*. Naples: R. Tipografia Francesco Giannini and Figli, 1898.

______. *The Book of Capri*. Naples: Emil Prass, 1906.

Vallardi, Giuseppe. *Itinerario d'Italia*. 20th ed. Milan: Pietro e Giuseppe Vallardi, 1832.

______. *Itinerario d'Italia*. 22th ed. Milan: Pietro e Giuseppe Vallardi, 1835.

11 Forgetting or Disguising?[1]

HIV/AIDS in the Italian Newspapers in the Twenty-First Century

Marco Rovinello

Introduction

The AIDS epidemic shaped the late twentieth century. However, data from the Joint United Nations Programme on HIV/AIDS (UNAIDS) show that it continues to have a significant impact in the twenty-first century. This is true both globally (38 million people with HIV, 1.7 million new infections and almost 700,000 deaths in 2019) and in the Western world (2.2 million people with HIV, 12,000 deaths and 65,000 new infections in 2020), though access to effective treatments has turned it into a chronic disease.[2] In Italy in 2020, although there were no longer 4,000–5,000 deaths and 3,000–4,000 verified new cases per year as in the 1990s, the Italian National Institute of Health (ISS) estimated in 2020 that there were still 130,000 people with HIV, 750 deaths and 2,500 new infections. These numbers explain why the issue has still been the subject of law proposals and informational campaigns in recent years.[3] It is also why here I chose to reconstruct narratives and representations of HIV/AIDS not in the emergency phase but in the postemergency phase between 2000, the year of the Durban Declaration and the session of the UN Security Council on HIV/AIDS,[4] and 2019, on the precipice of the spread of COVID-19 in Italy.

While aware of the growing importance and influence of other media on the press,[5] this first specifically historical reconstruction of the discourses about HIV/AIDS focuses on newspapers, examining five years (2000, 2005, 2010, 2015 and 2019) of national, local and online editions of five of Italy's major national newspapers, each with its own orientation and ownership structure: *Avvenire*, the most widely read Catholic daily newspaper; *l'Unità*, the historical press organ of the far left; *la Repubblica*, the most widely read center-left newspaper; *La Stampa*, tied to the financial and business world of Northern Italy; and *Corriere della Sera*, the most widely read and balanced Italian newspaper.

The purpose of this in-depth analysis is threefold. The first aim is to contribute to the emerging thread of historical studies of HIV/AIDS in Italy from the discursive perspective, as several studies have shown the crucial role played everywhere by discourses on AIDS in shaping public policies

DOI: 10.4324/9781003382805-11

and health strategies dealing with the epidemic.[6] Second, I want to assess whether the "post-problem stage" of the issue-attention cycle actually leads to the forgetting that has been widely perceived and denounced by experts and readers since 2000.[7] Third, I want to consider where, how and referring to which phenomena and contexts the newspapers talk about HIV/AIDS in the twenty-first century and highlight continuity, discontinuity and transfers from the emergency phase in Italy and other countries around the world.[8] I hypothesize that the disease becoming chronic amid new domestic and international contexts led neither to a drop in attention nor to a complete break from the narratives of the emergency phase, but rather that the issue was marginalized and repurposed with different positioning in the newspapers, and the rhetorical style about it was remodulated.

The Numbers

The media in much of the world treated HIV/AIDS with constant attention that verged on hysteria from the mid-1980s to the end of the twentieth century, though at various paces and intensities. This happened in Italy, as well, where private and public TV and radio stations,[9] advertisements[10] and the newspaper press helped construct HIV/AIDS as a sociocultural phenomenon. They covered the issue even before it became a serious problem in Italy and gradually intensified their coverage (Figures 11.1, 11.2).

The decline in deaths and infections shown by ISS from 1997–98 to the 2000s–2010s did not correspond to a comparable decline in media coverage. Thousands of TV and radio broadcasts at least mentioned HIV/AIDS.[11] Meanwhile, the newspapers I studied contained all together more than 25,000 mentions. In the last 15 years, against the epidemiological trends,

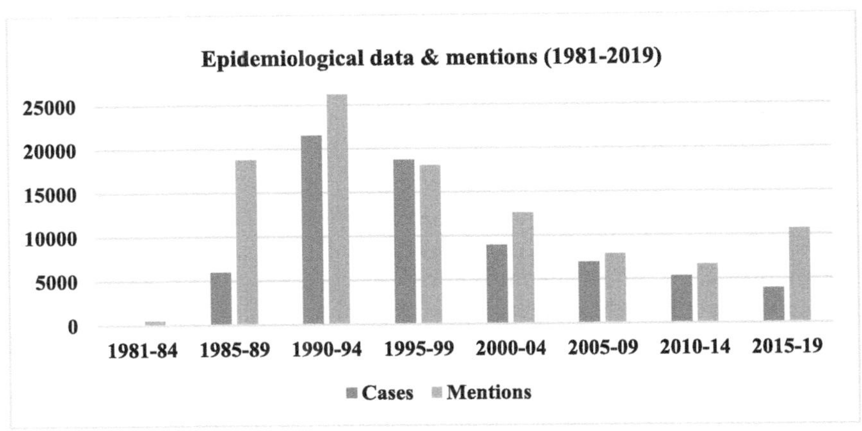

Figure 11.1 Epidemiological data and mentions (1981–2019).

Source: Chart created by author based on newspaper sources described in the chapter.

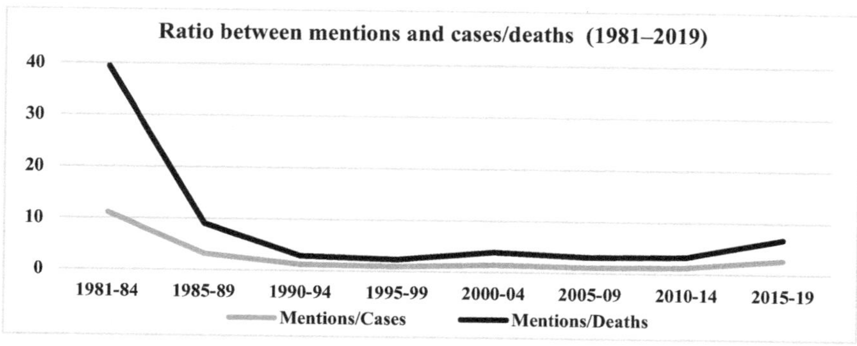

Figure 11.2 Ratio between mentions and cases/deaths (1981–2019).

Source: Chart created by author based on newspaper sources described in the chapter.

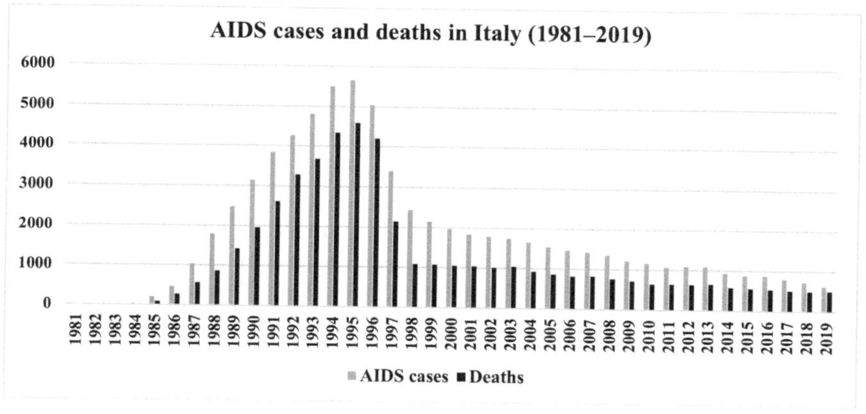

Figure 11.3 AIDS cases and deaths in Italy (1981–2019).

Source: Chart created by author based on newspaper sources described in the chapter.

mentions of HIV/AIDS started to increase, showing the second highest relationship between mentions and deaths/cases. This is without there being an explanation seen in the epidemic's global outlook, which had been constantly and markedly improving, especially in the 2010s (Figure 11.3).

In short, in the new millennium, AIDS was still discussed in Italy. The news blurbs common in the 1980s–1990s accounted for only 15–20% of the pieces mentioning it in the 2000s–2010s. However, a few considerations attenuate the impression these numbers give of great attention to the disease. First, many mentions were little more than mentions of services (toll-free numbers, contact details of associations etc.). Second, the issue rarely made the front page of national editions. Third, there are few pages completely or primarily about it, and the articles were often in secondary placements. HIV/AIDS was also frequently mentioned only as a comparison, a sign of a distant time, a biographical note or a decisive (not necessarily negative) aspect of entire lives, and not only for those for whom the syndrome was well-known parts of their lives, like actor Rock Hudson or rockstar Freddie Mercury. All this confirms that for the period considered, HIV/AIDS had a presence in the Italian press that was substantial but marginal in the realm of current event news.

News

HIV/AIDS's "marginal omnipresence" in the national news sections had a particular expression that marked a quite clear difference from the emergency period. Of course, especially in the early 2000s, there were news pieces and references to similar matters or those from previous years.[12] On other occasions, the references to HIV/AIDS were tied to issues traditionally connected to it. The first among these was prostitution. Though the ISS underscored the still important role of prostitution in spreading the virus, the issue was brought back up almost exclusively when the spotlight was shone on a particular personality.[13] The second issue was the "prison emergency," though even the still alarming data on HIV-positive/ill inmates (6.7% between 2003 and 2012, about 5% in 2015 and 2% in 2019) only earned just a few short news blurbs.[14] The newspapers returned to the issue only after a few powerful protests by inmates in the early 2000s. While conservative newspapers highlighted the link between HIV/AIDS and crime, leftist publications were more inclined to highlight the connections between social disadvantage and HIV positivity.[15]

In the pages of national news, there was still less discussion of HIV/AIDS than in the past. This was not because there were no stories worth coverage. The ISS was also still concerned about the disease's incidence, which was far below the peak in 1987 (26.8 per 100,000 people) but above any other infectious disease monitored by the authorities except for influenza (an average of 6–7 new cases per 100,000 people between 2000 and 2019). There were several other possible reasons for this lack of attention. The first was that AIDS in the 2000s–2010s affected mainly marginal groups, which the press in Italy and abroad have generally neglected.[16] The second reason was that there were no interconnections with other emergencies much covered in the 1980s–1990s, especially drugs,[17] as well as the political and legal scandals in Italy called *Tangentopoli*.

The local editions of newspapers spoke even less of HIV/AIDS, whereas in the past, "the newspapers focused on all the minute facts of current events."[18] However, when it was talked about, the newspapers often reengaged the set of stylistic templates that defined the emergency phase, such as alarmist tones,[19] stigmatizing mechanisms, equating HIV positivity and the full-blown disease[20] and the outdated concepts of HIV/AIDS as a "death sentence without reprieve."[21] Though these stylistic templates were well established and shared in all the newspapers considered, they never gave the impression of being able to reignite the social alarm and "hysteria in the Press" of the 1980s–1990s.[22] Though at times they even criticized the national press that "underscored non-existent dangers, such as the risk of the spread of Hepatitis C and AIDS,"[23] the more general tendency was to tone down some of the mechanisms typical of the emergency phase. The term "AIDS" was rarely used in the subject position, and when it was, it was often accompanied by a verb in the past tense. Relexicalization and overlexicalization were rarer than in the emergency phase, perhaps overshadowed by a vocabulary already well established at this time. Most pieces rarely used the rhetoric of quantification, key to creating the " 'us/them' dichotomy in which 'ordinary folk' have the role *patient* [*sic*], terrorized by a deviant out-group of 'thugs.' "[24] Finally, none of these news items was covered for more than one to two days, even if the syndrome was a key factor in strategies and major criminal episodes.[25] In other words, AIDS could easily return to being an alarming, stigmatizing current issue if taken on the local scale. Nevertheless, even though there was still an epidemic in these years, in the 2000s–2010s the Italian press failed to make news of it and present it as a general problem, especially nationally.

Research, Medicine and Health

HIV/AIDS was given more room in the health, science and medicine sections of newspapers. The *Corriere della Sera* has long had a series of news blurbs focused on it. Especially in the 2000s, all the considered newspapers had no lack of articles and short pieces about research in which any potential contribution to curing AIDS was made into an argument giving legitimacy to entire sectors, such as biotech.[26] Rather than the actual space given the issue, it was when and how it was discussed that marginalized the matter and marked a profound difference from the emergency phase.

First, there was still no cure. AIDS continued to claim millions of lives worldwide, and Italy still had a not insignificant amount of infections. However, it was not presented as a current problem though lesser and different than in the 1990s. Data were almost never provided. Scientists and specialists were given little voice. The still numerous denialist theories were not mentioned nor countered. With few exceptions,[27] the language became less explanatory, and there was a decreasing usage of images, explanations and tips. It appeared taken for granted that there was already knowledge of the virus, how it spread and tests available, notwithstanding late presenters of the disease and the ignorance that the ISS and some doctors had been decrying since the early 2000s, especially among the youth.[28]

Second, the issue was made current again only in unison with especially salient international events, such as when at the Durban Conference the emphasis given to the need for a vaccine led to a peak of attention for the trials started in Italy.[29] But here, too, the focus was more on the event in and of itself and international relations that shaped the strategies for fighting the pandemic, often merely skimming over the central question of drug prices and patents.[30]

Third, aside from major events, HIV/AIDS was talked about again with laudatory intent. This was in part directed at Italian research, such as valiantly defending the "Italian vaccine" pursued by the director of the National HIV/AIDS Research Center, which was blocked and criticized even by the famous American virologist Robert Gallo.[31] The praise was also for individual research centers, about which the local editions took tones that were sometimes shamelessly flag-waving about "state-of-the-art treatments and research,"[32] or even "good results," thanks to which the "nightmare is ending."[33]

However, more often than not, HIV/AIDS was used for its dramatic power. Though the syndrome only caused 0.1–0.2 deaths per 10,000 people (much less than hepatitis, influenza, pneumonia and cardiovascular diseases), it still served as a term of comparison in 2019 to suggest the severity of other public health problems. In 2010, it was even mentioned when a parasite spread among palm trees, and some experts invoked "national coordination for an epidemic comparable to the early spread of AIDS."[34]

In all these circumstances, a central element of the discourse about HIV/AIDS was it not being part of the present and not mentioned for the problems it presented in the 2000s–2010s in the Global North or Global South. In some cases, HIV/AIDS was projected in a future of certain success for the progress of medicine, possibly thanks to an Italian. It more often constituted an impressionistic remote past presented in hypostatized terms. This was sometimes also a past of success when the identification of HIV and the pharmacological protocol based on the three virus inhibitors, known as Highly Active Antiretroviral Therapy, were mentioned as the greatest victories of medicine, despite other more decisive discoveries. At other times, it was a past made of frightening terror and the perfect metaphor of disease for what AIDS had represented in the collective Western imagination between the 1980s and the 1990s rather than for the millions of victims it still took worldwide in the new millennium.[35]

In the pages about science and health, HIV/AIDS continued to be discussed in the twenty-first century. However, this was often done in different terms than in the emergency phase or in the late 1990s, when triple therapy was already in existence; decontextualized, naturalized and otherized in terms of time, the syndrome seemed almost to shift from being a complex object of research and a current health problem to become an ultrafamiliar element of comparison or proof of the excellence of the beleaguered Italian national health system, sometimes in flag-waving tones.

Domestic Politics

HIV/AIDS had little presence in the newspaper sections about domestic politics. There was no coverage of the legal initiatives in this period. The topic was not part of the frequent debates on healthcare. It was also at the margins of the broader discussion of the civil rights of LGBTQ people. This was due to several factors: first, the syndrome's lesser capacity to mobilize in the postemergency phase, and second, LGBTQ groups' new (anti-)identity horizons as well as their ability to break the AIDS-homosexuality link, and to introduce a different agenda of issues in the public discourse.[36] Despite informational campaigns like "Would you vote for me if I were HIV-positive?"[37] the issue almost disappeared from the election campaigns in 2000. It did not create consensus even in regions where the newspapers announced there was "still an emergency . . . even if cases are dropping."[38]

The issue did appear on the margins of radicals' antiprohibitionist battles and the hot-button issue of immigration. It was used at times to decry the social disadvantage suffered by immigrants.[39] At other times, it was employed to foment alarmism and xenophobia.[40] However, it was almost always a matter of statements by individual representatives and local administrators that national leaders did not echo.[41] They did not become full-fledged communication strategies, despite the growing percentage of foreigners among the ill/HIV-positive (20–30%).

Other situations brought HIV/AIDS back to the pages of domestic politics. On the one hand, it was used at times as a tool of political attacks, such as when the Center-Right leader Silvio Berlusconi told an off-color joke about AIDS patients in April 2000, sparking heated controversy. The *Corriere della Sera* and *La Stampa* printed some who defended him,[42] whereas the leftist publications condemned him unequivocally. Yet, even in such cases, little space was given to LGBTQ voices and associations that sought to focus on the HIV/AIDS problems. The syndrome at most served as proof of other accusations long lodged against Berlusconi.[43]

On the other hand, HIV/AIDS garnered attention when the Catholic Church made pronouncements, such as when Walter Veltroni, the secretary of the Left Democratics, suggested that the Pope reconsider his position on condoms to fight the syndrome in Africa. In the newspapers, a controversy ignited with some accusing him of playing politics "with charity"[44] and others who praised his attention to the "enduring enormity of a drama that ultimately also involves our politics."[45] The discussions and data on the spread of AIDS in the world that came with the reports on Veltroni's mission disappeared before the end of his trip. The issue was never connected to other flagship issues of the left, such as privatization/underfinancing of the national health services, the civil rights of LGBTQ people, the split between the Global North and South and so forth. Moreover, it was subjected to a normalization that led the *Corriere della Sera* to talk about it together with other problems, apparently much less dire, such as "the difficulty between the governments in Pretoria and Rome to agree on the importing in Europe of South African grappa."[46]

In the political pages, HIV/AIDS seldom emerged as a topic in and of itself. Only in the early 2000s was it occasionally and briefly brandished as a political weapon. Nonetheless, when the topic emerged, it still had a powerful capacity to polarize positions on the left/right and especially between secular/Catholic lines, focusing not on the more current health, socioeconomic and legal issues discussed internationally but more on the ethical matters that were linked to the emergency over the years. The newspapers preferred an approach, vocabulary and opinions about moral bases rather than more operational and technical perspectives of associations and experts that had been decisive in defining and legitimizing the directions of political and governmental powers in Italy as elsewhere during the AIDS crisis.[47]

World News

The emergency phase, having been overcome in Italy, almost naturally led to a large part of the articles about HIV/AIDS moving to the world news pages with a focus increasingly shifted away from the Western world, especially the United States, to the rest of the world, especially Africa. Though almost 70% of HIV-positive people were in Africa in the mid-2010s,[48] the fact that in the newspapers AIDS became essentially synonymous with Africa raised several issues. The first was the impact on the coverage of the pandemic, which was affected by the scant attention that the Italian press usually gives to areas outside of Europe and North America. The second was the silence about other regions where the cases were steady or rising, such as Eastern Europe, the former USSR and Latin America. The third problem was the tendency to associate AIDS with an Africa lacking in internal distinctions and tacitly "stacked upon the previously established concept of black Africa."[49] Most success stories were ignored as a result, with only a brief aside during the 2010 soccer World Cup about South Africa, which was the country most affected in Africa, but which is also its whitest and most Westernized country.[50] This was explained by the general tendency of the press to prefer bad news to good news and not to follow closely the real changes in epidemiological data. Nevertheless, there were other two crucial factors: the established interpretative and narrative patterns of HIV/AIDS and the function attributed to the syndrome in many articles.[51]

In effect, especially in the leftist and Catholic newspapers, talking about HIV/AIDS seems to have mainly served to otherize, naturalize and dehistoricize it, making it the most evocative of the many factors tied to the backwardness and suffering of Africa, an ideal complement to other images rooted in the Western collective imagination. This frequently was expressed in generic, dramatic terms. Reporters gave voice to volunteers and missionaries rather than doctors and scholars and presented stereotypical stories of women and children. Photographs showed generalized poverty and suffering more than patients or the consequences of the pandemic. In addition, AIDS was mentioned much more than the other diseases afflicting Africa (Figure 11.4), an exception to the lack of interest in the Italian media for humanitarian crises lamented by Doctors Without Borders.[52] However, this attention was aimed

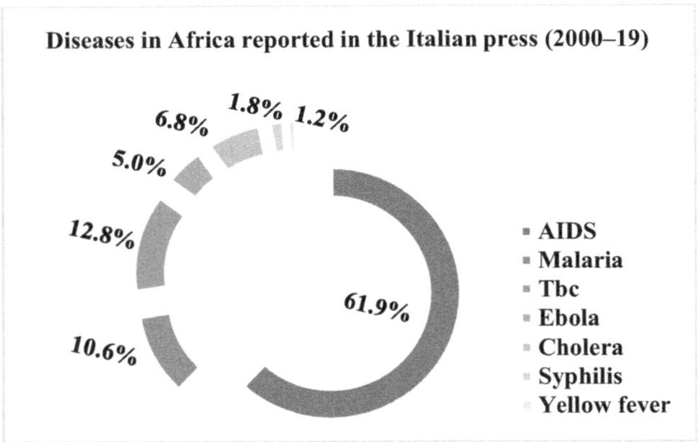

Figure 11.4 Diseases in Africa reported in the Italian press (2000–19).

Source: Chart created by author based on newspaper sources described in the chapter.

almost exclusively at making HIV/AIDS an effective argument in discussions about other matters.

The instrumental references and discursive models from the emergency era defined the discourse about Africa and those praising or attacking individuals. Commitment to fighting the pandemic seemed a must-have in articles meant to laud artists like Elton John and political leaders like Bill Clinton and Nelson Mandela, while glossing over their responsibilities.[53] On the other hand, references to the spread of HIV/AIDS were often used to bolster negative opinions on controversial figures, such as the South African presidents Thabo Mbeki[54] and Jacob Zuma,[55] the Russian president Vladimir Putin[56] and the Spanish president José Luis Zapatero, which *Avvenire* blamed for the many contagions despite the promised "million free condoms."[57]

Only limitedly and sporadically was the newspapers' attention on HIV/AIDS more focused on the issue and also more global. There were, of course, some important international meetings devoted to the issue. On these occasions, syntactic-lexical patterns of the past were used to raise alarms for a world that was "dying of AIDS"[58] of an "Africa depopulated by AIDS."[59] Nevertheless, most articles quickly returned to diluting the specificities of the AIDS emergency into the vaguer situation of the problems of underprivileged countries.[60]

Likewise, there were dramatic reports, such as the CIA calling AIDS "a threat to humanity" and a "threat to the world's security.[61]" The newspaper described it as a "new evil empire that . . . could silently do what not even the Soviet Union and its armies ever managed to do."[62] But this did not mean that they delved further into the matter or connected it to the problems that AIDS still posed in Italy, even though the disease has become chronic.

In general, in the world news pages, too, the main boosters of interest in AIDS were news related to the Church and commemorative events. The first of these sparked the polarization of positions seen in the domestic politics pages and the different contexts not mitigating the conflict or tones. Examples suffice in the controversy that ignited in 2010 about the confidential pro-condom memorandum of the Foreign Office published by the British press,[63] or the attention with which *la Repubblica* and *Avvenire* covered the heated debates about the opening of the Spanish Episcopal Conference regarding the use of condoms as a means of prevention.[64]

Despite the numerous initiatives and projects that continued to fill the calendar, the discussions effectively coincided with the single World AIDS Day. It was on December 1 that the newspapers took stock of the situation by sifting through data, photographs, articles, interviews and long lists of charity events. Not only was this media coverage ephemeral, but the very fact that the issue was being covered in the world news pages shows how it was presented in a way to replicate the generic, pitying, paternalistic attitudes to the suffering of others rather than investigate if and how the problem was situated or reverberated in Italy. The conversation was kept on a global level without understanding or comparing the statistics or analyses to the situation back home.

The prevalence of verbs in the present tense instead of the past tense used in the national/local news pages and passages about the West underscored the sense of distance, constructing dual levels in terms of time, too. There were exceptions, such as in 2005 when the Pope's exhortations to combat the epidemic with "chastity, promotion of fidelity in marriage, the importance of family life, education and care for the poor"[65] served to raise controversy and keep longer attention on the issue. In these cases, the newspapers tended to bring the discussion back to Italy but again differed greatly amongst themselves: the online edition of *la Repubblica* published the article with a photo of Buenos Aires's obelisk covered by a condom[66]; *Avvenire.it* glossed over the data while lauding the Church's charity actions for patients; the *Corriere della Sera* sought a balance by juxtaposing articles mentioning the many new HIV-positive infections every year and the pro-condom positions with interviews with hard-liner Catholics, which were, not incidentally, voices that had been oft-heard during the emergency years.[67]

AIDS becoming a chronic disease in the West and the shift of the epidemic's epicenter to sub-Saharan Africa explain the marked change. From the start, AIDS has always been "a disease of 'them', not 'us,'"[68] as well as an accusation directed toward other groups.[69] Newspapers of the twenty-first century essentially replicated well-worn mechanisms. It was only in 2000s–2010s that the evocative power of AIDS was used not only to reinforce stereotypical, paternalistic conceptions of Africa but also to suggest the idea of the threat's definitive disappearance from the West – and Italy, in particular – even though the same articles might mention international initiatives and institutions that emphasized the global scope and effects of the crisis.

Letters to the Editor

The letters to the editors show that the dichotomy of healthy Italians/poor and sick Africans did not lead to overcoming either the dichotomy within the national community or the stereotypes and stigmas constructed in the emergency phase between healthy and HIV-positive/patients.

These letters were not statistically representative nor without filters or (self-)censorship.[70] Several factors showed them to be part of the " 'reciprocity' between writers and readers."[71] They were mostly spurred by international events, World AIDS Day and the Church's taking of positions. They tended to avoid apparently taboo topics in the articles, such as the cost of HIV/AIDS medicine and the low transparency in fundraising.[72] They also shared their prevalent tones and attitudes: the otherization and Africanization of the issue; paternalistic, condescending language; inserting HIV/AIDS into more general discussions of poverty in the Global South; and the dichotomizing and harsh tones when the Church spoke on the subject and their ban on condoms, which was considered by many the most unacceptable form of the "invasiveness of the Italian Catholic Church."[73]

For the most part, those who wrote were often people dealing with HIV firsthand. Among these were associations otherwise given little room and made use of it to publicize initiatives or criticize delays and shortcomings.[74] There were young people seeking information, evidence of a general lack of knowledge and the trouble that the agencies in charge had in becoming trusted sources of information.[75] There were supporters of antiprogress and antiscientific ideas who took advantage of the greater evocative power of persistent conspiracy theories about AIDS compared to those of other epidemics, such as SARS.[76] There were, in particular, people living with HIV lamenting the prevailing imprudence,[77] seeking to reignite attention by connecting "this pandemic" to what "is not actually so far from all of us" but seemed in itself ignored or inadequate to generate interest.[78]

Nevertheless, these letters also had many elements of continuity with the emergency phase. The first was the persistence of connecting HIV/ AIDS and homosexuality, an entrenched stereotype originating from the United States rather than actual ISS data – not even mentioned in these letters – about the growing proportion of men who have sex with men among the new infections. For example, in 2000, a double-page spread in the *Corriere della Sera* printed a survey on positive and negative attitudes about homosexuals, accompanied by a photo of the actor Tom Hanks in *Philadelphia*, suggesting a particularly close relationship between AIDS and gays, and the letter of a woman who wrote, "AIDS is among the homosexuals. That's why I don't really accept them."[79] And even in 2010, a nurse still felt the need to note that "the international scientific community has established for twenty years that are no categories at greater risk for spreading AIDS,"[80] criticizing those who supported the rejection of homosexual blood donors in Lombardy.[81]

The second factor was the stigma was still tied to the syndrome as much in 2000,[82] as well as in letters from later years, including one from a student at Bocconi University published in 2010 on the front page of the local Milan edition of the *Corriere della Sera*.[83] As in the past, the stigma was still about the attitude of others, as seen in the student's lament, "I wish that people would at least not look at me badly because of my illness."[84] This was just as much about self-representation, as the same letter writer felt the need to clarify: "I am not a drug addict, a loose woman, or a sexually deviant person; I'm a normal girl."[85] This showed both the lack of effectiveness of campaigns starting in the 1990s that sought to foster inclusion[86] and the persistence in the collective imagination of epidemiological connections that were marginal at this point, such as between HIV/AIDS and drug addiction.

Reactions to the letter also made clear connections to the discussions of the emergency phase. On the one hand, there was a burst of sudden alarmism, especially but not limited to groups that had been focused on the 1980s–1990s: doctors who illegally tested their patients,[87] dentists who argued against privacy guarantees for HIV-positive people,[88] readers who wanted to "go back to the past" and those who wanted mandatory tests and "coercive rules" needed for "the social emergencies" that AIDS quickly brought back up.[89] On the other hand, even those who wished to express solidarity seemed to be thinking of HIV/AIDS that had not yet become chronic, often using terms that had long been discouraged ("victim," "normal girl," "not belonging to at-risk groups").[90] When it was experts writing, they abandoned the calm approach of their contributions to other sections and took back up the polemical tones of twenty years ago against proposals deemed unfairly discriminatory. Meanwhile, the *Corriere della Sera* dusted off articles that associated the AIDS emergency with other emergencies traditionally connected to it (prisons and health system failings) rather than reflecting on the current terms of the problem and hired the advertising agency that had written the first governmental campaigns for its awareness-raising initiatives.[91]

In the letters to the editors in the 2000s–2010s, HIV/AIDS was still part of a past that could be easily inflamed, and they tended to return to the traits typical of the emergency phase. Yet, even stories that were appealing in journalistic terms, like that of the Bocconi student, lasted no more than a few days and were also not taken up by other publications, reactivating the "generative mechanism" that had been crucial for self-fueling news about AIDS for long periods.[92]

Conclusion

This first, partial analysis of the Italian press in the early twenty-first century presents a situation consistent with my hypotheses, at least in part. First, the analysis contradicts the common, widespread belief and oft-repeated lament about the silence that is said to have shrouded the issue. In contrast, HIV/AIDS appears almost omnipresent, highlighting a not-always-linear relationship between the evolution of the epidemic in Italy and the rest of the world. In the absence of comparable historical analyses for other countries (much more research has been carried out by sociologists and media scholars), this may not make Italy a "strange country" in which "even emergencies . . . follow fashions,"[93] but it proves that "any problems that have gone through the cycle almost always receive a higher average level of attention."[94] However, the frequency of mentions of HIV/AIDS is often paired with the marginalization of the issue that may be reduced to a mere biographical reference, a term of comparison, a sign of a distant era or the subject of side articles in pages on topics traditionally tied to HIV/AIDS.

Second, the analysis shows how the issue has shifted from the sections on domestic politics and local/national news, where it dominated in the 1980s–1990s, to the world news pages. This is likely owed to several factors: the pandemic's evolution, the lack of emergencies and scandals connected to AIDS in the 1980s–1990s, its new ineffectiveness as a tool of political consensus or attack, the irrelevance attributed to it even in discussions around public health issues and the civil rights of LGBTQ people.

Third, the otherization of HIV/AIDS is a common tendency. In the pages on world news, this approach takes the form of the Africanization of the problem, which seems not to have the racist and finger-pointing function common in such discussions in the 80s–90s but still has at least two effects. First, it loses sight of the pandemic's global dimension. Second, it replicates and reinforces superficial, homogenizing conceptions of Africa, such as coinciding with an equally vaguely understood notion of "black Africa." Naturalized and dehistoricized, AIDS has become an element of especially evocative power within paternalistic and generalizing discussions of the poverty and backwardness of African peoples. In the sections on science and health, the otherization is mostly chronological. HIV/AIDS is talked about as if no longer needing explanations or warnings about its risks. It is presented as not current, either placed in an optimistic future of success and progress of medicine or an impressionistic, imagined distant past before triple therapy, and turned into a conceptual bogeyman and point of comparison when trying to create alarmism on public health issues.

My analysis also shows that HIV/AIDS still has considerable evocative power and a remarkable capacity to polarize positions and reactivate dynamics, dialectics and discourses belonging to the emergency phase. This happens especially in two circumstances. First, when the issue is intertwined with sensitive political and economic issues (globalization, multinationals etc.) or ethical and social issues (health, morality, prostitution, [homo]sexuality etc.) on which the Church takes a stance. Whether the issue is covered in the pages of domestic or world politics, heated controversies set newspapers of different orientations and political exponents against each other, many of whom were, not incidentally, key voices in the discussion in the 1980s–1990s, whereas less space is given to experts and associations. Second, when HIV/AIDS is made current and situated in real proximity to the readers, especially in the pages of local news and letters to the editors then – though they remain fleeting bursts – the press reverts to the alarmism, stigma and stories that draw from a stock of images and discussions built transnationally during the emergency years.

This is why I could conclude that to the question of whether HIV/AIDS was forgotten or disguised by the Italian press in the twenty-first century, the most convincing answer may be "neither." Despite the well-known cycles of media attention, overcoming the emergency phase did not lead to AIDS falling into oblivion or being intentionally disguised. Instead, it is given a different slant, otherized in space and time; sometimes, it is cut to fit better into broader discussions; sometimes, it is repurposed to become a point for use in partisan arguments. Yet, it remains a latent issue for the entire period, capable of so much evocative power and polemical charge that it can ignite and suddenly bring into the twenty-first century flashes of the last twenty years of the twentieth century, if only for a few days.

Notes

1 This chapter is a product of the PRIN 2022 titled Historicizing AIDS. Policies, rights, discourses, and memories in the Italian case (2022CY2J5S).
2 Elizabeth Fee and Daniel M. Fox, eds., *AIDS: The Making of a Chronic Disease* (Berkeley: University of California Press, 1992).
3 Gevisa La Rocca, "Dall'allarmismo alla prevenzione. Una riflessione sulle campagne di comunicazione sociale contro la diffusione dell'HIV/AIDS degli ultimi trent'anni," *Mediascapes Journal*, no. 8 (2017): 219–52.
4 Alan Whiteside, *HIV & AIDS: A Very Short Introduction*, 2nd ed. (Oxford: Oxford University Press, 2016).
5 Valerio Castronovo and Nicola Tranfaglia, eds., *La stampa italiana nell'età della TV. Dagli anni Settanta a oggi* (Rome and Bari: Laterza, 2008); Richard A. Grusin, *Premediation. Affect and Mediality After 9 11* (Basingstoke: Palgrave Macmillan, 2010).
6 Cindy Patton, *Inventing AIDS* (New York: Routledge, 1990).
7 Anthony Downs, "Up and Down with Ecology–'The Issue Attention Cycle'," *The Public Interest*, no. 28 (1972): 40; and Alt 76 [pseud.], "Di Aids si parla meno ma c'è ancora," *La Stampa*, December 3, 2000.
8 For Italy, see Agnese Giacchetta, Andrea Caputo, and Viviana Langher, "La "peste del secolo" nella stampa italiana: le rappresentazioni dell'AIDS negli anni '80 e 2000 a confronto," *Psicologia della salute* 1 (2016): 90–110; and Fabio Guidali, "I media e la rappresentazione dell'AIDS negli anni Ottanta," in *L'AIDS in Italia (1982–1996). Istituzioni, società, media*, ed. Fiammetta Balestracci, Fabio Guidali, and Enrico Landoni (Pisa: Pacini, 2022). For the rest of the world, see Nicolas Mauriac, *Le mal entendu: Le sida et les médias* (Paris: Plon, 1990); James Kinsella, *Covering the Plague: AIDS and the American Media* (New Brunswick: Rutgers University Press, 1992); Deborah Lupton, *Moral Threats and Dangerous Desires. AIDS in the News Media* (London and New York: Routledge, 1994); Virginia Berridge, *AIDS in the UK. The Making of Policy, 1981–1994* (Oxford: Oxford University Press, 1996); and Johanna Hood, *HIV/AIDS, Health and the Media in China: Imagined Immunity Through Racialized Disease* (London: Routledge, 2011).

 9 Guidali, "I media e la rappresentazione dell'AIDS negli anni Ottanta."
10 Fiammetta Balestracci, "AIDS, sessualità e corpi nelle campagne informative del Ministero della Sanità (1982–1992/1996)," in *L'AIDS in Italia (1982–1996). Istituzioni, società, media*, ed. Fiammetta Balestracci, Fabio Guidali, and Enrico Landoni (Pisa: Pacini, 2022).
11 I would like to thank RAI Teche and the RAI Regional Center for Calabria for having given me access to its data and Dr. Sara Dente for her material research.
12 "Contagiò la moglie che morì di Aids: condanna a 14 anni," *la Repubblica*, July 4, 2000.
13 Silvana Mazzocchi, "La nostra vita sulla strada con trenta clienti a notte," *la Repubblica*, July 19, 2000.
14 "Penitenziari, dossier della Lila," *Corriere della Sera*, February 12, 2000; and Agi [pseud.], "Carceri e malati Aids, leggi inapplicate," *La Stampa*, February 12, 2000.
15 Giantomano De Matteis, "Poggioreale, stato d'allerta 'Una bomba a orologeria,'" *la Repubblica*, June 27, 2000; and "Carceri, nel Lazio record di malati di Aids" *Corriere della Sera*, February 12, 2010.
16 Claudine Herzlich and Pierret Janine, "The Construction of a Social Phenomenon: AIDS in the French Press," *Social Science & Medicine* 29, no. 11 (1989): 1235–42; Dorothy Nelkin, "AIDS and the News Media," *The Milbank Quarterly* 2, no. 69 (1991): 293–307; Roger Fowler, *Language in the News. Discourse and Ideology in the Press* (London: Routledge, 1991); Berridge, *AIDS in the UK*; and Guidali, "I media e la rappresentazione dell'AIDS negli anni Ottanta."
17 Maria Elena Cantilena, *Una storia disonesta? Il consumo di droghe nell'Italia dei lunghi anni Settanta* (Pisa: Pacini, 2022).
18 Guidali, "I media e la rappresentazione dell'AIDS negli anni Ottanta," 150.
19 Federica Angeli, "Una siringa per venti rapine," *la Repubblica*, February 6, 2000; and Lorenza Pleuteri, "Il rapinatore che perseguita le donne," *la Repubblica*, May 15, 2005.
20 Michele Focarete and Gianni Santucci, "'Hai l'Aids,' lei lo rifiuta e lui cerca di stuprarla," *Corriere della Sera*, January 24, 2010.
21 M. Peg, "Violenta la prostituta che gli dice: 'Ho l'Aids'," *La Stampa*, January 4, 2000.
22 Fowler, *Language in the News*, 148.
23 Achille Conte di Laviano, "La corporazione dei dentisti," *la Repubblica*, January 2, 2010.
24 Fowler, *Language in the News*, 140.
25 Francesco Cucinotta, "Faida d'onore, poliziotto in manette," *la Repubblica*, February 9, 2000.
26 Nicoletta Manuzzato, "AIDS, ecco l'anticorpo che protegge dal virus," *l'Unità*, March 10, 2000; Giovanni Maria Pace, "AIDS, una cellula lo blocca il vaccino ora è più vicino," *la Repubblica*, March 30, 2000; Mario Pappagallo, "Vaccino nasale contro l'AIDS," *Corriere della Sera*, June 12, 2000; "AIDS, così il virus si propaga nelle cellule," *la Repubblica*, February 1, 2010; "Un antibiotico low-cost contro l'AIDS, 'con terapia combinata dimezza i morti,'" *Repubblica.it*, March 29, 2010, www.repubblica.it/salute/medicina/2010/03/29/news/un_antibiotico_low-cost_contro_l_aids_con_terapia_combinata_dimezza_i_morti_-5584459/?ref=search. For its relation to biotech, see Adriana Bazzi, "'Terapia biotech per tornare l'Aids,'" *Corriere della Sera*, May 27, 2000.
27 "Il virus bloccato dagli anticorpi," *Corriere del Sera*, April 23, 2000.
28 Alessandra Paolini, "L'AIDS? È colpa delle zanzare," *la Repubblica*, May 26, 2005.
29 Giovanni Maria Pace, "AIDS, il sogno di un vaccino," *la Repubblica*, July 12, 2000.
30 Peter Piot, *AIDS. Between Science and Politics* (New York: Columbia University Press, 2015).

31 Margherita De Bac, "AIDS, bloccato il vaccino italiano," *Corriere del Sera*, June 18, 2000; and De Bac, "AIDS, Gallo critica il vaccino italiano: dannoso per l'uomo," *Corriere del Sera*, April 6, 2000.

32 "Analisi, cure e ricerca d'avanguardia," *La Stampa*, December 30, 2000.

33 Lucia Zambelli, "AIDS, l'incubo finisce a Pisa," *la Repubblica*, February 13, 2000.

34 Claudia Voltattorni, "La strage delle palme cambia volto all'Italia," *Corriere del Sera*, May 1, 2010.

35 Susan Sontag, *AIDS and its Metaphors* (New York: Farrar, Straus and Giroux, 1989).

36 Maya De Leo, *Queer. Storia culturale della comunità LGBT+* (Torino: Einaudi, 2021).

37 Gevisa La Rocca, "Dall'allarmismo alla prevenzione. Una riflessione sulle campagne di comunicazione sociale contro la diffusione dell'HIV/AIDS degli ultimi trent'anni," *Mediascapes journal*, no. 8 (2017)

38 Claudio Lazzaro, "Aids nel Lazio: situazione grave, ma casi in diminuzione," *Corriere della Sera*, April 14, 2000.

39 Daniela Daniele, "'Consumisti e poco capaci': Gli immigrati ci vedono così," *La Stampa*, December 14, 2000.

40 Giuseppe Spatola, "Sposa-bambina prigioniera del marito: ho paura, ha l'Aids," *Corriere della Sera*, February 4, 2010.

41 Marisa Fumagalli, "Io, un modello per Haider," *Corriere della Sera*, March 6, 2000.

42 Roberto Zuccolini, "Barzelletta sull'Aids, tutti contro Berlusconi," *Corriere della Sera*, April 5, 2000; and Maria Teresa Meli, "Accuse a Berlusconi: offende i malati," *La Stampa*, April 5, 2000.

43 Alessandra Longo, "Berlusconi nella bufera per la barzelletta sull'Aids," *la Repubblica*, April 5, 2000; and N. L., "Aids, bufera su Berlusconi," *l'Unità*, April 5, 2000.

44 Filippo Ceccarelli, "E adesso la politica si fa con la carità," *La Stampa*, February 28, 2000.

45 "Veltroni in Africa," *Corriere della Sera*, March 3, 2000.

46 Gianna Fregonara, "La proposte di Veltroni 'Allarghiamo il G-8 ad Africa e Sud America,'" *Corriere della Sera*, March 1, 2000.

47 Peter Baldwin, *Disease and Democracy. The Industrialized World Faces AIDS* (Berkeley, Los Angeles and London: University of California Press, 2005).

48 Whiteside, *HIV & AIDS*, 33.

49 Sydney Bryn Austin, "AIDS and Africa: United States Media and Racist Fantasy," *Cultural Critique* 1, no. 14 (1989): 142.

50 Samira Shackle, "Proviamo a divertirci anche se questo calcio è solo un grande circo," *la Repubblica*, June 8, 2010; and Igiaba Scego, "Due donne per il Sud Africa," *l'Unità*, June 26, 2010.

51 Fowler, *Language in the News*.

52 Carlo Ciavoni, "Msf contro il sistema dei tg 'Più tempo per i saldi che per la fame,'" *Repubblica.it*, April 20, 2010, www.repubblica.it/esteri/2010/04/20/news/msf_per_i_tg_valgono_pi_i_saldi_di_fine_stagione_che_le_grandi_crisi_umanitarie_in_tutto_il_mondo-3497690/?ref=search.

53 Alfio Bernabei, "Nozze gay, Elton John sposa il suo partner," *l'Unità*, December 22, 2005; and Ennio Caretto, "Clinton: 'America, sei sulla vetta,'" *Corriere della Sera*, January 29, 2000.

54 "Aids, il Sudafrica non crede all'Hiv come causa," *Corriere della Sera*, April 20, 2000.

55 Monica Ricci Sargentini, "Zuma alla ventesima figlia ma non dalle sue tre mogli," *Corriere della Sera*, February 2, 2010.

56 Klaus Davi, "Vladimir, il declino del macho," *La Stampa*, March 10, 2005.

57 Davide Rondoni, "Il preservativo anziché le politiche," *Avvenire.it*, March 29, 2009, www.avvenire.it/opinioni/pagine/irresponsabile-leggerezza-dei-governanti-europei_20090320083220950000.

58 Adriana Bazzi, "Farmaci costosi, l'Africa muore di Aids," *Corriere della Sera*, July 9, 2000.

59 Giovanni Maria Pace, "L'Africa spopolata dall'Aids" *Repubblica.it*, July 11, 2000, https://quotidiano.repubblica.it/edicola/searchdetail?id=http://archivio.repubblica.extra.kataweb.it/archivio/repubblica/2000/07/11/africa-spopolata-dall-aids.html&hl=&query=%22L%E2%80%99Africa+spopolata+dall%E2%80%99Aids%22&field=nel+testo&testata=repubblica&newspaper=REP&edition=nazionale&zona=sfoglio&ref=search.

60 "Nel mondo 600 milioni di bambini poveri," *Repubblica.it*, July 12, 2000, www.repubblica.it/online/mondo/unice/unice/unice.html?ref=search.

61 Ennio Caretto, " 'Dall'Aids rischio di crisi mondiale,' " *Corriere della Sera*, May 1, 2000.

62 Vittorio Zucconi, "L'Aids minaccia la democrazia," *la Repubblica*, May 1, 2000.

63 Fabio Cavalera, " 'Il Papa promuova i condom': Londra costretta a scusarsi," *Corriere della Sera*, April 26, 2010.

64 Alessandro Oppes, "Spagna, la svolta della Chiesa. Contro l'Aids sì al preservativo," *la Repubblica*, January 19, 2005; "Il portavoce dei vescovi spagnoli: mai consigliato il preservativo," *la Repubblica*, January 21, 2005; and Gianni Gennari, "Angosce e manie: religione dell'antireligione," *Avvenire.it*, January 28, 2005, www.avvenire.it/rubriche/pagine/angosce-e-manie-br–religione-dell-antireligione_20050128.

65 Margherita De Bac, "Aids, il Papa e l'Europa divisi sulla castità," *Corriere della Sera*, December 2, 2005.

66 "Aids, celebrata giornata mondiale Benedetto XVI: 'La castità aiuta,' " *Repubblica.it*, December 1, 2005, www.repubblica.it/2005/b/sezioni/scienza_e_tecnologia/aids/riepilogogiorn/riepilogogiorn.html?ref=search.

67 Guidali, "I media e la rappresentazione dell'AIDS negli anni Ottanta."

68 Sontag, *AIDS and its Metaphors*, 56.

69 Austin, "AIDS and Africa"; and Paul Farmer, *AIDS & Accusation. Haiti and the Geography of Blame*, 2nd ed. (Berkeley: University of California Press, 2006).

70 Fowler, *Language in the News*.

71 Ibid., 48.

72 "Lettere," *la Repubblica*, July 19, 2000; and "Lettere," *la Repubblica*, March 13, 2005.

73 Paolo Cavallo, "Le scuse tardive della Chiesa," *La Stampa*, December 3, 2000.

74 "Un telefono per 'amico,' " *Corriere della Sera*, April 23, 2000; and Fernando Aiuti, "Come boicottare i giovani medici," *la Repubblica*, February 10, 2000.

75 Massimo De Martino, "Un bacio non vale il contagio. Hiv, come si trasmette la malattia," *Repubblica.it*, March 4, 2010, www.repubblica.it/salute/esperti/andrologia/2010/03/04/news/un_bacio_non_vale_il_contagio_hiv_come_si_trasmette_la_malattia-5584531/?ref=search.

76 Luciano Gallini, "Ancora sui transgenici," *La Stampa*, January 31, 2000.

77 "L'amore ai tempi del virus," *La Stampa*, December 2, 2000.

78 "Io, 21 anni, bocconiana sono sieropositiva. Non chiudete gli occhi l'Aids non è lontano da noi," *Corriere della Sera*, January 5, 2010.

79 "Fiduciosi, consumisti, poco integrati," *La Stampa*, February 18, 2000.

80 Maria Luisa Canna, "I rischi di trasmissione," *Corriere della Sera*, July 26, 2010.

81 "Sangue donato da omosessuali. Fazio chiede parere agli esperti," *Corriere della Sera*, July 24, 2010.

82 Luca Lucente, "Lettere," *la Repubblica*, April 4, 2000.

83 "Io, 21 anni, bocconiana sono sieropositiva."

84 Ibid.
85 Ibid.
86 Emanuele Gabardi, *Stop Aids. I linguaggi della pubblicità contro l'Aids in Italia e nel mondo* (Milan: FrancoAngeli, 2017).
87 Alessandro Capponi, "Il test dell'Aids ai minorenni: io lo faccio," *Corriere della Sera*, February 10, 2010.
88 Margherita De Bac, "Il dentista non può chiedere se il paziente ha l'Aids," *Corriere della Sera*, January 14, 2010.
89 Francesco Milazzo, "Tornare al passato," *Corriere della Sera*, January 8, 2010.
90 Simona Ravizza, "La sfida della bocconiana malata di Aids: 'Mia madre non sa, mi curo in segreto,'" *Corriere della Sera*, January 8, 2010.
91 "Il 'tris' del Corriere contro l'Aids," *Corriere della Sera*, January 10, 2010.
92 Fowler, *Language in the News*, 174.
93 Beppe Severgnini, "Se una sieropositiva ci fa pensare," *Corriere della Sera*, January 14, 2010.
94 Downs, "Up and Down with Ecology – The Issue Attention Cycle," 41.

References

Agi. "Carceri e malati AIDS, leggi inapplicate." *La Stampa*, February 12, 2000.

"AIDS, bufera su Berlusconi," *l'Unità*, April 5, 2000.

"AIDS, celebrata giornata mondiale Benedetto XVI: 'La castità aiuta.'" *Repubblica. it*, December 1, 2005. www.repubblica.it/2005/b/sezioni/scienza_e_tecnologia/aids/riepilogogiorn/riepilogogiorn.html?ref=search.

"AIDS, così il virus si propaga nelle cellule." *la Repubblica*, February 1, 2010.

"AIDS, il Sudafrica non crede all'Hiv come causa." *Corriere della Sera*, April 20, 2000.

Aiuti, Fernando. "Come boicottare i giovani medici." *la Repubblica*, February 10, 2000.

Alt 76. "Di AIDS si parla meno ma c'è ancora." *La Stampa*, December 3, 2000.

"Analisi, cure e ricerca d'avanguardia." *La Stampa*, December 30, 2000.

Angeli, Federica. "Una siringa per venti rapine." *la Repubblica*, February 6, 2000.

Austin, Sydney Bryn. "AIDS and Africa: United States Media and Racist Fantasy." *Cultural Critique* 14, no. 1 (1989–90): 129–52.

Baldwin, Peter. *Disease and Democracy: The Industrialized World Faces AIDS*. Berkeley: University of California Press, 2005.

Balestracci, Fiammetta. "AIDS, sessualità e corpi nelle campagne informative del Ministero della Sanità (1982–1992/1996)." In *L'AIDS in Italia (1982–1996): Istituzioni, società, media*, edited by Balestracci, Fabio Guidali, and Enrico Landoni, 157–222. Pisa: Pacini, 2022.

Bazzi, Adriana. "Terapia biotech per tornare l'AIDS." *Corriere della Sera*, May 27, 2000a.

———. "Farmaci costosi, l'Africa muore di AIDS." *Corriere della Sera*, July 9, 2000b.

Bernabei, Alfio. "Nozze gay, Elton John sposa il suo partner." *l'Unità*, December 22, 2005.

Berridge, Virginia. *AIDS in the UK: The Making of Policy, 1981–1994*. Oxford: Oxford University Press, 1996.

Canna, Maria Luisa. "I rischi di trasmissione." *Corriere della Sera*, July 26, 2010.

Cantilena, Maria Elena. *Una storia disonesta? Il consumo di droghe nell'Italia dei lunghi anni Settanta*. Pisa: Pacini, 2022.

Capponi, Alessandro. "Il test dell'AIDS ai minorenni: io lo faccio." *Corriere della Sera*, February 10, 2010.

"Carceri, nel Lazio record di malati di AIDS." *Corriere della Sera*, February 12, 2010.

Caretto, Ennio. "Clinton: 'America, sei sulla vetta.'" *Corriere della Sera*, January 29, 2000a.

______. "'Dall'AIDS rischio di crisi mondiale." *Corriere della Sera*, May 1, 2000b.

Castronovo, Valerio, and Nicola Tranfaglia, eds. *La stampa taliana nell'età della TV: Dagli anni Settanta a oggi*. Rome and Bari: Laterza, 2008.

Cavalera, Fabio. "'Il Papa promuova i condom': Londra costretta a scusarsi." *Corriere della Sera*, April 26, 2010.

Cavallo, Paolo. "Le scuse tardive della Chiesa." *La Stampa*, December 3, 2000.

Ceccarelli, Filippo. "E adesso la politica si fa con la carità." *La Stampa*, February 28, 2000.

Ciavoni, Carlo. "Msf contro il sistema dei tg 'Più tempo per i saldi che per la fame.'" *Repubblica.it*, April 20, 2010. www.repubblica.it/esteri/2010/04/20/news/msf_per_i_tg_valgono_pi_i_saldi_di_ fine_stagione_che_le_grandi_crisi_umanitarie_in_tutto_il_mondo-3497690/?ref=search

"Contagiò la moglie che morì di AIDS: condanna a 14 anni." *la Repubblica*, July 4, 2000.

Conte di Laviano, Achille. "La corporazione dei dentisti." *la Repubblica*, January 2, 2010.

Cucinotta, Francesco. "Faida d'onore, poliziotto in manette." *la Repubblica*, February 9, 2000.

Daniele, Daniela. "'Consumisti e poco capaci': Gli immigrati ci vedono così." *La Stampa*, December 14, 2000.

Davi, Klaus. "Vladimir, il declino del macho." *La Stampa*, March 10, 2005.

De Bac, Margherita. "AIDS, Gallo critica il vaccino italiano: dannoso per l'uomo." *Corriere del Sera*, April 6, 2000a.

______. "AIDS, bloccato il vaccino italiano." *Corriere del Sera*, June 18, 2000b.

______. "AIDS, il Papa e l'Europa divisi sulla castità." *Corriere della Sera*, December 2, 2005.

______. "Il dentista non può chiedere se il paziente ha l'AIDS." *Corriere della Sera*, January 14, 2010.

De Leo, Maya. *Queer: Storia culturale della comunità LGBT+*. Torino: Einaudi, 2021.

De Martino, Massimo. "Un bacio non vale il contagio. Hiv, come si trasmette la malattia." *Repubblica.it*, March 4, 2010. www.repubblica.it/salute/esperti/andrologia/2010/03/04/news/un_bacio_non_vale_il_contagio_hiv_come_si_trasmette_la_malattia-5584531/?ref=search.

De Matteis, Giantomano. "Poggioreale, stato d'allerta 'Una bomba a orologeria.'" *la Repubblica*, June 27, 2000.

Downs, Anthony. "Up and Down with Ecology: The 'Issue Attention' Cycle." *Public Interest* 28 (1972): 38–50.

Farmer, Paul. *AIDS & Accusation: Haiti and the Geography of Blame*. 2nd ed. Berkeley: University of California Press, 2006.

Fee, Elizabeth, and Daniel M. Fox, eds. *AIDS: The Making of a Chronic Disease*. Berkeley: University of California Press, 1992.

"Fiduciosi, consumisti, poco integrati." *La Stampa*, February 18, 2000.

Focarete, Michele, and Gianni Santucci. "'Hai l'AIDS,' lei lo rifiuta e lui cerca di stuprarla." *Corriere della Sera*, January 24, 2010.

Fowler, Roger. *Language in the News: Discourse and Ideology in the Press*. London: Routledge, 1991.

Fregonara, Gianna. "La proposte di Veltroni 'Allarghiamo il G-8 ad Africa e Sud America.'" *Corriere della Sera*, March 1, 2000.

Fumagalli, Marisa. "Io, un modello per Haider." *Corriere della Sera*, March 6, 2000.

Gabardi, Emanuele. *Stop AIDS: I linguaggi della pubblicità contro l'AIDS in Italia e nel mondo*. Milan: FrancoAngeli, 2017.

Gallini, Luciano. "Ancora sui transgenici." *La Stampa*, January 31, 2000.

Gennari, Gianni. "Angosce e manie: religione dell'antireligione." *Avvenire.it*, January 28, 2005. www.avvenire.it/rubriche/pagine/angosce-e-manie-br-religione-dell-antireligione_20050128.

Giacchetta, Agnese, Andrea Caputo, and Viviana Langher. "La 'peste del secolo' nella stampa italiana: Le rappesentazioni dell'AIDS negli anni '80 e 2000 a confronto." *Psicologia della salute* 1 (2016): 90–110.

Grusin, Richard A. *Premediation: Affect and Mediality after 9/11*. Basingstoke: Palgrave Macmillan, 2010.

Guidali, Fabio. "I media e la rappresentazione dell'AIDS negli anni Ottanta." In *L'AIDS in Italia (1982–1996): Istituzioni, società, media*, edited by Guidali Balestracci and Enrico Landoni, 85–156. Pisa: Pacini, 2022.

Herzlich, Claudine, and Janine Pierret. "The Construction of a Social Phenomenon: AIDS in the French Press." *Social Science & Medicine* 29, no. 11 (1989): 1235–42.

Hood, Johanna. *HIV/AIDS, Health and the Media in China: Imagined Immunity Through Racialized Disease*. London: Routledge, 2011.

"Il portavoce dei vescovi spagnoli: mai consigliato il preservativo." *la Repubblica*, January 21, 2005.

"Il 'tris' del Corriere contro l'AIDS." *Corriere della Sera*, January 10, 2010.

"Il virus bloccato dagli anticorpi." *Corriere del Sera*, April 23, 2000.

"Io, 21 anni, bocconiana sono sieropositiva. Non chiudete gli occhi l'AIDS non è lontano da noi." *Corriere della Sera*, January 5, 2010.

Kinsella, James. *Covering the Plague: AIDS and the American Media*. New Brunswick, NJ: Rutgers University Press, 1992.

"L'amore ai tempi del virus." *La Stampa*, December 2, 2000.

La Rocca, Gevisa. "Dall'allarmismo alla prevenzione: Una riflessione sulle campagne di comunicazione sociale contro la diffusione dell'HIV/AIDS degli ultimi trent'anni." *Mediascapes Journal* 8 (2017): 219–52.

Lazzaro, Claudio. "AIDS nel Lazio: situazione grave, ma casi in diminuzione." *Corriere della Sera*, April 14, 2000.

"Lettere." *la Repubblica*, July 19, 2000.

"Lettere." *la Repubblica*, March 13, 2005.

Longo, Alessandra. "Berlusconi nella bufera per la barzelletta sull'AIDS," *la Repubblica*, April 5, 2000.

Lucente, Luca. "Lettere," *la Repubblica*, April 4, 2000.

Lupton, Deborah. *Moral Threats and Dangerous Desires: AIDS in the News Media*. London: Routledge, 1994.

Manuzzato, Nicoletta. "AIDS, ecco l'anticorpo che protegge dal virus," *l'Unità*, March 10, 2000.

Mauriac, Nicolas. *Le mal entendu: Le sida et les médias*. Paris: Plon, 1990.

Mazzocchi, Silvana. "La nostra vita sulla strada con trenta clienti a notte," *la Repubblica*, July 19, 2000.

Meli, Maria Teresa. "Accuse a Berlusconi: offende i malati", *La Stampa*, April 5, 2000.

Milazzo, Francesco. "Tornare al passato," *Corriere della Sera*, January 8, 2010.

Nelkin, Dorothy. "AIDS and the News Media." *Milbank Quarterly* 69, no. 2 (1991): 293–307.

"Nel mondo 600 milioni di bambini poveri." *Repubblica.it*, July 12, 2000. www.repubblica.it/online/mondo/unice/unice/unice.html?ref=search.

Oppes, Alessandro. "Spagna, la svolta della Chiesa. Contro l'AIDS sì al preservativo." *la Repubblica*, January 19, 2005.

Pace, Giovanni Maria. "AIDS, una cellula lo blocca il vaccino ora è più vicino." *la Repubblica*, March 30, 2000a.

———. "L'Africa spopolata dall'AIDS." *Repubblica.it*, July 11, 2000b. https://quotidiano.repubblica.it/edicola/searchdetail?id=http://archivio.repubblica.extra.

kataweb.it/archivio/repubblica/2000/07/11/africa-spopolata-dall-aids.html&hl=&
query=%22L%E2%80%99Africa+spopolata+dall%E2%80%99Aids%22&field
=nel+testo&testata=repubblica&newspaper=REP&edition=nazionale&zona=sfog
lio&ref=search.

———. "AIDS, il sogno di un vaccino." *la Repubblica*, July 12, 2000c.

Paolini, Alessandra. "L'AIDS? È colpa delle zanzare." *la Repubblica*, May 26, 2005.

Pappagallo, Mario. "Vaccino nasale contro l'AIDS." *Corriere della Sera*, June 12, 2000.

Patton, Cindy. *Inventing AIDS*. London: Routledge, 1990.

Peg, M. "Violenta la prostituta che gli dice: 'Ho l'AIDS'." *La Stampa*, January 4, 2000.

"Penitenziari, dossier della Lila." *Corriere della Sera*, February 12, 2000.

Piot, Peter. *AIDS: Between Science and Politics*. New York: Columbia University Press, 2015.

Pleuteri, Lorenza. "Il rapinatore che perseguita le donne." *la Repubblica*, May 15, 2005.

Ravizza, Simona. "La sfida della bocconiana malata di AIDS: 'Mia madre non sa, mi curo in segreto.'" *Corriere della Sera*, January 8, 2010.

Ricci Sargentini, Monica. "Zuma alla ventesima figlia ma non dalle sue tre mogli." *Corriere della Sera*, February 2, 2010.

Rondoni, Davide. "Il preservativo anziché le politiche." *Avvenire.it*, March 29, 2009. www.avvenire.it/opinioni/pagine/irresponsabile-leggerezza-dei-governanti-europei_20090320083220950000000.

"Sangue donato da omosessuali. Fazio chiede parere agli esperti." *Corriere della Sera*, July 24, 2010.

Scego, Igiaba. "Due donne per il Sud Africa." *l'Unità*, June 26, 2010.

Severgnini, Beppe. "Se una sieropositiva ci fa pensare." *Corriere della Sera*, January 14, 2010.

Shackle, Samira. "Proviamo a divertirci anche se questo calcio è solo un grande circo." *la Repubblica*, June 8, 2010.

Sontag, Susan. *AIDS and Its Metaphors*. New York: Farrar, Straus and Giroux, 1989.

Spatola, Giuseppe. "Sposa-bambina prigioniera del marito: ho paura, ha l'AIDS." *Corriere della Sera*, February 4, 2010.

"Un antibiotico low-cost contro l'AIDS, 'con terapia combinata dimezza i morti.'" *Repubblica.it*, March 29, 2010.

"Un telefono per 'amico.'" *Corriere della Sera*, April 23, 2000.

"Veltroni in Africa." *Corriere della Sera*, March 3, 2000.

Voltattorni, Claudia. "La strage delle palme cambia volto all'Italia." *Corriere del Sera*, May 1, 2010.

Whiteside, Alan. *HIV & AIDS: A Very Short Introduction*. 2nd ed. Oxford: Oxford University Press, 2016.

Zambelli, Lucia. "AIDS, l'incubo finisce a Pisa." *la Repubblica*, February 13, 2000.

Zuccolini, Roberto. "Barzelletta sull'AIDS, tutti contro Berlusconi." *Corriere della Sera*, April 5, 2000.

Zucconi, Vittorio. "L'AIDS minaccia la democrazia." *la Repubblica*, May 1, 2000.

12 The Italian National Health Service in a Time of Crisis

What Were the Responses for the Most Vulnerable People?

Marco Terraneo

The Healthcare System, Health and Vulnerable People

The healthcare system includes the set of institutions, people and resources (and their relationships) whose primary purpose is to contribute to the promotion, recovery and maintenance of health.[1] Within the framework of social determinants of health, the healthcare system is considered an intermediary determinant. I refer to determinants as the set of social, economic, cultural and political factors, both individual and contextual, that shape the health opportunities of social groups and individuals. One must distinguish between structural determinants and intermediary determinants. The terminological difference highlights a significant substantive difference – namely, the prioritization of structural determinants over intermediary determinants in the causal chain that produces health inequities.[2]

The healthcare system's significance lies in addressing disparities in exposure and vulnerability by facilitating access to care and promoting actions to improve health status.[3] Access to high-quality healthcare undeniably provides a substantial advantage in dealing with diseases, as it increases the likelihood of physical and social recovery. A high-quality healthcare system should not only facilitate health recovery but also strive to reduce inequalities by ensuring that individuals in lower social positions experience health conditions and disease risks similar to those in higher socioeconomic groups.[4]

Individuals in lower socioeconomic positions have a higher likelihood of being excluded from accessing and utilizing healthcare services. While fair utilization of available resources for the benefit of the entire population is the foundation of an equitable healthcare system, a more stringent definition is required to establish healthcare system equity.[5] I argue that the concept of equity in healthcare should be regarded as a multidimensional concept, although in this context I define a healthcare system as fair if it can guarantee equal access to care and equal utilization of services based on individual needs.

The World Health Organization recognizes the right to access healthcare as an essential aspect of human rights, and European healthcare systems are built on the principle of equity, aiming for equal care provision to individuals

DOI: 10.4324/9781003382805-12

with equal needs (horizontal equity) and tailored interventions for those with diverse needs (vertical equity).[6] However, despite the efforts of most countries to establish healthcare systems with universal and fair coverage, achieving equal access and utilization of healthcare services remains a challenge.[7] Persistent disparities in healthcare services utilization have been observed across sociodemographic and economic characteristics, such as income, education, social class and a combination of these factors, along with gender and ethnic background.[8]

An unfair healthcare system that disadvantages socially, economically and culturally deprived individuals exacerbates the harm experienced by vulnerable populations already at higher risk of illness. The policies and resources allocated by the healthcare system contribute to the heterogeneity in health outcomes, directly impacting citizens' lives through prevention, treatment and care. Consequently, the healthcare system has the potential to either widen or reduce health inequalities, although measuring its precise contribution to addressing unjust disparities in health conditions may be challenging.[9] Nonetheless, it is undeniable that the healthcare system plays a role in shaping health inequalities.

The Italian Healthcare System

The scope of this chapter does not allow me to explore the specific political, economic, cultural and social processes that have shaped the current form of the Italian healthcare system. However, I can present some of its actual relevant features to discuss if and to what extent it is able to respond to individual needs. The pivotal moment in illustrating the fundamental aspects of the Italian healthcare system is the year 1978, when Law 833/1978 was enacted, establishing the National Health Service (Servizio Sanitario Nazionale [SSN]). This reform represented a significant departure from the two previous phases. The first phase, lasting until the 1940s, relied on voluntary health insurance and placed the responsibility for health protection primarily on individual families and charitable organizations, particularly religious ones. The second phase, from around 1940 to 1977, witnessed the dominance of a social health insurance model, where nonprofit health funds collected contributions from workers and employers based on occupational or territorial categories. However, with the establishment of the SSN, healthcare shifted from being a benefit for workers to a fundamental right of citizenship.

Equity is a central principle underlying the SSN. It is a universal health service system that guarantees the right to healthcare for the entire population, irrespective of discrimination, time and cost constraints. The SSN aimed to promote equality of treatment, ensuring that all citizens receive equal care and find appropriate responses to their healthcare needs across the country. The system was designed to provide a comprehensive range of services, addressing a broad spectrum of health needs, not limited to disease treatment but also encompassing interventions that influence the health of individuals and the community. Furthermore, equitable financing was a key objective, with a significant reliance on general taxation. This ensured that everyone contributed based on their ability and received healthcare services based on their needs. However, the Italian healthcare system has undergone significant changes since its establishment more than forty years ago. Despite the initial promises, many of them have remained unfulfilled, and even the foundational principles have come under scrutiny, particularly following a series of reforms that have had a profound impact on its original core (Table 12.1).

One notable transformation resulting from the devolution processes (i.e., the processes by which a centralized state expands the legislative and administrative powers of territorial autonomies, granting them new functions) and fiscal federalism regulations is the configuration of the SSN as a federation of regional healthcare systems. This has resulted in a complex and heterogeneous healthcare system across Italian regions, in terms of both organizational and economic-financial aspects. Therefore, it is now more accurate to refer to the Italian healthcare system as twenty Regional Health Systems (RHSs). These changes have had far-reaching consequences, exacerbating preexisting

Table 12.1 The key stages of the Italian healthcare system reform starting from 1978

Year	Reform	Description
1978	Law 833/1978	Establishes the National Health Service (SSN) with universal coverage funded by general taxation.
1992-93	Law October 23, 1992, No. 421; Decree Law December 30, 1992, No. 502; Decree Law December 7, 1993, No. 517	Promote devolution of healthcare to the Regions. Grants managerial autonomy to local health authorities (ASL) and hospitals (AO) and introduces elements of internal market in healthcare (distinction between purchasers and providers of services to stimulate competition in terms of quality improvement and cost containment).
1999	Decree Law June 19, 1999, No. 229	Further promotes devolution; strengthens cooperation and regulation to partially reorient the internal market; establishes tools for defining Essential Levels of Care (Livelli Essenziali di Assistenza – LEA); introduces the practice of intramoenia; regulates the introduction of clinical guidelines for healthcare quality.
2001	Constitutional Law October 18, 2001, No. 3	Amends the second part of the Italian Constitution (Title V), granting increased powers to the Regions, including in healthcare matters.

inequalities and affecting the system's ability to effectively address the health needs of the Italian population.

A significant disparity can be observed in the levels of care provided by Italian regions to their citizens. The state–regions agreement of March 23, 2005, delegates the certification of compliance with the essential levels of assistance (LEA, i.e., the services and treatments that the National Health Service is required to provide to all citizens, either free of charge or with the payment of a copayment fee [ticket], using public resources collected through general taxation [taxes]) to the regions, utilizing indicators related to assistance activities in various settings, district-level care and hospital care.[10] In 2019, 17 regions were positively evaluated, scoring equal to or higher than 160 (the minimum acceptable score). However, four regions were found to be noncompliant, scoring below 160. It is important to note that among the 17 compliant regions, significant differences exist. Indeed, ten regions achieved a score above 200, whereas seven regions scored between 200 and 160. In some cases, the score was just above the compliance threshold.

Guido Giarelli and Giovanna Vicarelli identify four key distortions that have characterized the SSN since its establishment.[11] These include the distributive distortion, which encompasses social health inequalities; the cultural distortion, which emphasizes illness and the subsequent medicalization of health; the structural distortion, characterized by regional differentiation; and the functional distortion, where hospitals retain a central role within the healthcare system (hospital-centric approach). This situation has further deteriorated following the 2008 financial and social crisis, as I will explore in the next section.

Financial Crisis and Health: The Consequences of the Great Recession on the Italian Healthcare System

From a financial perspective, the relationship between the economic crisis and the healthcare system in Italy reveals two distinct yet strongly interconnected levels. First, the crisis significantly reduced the economic resources available to a large portion of individuals, resulting in severe consequences for their health and their ability to access both public and private healthcare services for treatment. Second, austerity measures aimed at controlling and reducing public spending due to limited resources have had a significant impact on the Italian healthcare system's capacity to address the healthcare needs of its citizens. It is useful to remember that the Italian GDP decreased by −1.2% in 2008 and even more markedly in 2009 (−5.5%).

Concerning the first aspect, economic crises – such as the one experienced by Western countries since 2008 – have exposed growing segments of the middle class to social and health vulnerabilities. These groups have faced increasing difficulties in meeting their healthcare needs, even within a public healthcare system like Italy's. In Italy, the number of people foregoing medical care due to economic reasons has significantly increased following the

2008 economic crisis, reaching more than four million individuals, which accounted for 7% of the population in 2018. This particularly affects individuals aged 45–54 and migrants, who often lack regular healthcare coverage. Additionally, approximately two million people, equivalent to 3.3% of the entire population, have been forced to forgo specialist visits or examinations due to waiting lists, making them unable to access private healthcare or noncontracted services (i.e., medical services or treatments that are not covered or reimbursed by the public healthcare system or insurance providers).

Despite the public nature of the SSN, there is a high level of private out-of-pocket healthcare expenditure as a percentage of total healthcare spending. In 2019, Italy's private out-of-pocket expenditure accounted for 23.3%, significantly higher than that of France (9.3%), Germany (12.7%) and the United Kingdom (15.9%), while aligning with Spain's figure (21.8%). Moreover, 8% of households in Italy experienced catastrophic healthcare expenses in 2018, surpassing the EU27 average of 6.6% (WHO Regional Office for Europe). Catastrophic healthcare expenditures are defined as the excessive impact of health expenditure on household budgets, such as those that account for more than 40% of the capacity to pay off families.

Regarding the second aspect, the chronic deficit of public financial resources in Italy, compounded by the 2008 financial crisis and subsequent economic and social recession, has severely impacted the healthcare system. This has led to significant budget cuts, reduced services, salary freezes for employees and a slowdown in technological investments, greatly affecting the ability of the healthcare system to deliver public healthcare services up to the expected standards.[12] The following data provide a clear picture of the challenges faced by the Italian healthcare system.

The public healthcare expenditure as a percentage of GDP indicates that the SSN is underfunded compared to other European countries. In 2019, Italy's percentage stood at 6.4%, in contrast to the Netherlands (8.4%), Sweden and France (9.3%) and Germany (9.9%). Furthermore, total public healthcare expenditure in Italy, including investments, intermediate consumption, research and development and other components, experienced a significant setback after the 2008 economic and financial crisis. From 2008 to 2018, the total public healthcare expenditure in nominal terms (accounting for inflation) increased by only 5.3%, while in Germany, it grew by 46.8%.

The control of public healthcare expenditure has been achieved primarily through minimal increases and, in some cases, reductions in funding, particularly in the standard national requirement of the SSN. These funds are allocated by the central government to the regions to finance the LEA provided throughout the country. In addition to the containment of the standard national requirement, austerity policies have focused on controlling specific sources of expenditure related to the acquisition of productive factors. Interventions have been implemented to rationalize pharmaceutical expenditure, reduce the hospitalization rate, redefine maximum reference rates for outpatient and inpatient specialized services, rationalize expenditure on goods and services and increase revenue through cost-sharing for citizens. Measures have also been taken to control expenditure and the number of personnel in the public healthcare sector, including gradual reduction of employees and containing salaries.[13]

The Effect of the Pandemic on Health and the Healthcare System

In 2020, the total number of deaths from all causes in Italy was the highest ever recorded since the postwar period: 746,146 deaths, which is 100,526 more deaths compared to the 2015–19 average, an excess mortality of 15.6%. The excess mortality is an indicator that allows us to measure the direct and indirect impacts of the pandemic by providing a more objective measure than deaths directly associated with COVID-19. It is calculated as the difference between the total number of deaths from all causes since the beginning of the pandemic and the expected trend of deaths based on the historical trend (the average for the period 2015–19) if the COVID-19 pandemic had not occurred. In 2021, the total number of deaths from all causes decreased compared to the previous year, although it remained at very high levels: 709,035 deaths, which is roughly 37,000 fewer than in 2020 (–5.0%), but 63,000 more than the 2015–19 average (+9.8%).[14]

A comprehensive analysis of the effects of the pandemic on health and healthcare must take into account the heightened risks faced by the most disadvantaged individuals in society and the extent to which these risks align with social determinants of health.[15] By framing the discussion within this conceptual background, I acknowledge significant variations among individuals regarding their likelihood of exposure to and contraction of the virus, as well as the consequences for those who have been exposed. Unequal exposure to risk factors can give rise to disparities in illness and mortality during the pandemic. Furthermore, we must not overlook the social, economic and psychological ramifications, such as forced isolation or economic crises, which can lead to long-term deterioration of the overall well-being of the population and exacerbate health inequities.

To illustrate this point, Figure 12.1 depicts the relationship between individuals' social position and the disparities associated with the virus that contribute to unequal levels of illness and mortality. It also represents the health, social and economic consequences of the pandemic that intensify health inequities within society. Additionally, the impact of social position can be influenced by intersecting factors within the social hierarchy, such as age, gender and ethnicity, which can either amplify or mitigate these effects.[16]

The relationship between social position and unequal levels of illness and mortality focuses on three specific areas of disparity.[17] These include:

1. Differences in exposure. The risk of exposure was higher for individuals with low-income and low-skilled occupations who had fewer opportunities to stay at home when one of the most effective strategies to avoid

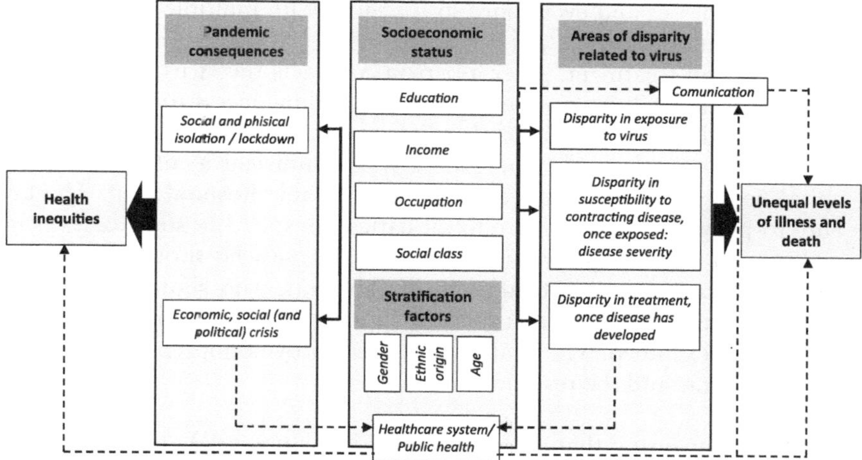

Figure 12.1 Framework for analyzing health inequalities during a pandemic. Note: Regarding the relationship between areas of disparity related to the virus and unequal levels of illness and mortality, the figure is an adaptation from Blumenshine et al. (2008) and Quinn and Kumar (2014).

contagion was to limit contact with others. These people held jobs that were less likely to be performed remotely, such as through smart-working, and required their physical presence in the workplace. Undocumented workers, also due to the lack of protections provided to regular employees, often had to choose between protecting their health or securing an income. Additionally, some workers were essential because they contributed to providing goods and services fundamental to the entire population (e.g., goods handling). Another factor that increased the risk of virus exposure was overcrowding. This risk is associated with negative social and economic characteristics within families, such as living in rental housing, having a low household income and being of foreign origin. People living in institutions such as Residenze Asistenziali Sanitarie (residential care facilities), prisons and residences for disabled individuals were particularly at risk of infection due to the close proximity that significantly increased the chances of contracting the virus.

2. Differences in susceptibility. Once exposed to the virus, the likelihood of falling ill and the severity of the illness can be influenced by a set of factors that make individuals more vulnerable. These risk factors are not evenly distributed among the population but vary based on the social position and health conditions of individuals. Moreover, there is a strong association between these two dimensions: the lower the availability of resources, the greater the health risks. One notable example is the susceptibility to the virus and the fatality rate, which was much higher for individuals with

chronic illnesses and even more so for those with multiple chronic conditions (multimorbidity).

3. Difference in treatment. After a person contracts the virus and the illness develops, inequalities can be observed regarding access to the healthcare system and the treatment of the disease. During the acute phase of the COVID-19 pandemic in Italy, there was insufficient availability of hospital beds, access to intensive care and available hospital staff. The failure to provide necessary care to all patients resulted in some cases being relegated to a position where one had to choose who should be deferred and treated at home instead of in the hospital, who should have access to potentially lifesaving therapies, such as respiratory support, and who should be excluded. The healthcare system proved unprepared to handle the pandemic and the resulting crisis.

Another dimension that comes into play is the potential amplifiers of disparities. The healthcare system (in its regional variants) appears to be a focal point in the ability to respond to health emergency. Among the RHSs, significant differences have emerged over time, in terms of both organization and the quality of services provided.[18] Therefore, it is not surprising that there have been varied responses in managing the pandemic depending on the pre-existing organizational framework.[19] RHSs based on community medicine, focusing on primary care and preventive services, and hospital-centric RHSs, which prioritize hospital admissions, had different capacities to intervene and promote health during the pandemic, with the former being more responsive to individuals' needs and better at protecting people than the latter.

The COVID-19 pandemic has also had (and continues to have) consequences that are not directly related to the spread of the virus and contagion. We cannot underestimate the social, economic and psychological repercussions that certain factors, such as forced isolation, job loss, school closures and the perception of risk, have caused and can continue to cause in the long term, leading to a deterioration in the overall well-being of the population and at the same time exacerbating health inequities.[20] Once again, individuals have found themselves dealing with inequality – in this case, an inequality in the face of the virus and its consequences.

The Most Vulnerable Individuals Among the Vulnerable

As observed, there have been significant inequalities among individuals in the face of the pandemic. It is important to acknowledge that the challenges associated with the COVID-19 emergency have been greater for certain vulnerable groups. Among the most exposed individuals are those living in overcrowded settings, such as nursing homes, prisons, administrative detention centers, informal settlements and reception centers, and all those who were homeless and thus forced to live on the streets or in shelters. These individuals often reside in overcrowded informal settlements, making it challenging to maintain proper hygiene practices and physical distancing measures, with limited access to protective measures. They typically face difficulties in accessing the public healthcare system and often resort to emergency rooms for medical assistance. These groups are particularly at risk for various health problems due to their precarious living conditions, low levels of education and employment and limited access to healthcare services. Moreover, their likelihood of being monitored for early symptoms of COVID-19 has been low, exposing both themselves and the community to associated risks.

I report here briefly a description of the most problematic dimensions that have affected these particularly vulnerable groups in their relationship with the health system during the pandemic.

1. Immigrants have proven to be particularly vulnerable to the coronavirus crisis for multiple reasons. Their vulnerable position stems from their work situation (concentration in essential sectors and in manual and precarious jobs), legal status (foreigners) and housing conditions (limited and overcrowded spaces). Socioeconomically and in terms of employment, they have been heavily impacted by unemployment, underemployment, deteriorating working conditions and impoverishment, once again due to various factors. These challenges are exacerbated by their strong presence in sectors affected by the health crisis (e.g., hospitality, food service and domestic work) that are also characterized by widespread informality and irregularity. Moreover, the majority of them have had to accept any working conditions to safeguard their jobs and, consequently, their residence permits. This has intensified job and professional disqualification and wage erosion, and in the context of unemployment and stricter migration policies, they have had to adapt to lower qualifications, lower wages, longer hours and more intense work rhythms to maintain or obtain employment necessary to obtain or renew their residence permits. In certain sectors, there have been instances of exacerbated labor exploitation, increased workplace discrimination and frequent outbreaks of infection (especially in slaughterhouses, logistics hubs and food companies). Moreover, the condition of irregularity, which is still widespread in Italy, leads to further social marginalization, inadequate prevention measures and overcrowding, all of which contribute to vulnerability.

2. Asylum seekers hosted in overcrowded reception centers have been identified as at-risk individuals. Despite a significant reduction in arrivals due to controversial agreements with Libya, Italy still lacks an effective reception system capable of managing new emergencies and drawing lessons from past experiences, particularly during the "refugee crisis" from 2015 to 2017.[21]

   Asylum seekers have experienced significant health and social consequences due to their preexisting structural social vulnerability. At times, reception centers and refugee detention camps have been unable to ensure physical distancing, hygiene and public health. In addition to overcrowding, infected individuals often have not been evacuated from these facilities, resulting in the spread of the virus throughout the entire structure. Within these centers, asylum seekers who have permission to work outside become potential carriers of the virus. In the management of positive cases, diverse and improvised measures have been implemented on more than one occasion.

Many asylum seekers have lost their jobs or witnessed an increase in irregular work, leading to higher levels of inactivity and monotony for those residing in reception centers, especially during lockdowns. Forced overcrowding, feelings of abandonment and a sense of despair have grown during these periods. Added to this are uncertainties regarding asylum seekers' residency status due to the suspension of asylum applications and permits, the weakened legal standing resulting from the state of emergency, border closures and the lack of humanitarian corridors, as well as the disruption of reception and integration services.

All of this has worsened an already compromised and deteriorating situation, burdened by the hardships of migration, poor psychophysical conditions from travel and life in camps and the prevailing anti-immigrant sentiment in many parts of the world, such as in Italy. These factors have negatively impacted both virus exposure and social integration, leaving thousands of people in limbo. This has particularly affected those who have not received humanitarian protection or asylum, as well as those who have exited international reception and protection systems, commonly referred to as "irregular" individuals. They have often been subjected to blame and stigmatization, with reception facilities and their residents being labeled as carriers of disease. In addition to the distorted public perception of asylum seekers as lazy, freeloaders and backward, the element of them being a so-called health hazard has further perpetuated situations of exclusion and racism.

3. In Italy, as specified in the National Action Plan against Trafficking and Severe Exploitation 2016–2018,

The Ministry of Health plays a guiding role aimed at ensuring uniform assistance to victims of trafficking throughout the national territory, concerning the medical care that our country is able to provide and the modalities through which it is delivered, with particular attention to vulnerable individuals and taking into account gender-related issues (e.g., pregnant women or victims of violence, minors and so on)

(Legislative Decree 286/98, Article 35, Paragraph 3)

Therefore, all individuals enrolled in recovery and social integration programs have the right to be registered with the SSN. Having a primary care physician was more essential than ever in the health emergency we faced. However, it was one of the most difficult challenges and the main obstacle to integration for the victims, both in the reception phase and when they are already self-sufficient. Undoubtedly, sex workers, especially migrants, have been one of the most affected and least protected marginalized communities. Isolation and the inability to work have further intensified the precarious conditions experienced by many sex workers, leaving them with limited resources. Those who continue to engage in street-based sex work face numerous risks. In addition to the risk of contagion, they are exposed to forms of violence, control and sanctions, which disproportionately affect sex workers without proper documentation. On January 21, 2021, the European Parliament also emphasized the need to guarantee and protect the human rights of sex workers, acknowledging the lack of a comprehensive legal framework. During the initial months of the Italian national lockdown, the suspension of many local services and the minimal functioning of courts, territorial commissions and police headquarters made it more challenging to identify the most vulnerable individuals engaged in sex work, particularly those facing exploitation and uncertain legal status.

4. Individuals deprived of their liberty, such as those in prisons and other detention facilities, are particularly susceptible to coronavirus disease compared to the general population. This heightened vulnerability is due to the confined living conditions in which they reside for extended periods. Moreover, historical evidence indicates that prisons, jails and similar settings where people are closely gathered can serve as sources of infection, amplification and spread of infectious diseases within and beyond their confines. In addition to demographic disparities, individuals deprived of their liberty often carry a heavier burden of underlying diseases and experience poorer health conditions than the general population. They are frequently exposed to higher risks, such as smoking, inadequate hygiene and weakened immune defenses resulting from stress, substandard nutrition and the prevalence of coexisting ailments like bloodborne viruses, tuberculosis and drug-use disorders.[22] Prisons and detention facilities are enclosed environments where people, including staff, live in close proximity. Therefore, preventing the introduction of the virus into these settings is crucial to mitigate the occurrence of infections and serious outbreaks within these facilities and beyond.

The response to the COVID-19 outbreak must adhere to the guiding principles of the human rights framework. The rights of all affected individuals must be upheld, and all public health measures should be implemented without any form of discrimination. People in prisons and other places of detention not only face heightened vulnerability to COVID-19 but are also particularly susceptible to human rights violations. In Italy, the penitentiary system has also experienced the effects of the pandemic and had to adapt to a new normality characterized by closures to the outside world and even greater isolation of incarcerated individuals.

Recognizing the risks that infectious diseases pose to incarcerated individuals, proposals were made to implement measures aimed at reducing the prison population (it stood at around 61,230 detainees for 50,931 available places), preventing contagion within the institutions through the distribution of sanitary supplies and environment sanitization and alleviating the isolation of detainees by allowing more frequent phone calls, video calls and the use of electronic mail.

An important development concerned the vaccination of the incarcerated population against COVID-19. Numerous international institutions, including the WHO and the European Commission, have identified individuals living in places of deprivation of liberty as priority groups for COVID-19 vaccination. Among the various reasons for prioritizing the vaccination of detainees, the following stand out. First, there is the impossibility of maintaining physical distancing due to overcrowding. Additionally, there are health-related reasons, including the rapid spread of infectious diseases and pathogens within correctional institutions, as well as a high prevalence of preexisting medical conditions among the incarcerated.

5. Homeless individuals have been among the most vulnerable and exposed social groups during the health emergency. Scientific literature has long emphasized the health risks faced by homeless individuals living on the streets and utilizing low-threshold services, which further magnify their vulnerability during pandemics.[23]

The latest national census of homelessness in Italy identified more than 96,000 people in this situation, with more than half residing in only six municipalities, particularly in large metropolitan areas. Almost 38% of them are of foreign nationality.[24] For this segment of the population, the challenges related to the disease are magnified and prolonged. In addition to the increased exposure to risk factors for infection and the consequences of the disease during the first wave, they also faced the issue of cold weather during the winter months of the second wave. These individuals generally have unhealthy lifestyles, multiple chronic conditions, mental distress, dependency issues, relational fragility and difficulties accessing healthcare services and shelter facilities. As a result, prevention measures to contain the spread of the virus have been practically unattainable for them. Besides lacking a home for self-isolation, homeless individuals have had to rely on crowded and communal places, such as soup kitchens and shelters, for meals and accommodation, where maintaining the minimum distance is often not feasible. Moreover, those without housing, despite understanding the gravity of the situation and making earnest efforts to comply with hygiene regulations, face significant challenges in adhering to basic sanitary practices prescribed by the authorities, to which were added difficulties in acquiring protective equipment due to financial limitations. Simultaneously, those living on the streets have experienced the consequences of the lockdown more acutely: with the closure of activities and deserted cities, they have been unable to rely on the solidarity of citizens and businesses, exacerbating their primary needs for food and hygiene and increasing loneliness and isolation.

The lack of targeted prevention strategies to address the spread of contagion and facilitate access to healthcare services for homeless individuals and other socially excluded groups poses a significant public health concern. In many cities, clinics established by religious institutions and volunteer organizations have played a crucial role in providing essential medical care. These clinics often serve as the only available healthcare facilities for marginalized individuals.

Reconsidering the Needs of the Italian Healthcare System

Giarelli and Vicarelli identify some strategic guidelines that they evaluate as essential for the revitalization of the SSN, which are fully expressed in four guiding principles.[25] These are a universal SSN that promotes equality, fairness and personalization; a salutogenic (à la Antonovsky) SSN that places the individual citizen and their associations at the center; a community-based SNN, based on responsible and supportive regionalism; and a networked SSN, founded on territorial and sociohealth integration.

In a similar vein, Gavino Maciocco emphasized the necessity of a profound overhaul of the Italian healthcare system.[26] He underscored that the SSN should not be reduced to a mere healthcare factory; rather, it should prioritize the protection and promotion of people's health while equipping itself to effectively tackle the epidemic of chronic diseases and the subepidemic of multimorbidity. According to Maciocco, the key to this transformation lies in adopting a new paradigm centered on anticipatory healthcare, which includes prevention efforts and addressing socioeconomic inequalities that disproportionately impact the health of the most disadvantaged sections of the population. This paradigm shift necessitates a strengthening of primary care and community services.

It is evident that our healthcare system is currently facing profound difficulties. The outbreak of the pandemic has exacerbated well-known structural weaknesses and organizational limitations. However, the attention toward the SSN, not only from healthcare professionals but also from the public, is now higher, especially considering the significant resources that will be allocated to it through the National Recovery and Resilience Plan. This includes initiatives such as the development of local proximity networks (community houses) and telemedicine.

The Italian healthcare system finds itself confronted with a challenge for its own survival, at least if one defines the SSN as an institution that intends to uphold the principles that guided its establishment. Despite the changing social, economic and cultural conditions since its inception, the question is: Will the SSN be able to achieve a balance amidst conflicting forces (homogeneity/heterogeneity of service quality at the territorial level, public/private provision and delivery of services, public funding/out-of-pocket expenses) that could potentially lead it to collapse?

The answer, according to Emanuele Pavolini and colleagues, lies in the ability to achieve four objectives that they define as the "quadrilemma" of healthcare policy.[27] The first objective of healthcare systems is equal access to healthcare for all. The second objective is medical in nature, ensuring the system's capacity to provide the highest possible quality of care and optimal health conditions for the population. The third objective is of an economic nature, as all healthcare systems must tackle the thorny issue of financing. This involves controlling costs and managing the increase in healthcare expenditure, such as due to population aging. Lastly, the fourth objective is of a political nature and relates to the system's ability to be responsive and sensitive to the demands and needs of patients and professionals, ensuring their satisfaction, freedom and comfort.

I do not know if the Italian healthcare system will be able to overcome this challenge. However, what I do know, as the pandemic has taught us, is that evading these evident problems is not a viable solution for citizens, public policymakers or scholars in the field. If change is indispensable, it will be crucial, at least for the author, to strive to preserve the principles of one of the most significant, if not the most important, reforms that have ensured the health and well-being of Italian citizens from the post–Second World War period to the present day.

Notes

1 World Health Organization (WHO), "The World Health Report, 2000: Health System; Improving Performance" (Geneva: World Health Organization, 2000), www.who.int/iris/handle/10665/42281.
2 Göran Dahlgren and Margaret Whitehead, *Policies and Strategies to Promote Social Equity in Health* (Stockholm: Institute for Futures Studies, 1991).
3 Orielle Solar and Alec Irwin, "A Conceptual Framework for Action on the Social Determinants of Health," in *Social Determinants of Health Discussion Paper*, no. 2 (Policy and Practice) (Geneva: WHO, 2010), https://apps.who.int/iris/bitstream/handle/10665/44489/9789241500852_eng.pdf.
4 Johan P. Mackenbach, "An Analysis of the Role of Health Care in Reducing Socioeconomic Inequalities in Health: The Case of the Netherlands," *International Journal of Health Services: Planning, Administration, Evaluation* 33, no. 3 (2003): 523–41, https://doi.org/10.2190/C12H-NBA4-7QWE-6K3T.
5 Margaret Whitehead, "The Concepts and Principles of Equity and Health," *Health Promotion International* 6, no. 3 (1991): 217–28.
6 Edward Kelley and Jeremy Hurst, "Health Care Quality Indicators Project: Conceptual Framework Paper," *OECD Health Working Papers*, no. 23 (Paris: OECD Publishing, 2006).
7 European Commission, *Joint Report 2008 on Social Protection and Social Inclusion.* (Luxembourg: Office for Official Publications of the European Communities, 2008).
8 Enrique Regidor et al., "Socioeconomic Patterns in the Use of Public and Private Health Services and Equity in Health Care," *BMC Health Services Research* 8 (2008), https://doi.org/10.1186/1472-6963-8-183; Marco Carme

et al., "Social Class Inequalities in the Utilization of Health Care and Preventive Services in Spain, a Country with a National Health System," *International Journal of Health Services* 40, no. 3 (2010): 525–42; Marion Devaux, "Income-Related Inequalities and Inequities in Health Care Services Utilisation in 18 Selected OECD Countries," *European Journal of Health Economics* 16, no. 1 (2015): 22–33; and Marco Terraneo, "Inequities in Health Care Utilization by People Aged 50+: Evidence from 12 European Countries," *Social Science & Medicine* 126 (February 2015): 154–63, http://dx.doi.org/10.1016/j.socscimed.2014.12.028.

 9 Agnès Couffinhal et al., "Policies for Reducing Inequalities in Health, What Role Can the Health System Play? A European Perspective. Part I: Determinants of Social Inequalities in Health and the Role of the Healthcare System," *Issues in Health Economics* 92 (February 2005).

10 Ministero della Salute, *Monitoraggio dei LEA attraverso la cd: Griglia LEA; Metodologia e Risultati dell'anno 2019* (Direzione Generale della Programmazione Sanitaria–Ufficio VI, 2021), www.salute.gov.it/imgs/C_17_pubblicazioni_3111_allegato.pdf.

11 Guido Giarelli and Giovanna Vicarelli, eds., *Libro bianco: Il servizio sanitario nazionale e la pandemia da COVID-19; Problemi e proposte* (Milan: FrancoAngeli, 2021).

12 Walter Ricciardi, *La battaglia per la salute* (Rome: Laterza, 2019).

13 Stefano Neri and Anna Mori, "Crisi economica, politiche di austerità e relazioni intergovernative nel SSN: Dalla regionalizzazione al federalismo differenziato?," *Autonomie Locali e Servizi Sociali* 2 (2017): 201–20.

14 Instituto Nazionale di Statistica (ISTAT), "Impatto dell'epidemia Covid-19 sulla mortalità totale della popolazione residente," March 2, 2022, www.istat.it/it/files//2022/03/Report_ISS_ISTAT_2022_tab3.pdf.

15 Tracey L. O'Sullivan and Karen P. Phillips, "From SARS to Pandemic Influenza: The Framing of High-Risk Populations," *Natural Hazards* 98, no. 1 (2019): 103–17, https://doi.org/10.1007/s11069-019-03584-6.

16 Marco Terraneo, "Studiare le disuguaglianze di salute in tempo di pandemia: Una cornice teorica," *Sociologia italiana*, no. 16 (2020): 87–97, https://doi.org/10.1485/2281-2652-202016-6.

17 Philip Blumenshine et al., "Pandemic Influenza Planning in the United States from a Health Disparities Perspective," *Emerging Infectious Diseases* 14, no. 5 (2008): 709–15, https://doi.org/10.3201/eid1405.071301; and Sandra Crouse Quinn and Supriya Kumar, "Health Inequalities and Infectious Disease Epidemics: A Challenge for Global Health Security," *Biosecurity and Bioterrorism: Biodefense Strategy, Practice, and Science* 12, no. 5 (2014): 263–73, https://doi.org/10.1089/bsp.2014.0032.

18 Mattia Casula, Andrea Terlizzi, and Federico Toth, "I servizi sanitari regionali alla prova del COVID-19," *Rivista italiana di politiche pubbliche* 3 (2020): 307–36, https://doi.org/10.1483/98732.

19 Giovanna Vicarelli, "Regionalismo sanitario e COVID-19: Punti di forza e di debolezza," in Giarelli and Vicarelli, *Libro bianco*, 23–30.

20 Marco Terraneo, Linda Lombi, and Hannah Bradby, "Depressive Symptoms and Perception of Risk during the First Wave of the COVID-19 Pandemic: A Web-Based Cross-Country Comparative Survey," *Sociology of Health & Illness* 43, no. 7 (2021): 1660–68.

21 Hanne Beirens, "The COVID-19 Pandemic Suggests the Lessons Learned by European Asylum Policymakers after the 2015 Migration Crisis Are Fading," Migration Policy Institute, April 2020, www.migrationpolicy.org/news/pandemic-lessons-learned-europe-asylum-fading.

22 Stuart A. Kinner and Jesse T. Young, "Understanding and Improving the Health of People Who Experience Incarceration: An Overview and Synthesis," *Epidemiologic Reviews* 40, no. 1 (2018): 4–11, https://doi.org/10.1093/epirev/mxx018.
23 Silvia Stefani, "L'isolamento impossibile delle persone senza dimora," *Percorsi di Secondo Welfare*, April 8, 2020, www.secondowelfare.it/povert-e-inclusione/lisolamento-impossibile-delle-persone-senza-dimora/.
24 ISTAT, "Le persone senza fissa dimora," December 15, 2022, www.istat.it/it/files//2022/12/CENSIMENTO-E-DINAMICA-DEMOGRAFICA-2021.pdf.
25 Giarelli and Vicarelli, *Libro bianco*, 117–23.
26 Gavino Maciocco, "SSN: Solo un cambio di paradigma lo salverà," *Sistema salute* 62, no. 4 (2018): 468–75.
27 Emanuele Pavolini, Bruno Palier, and Ana M. Guillén, "The Health Care Policy Quadrilemma and Comparative Institutional Reforms," in *Health Care Systems in Europe under Austerity: Work and Welfare in Europe*, ed. Pavolini and Guillén (London: Palgrave Macmillan, 2013), 193–221.

References

Beirens, Hanne. "The COVID-19 Pandemic Suggests the Lessons Learned by European Asylum Policymakers After the 2015 Migration Crisis are Fading." *Migration Policy Institute*, April 2020. www.migrationpolicy.org/news/pandemic-lessons-learned-europe-asylum-fading.
Blumenshine, Philip, Arthur Reingold, Susan Egerter, Robin Mockenhaupt, Paula Braveman, and James Marks. "Pandemic Influenza Planning in the United States from a Health Disparities Perspective." *Emerging Infectious Diseases* 14, no. 5 (2008): 709–15. https://doi.org/10.3201/eid1405.071301.
Carme, Marco, Carme Borrell, Laia Palència, Albert Espelt, Maica Rodríguez-Sanz, M. Isabel Pasarín, and Anton Kunst. "Social Class Inequalities in the Utilization of Health Care and Preventive Services in Spain, a Country with a National Health System." *International Journal of Health Services* 40, no. 3 (2010): 525–42.
Casula, Mattia, Andrea Terlizzi, and Federico Toth. "I servizi sanitari regionali alla prova del COVID-19." *Rivista italiana di politiche pubbliche* 3 (2020): 307–36. https://doi.org/10.1483/98732.
Couffinhal, Agnès, Paul Dourgnon, Pierre-Yves Geoffard, Michel Grignon, Florence Jusot, John Lavis, Florence Naudin, and Dominique Polton. "Policies for Reducing Inequalities in Health, What Role Can the Health System Play? A European Perspective. Part I: Determinants of Social Inequalities in Health and the Role of the Healthcare System." *Issues in Health Economics* 92 (February 2005).
Dahlgren, Göran, and Margaret Whitehead. *Policies and Strategies to Promote Social Equity in Health*. Stockholm: Institute for Futures Studies, 1991.
Devaux, Marion. "Income-Related Inequalities and Inequities in Health Care Services Utilisation in 18 Selected OECD Countries." *European Journal of Health Economics* 16, no. 1 (2015): 22–33. http://dx.doi.org/10.1007/s10198-013-0546-4.
European Commission. *Joint Report 2008 on Social Protection and Social Inclusion: Social Inclusion, Pensions, Healthcare and Long-Term Care*. Luxembourg: Office for Official Publications of the European Communities, 2008.
Giarelli, Guido, and Giovanna Vicarelli, eds. *Libro bianco: Il servizio sanitario nazionale e la pandemia da COVID-19; Problemi e proposte*. Milan: FrancoAngeli, 2021.
Instituto Nazionale di Statistica (ISTAT). "Impatto dell'epidemia Covid-19 sulla mortalità totale della popolazione residente." March 2, 2022a. www.istat.it/it/files//2022/03/Report_ISS_ISTAT_2022_tab3.pdf.

______. "Le persone senza fissa dimora." December 15, 2022b. www.istat.it/it/files//2022/12/CENSIMENTO-E-DINAMICA-DEMOGRAFICA-2021.pdf.

Kelley, Edward, and Jeremy Hurst. "Health Care Quality Indicators Project: Conceptual Framework Paper." OECD Health Working Papers no. 23. Paris: OECD Publishing, 2006. https://doi.org/10.1787/440134737301.

Kinner, Stuart A., and Jesse T. Young. "Understanding and Improving the Health of People Who Experience Incarceration: An Overview and Synthesis." *Epidemiologic Reviews* 40, no. 1 (2018): 4–11. https://doi.org/10.1093/epirev/mxx018.

Maciocco, Gavino. "SSN: Solo un cambio di paradigma lo salverà." *Sistema salute* 62, no. 4 (2018): 468–75.

Mackenbach, Johan. "An Analysis of the Role of Health Care in Reducing Socioeconomic Inequalities in Health: The Case of the Netherlands." *International Journal of Health Services: Planning, Administration, Evaluation* 33, no. 3 (2003): 523–41. https://doi.org/10.2190/C12H-NBA4-7QWE-6K3T.

Ministero della Salute. *Monitoraggio dei LEA attraverso la cd: Griglia LEA; Metodologia e risultati dell'anno 2019*. Rome: Direzione Generale della Programmazione Sanitaria–Ufficio VI, 2021. www.salute.gov.it/imgs/C_17_pubblicazioni_3111_allegato.pdf.

Neri, Stefano, and Anna Mori. "Crisi economica, politiche di austerità e relazioni intergovernative nel SSN: Dalla regionalizzazione al federalismo differenziato?" *Autonomie locali e servizi sociali* 2 (2017): 201–20.

O'Sullivan, Tracey L., and Karen P. Phillips. "From SARS to Pandemic Influenza: The Framing of High-Risk Populations." *Natural Hazards* 98 (2019): 103–17. https://doi.org/10.1007/s11069-019-03584-6.

Pavolini, Emanuele, Bruno Palier, and Ana M. Guillén. "The Health Care Policy Quadrilemma and Comparative Institutional Reforms." In *Health Care Systems in Europe Under Austerity: Work and Welfare in Europe*, edited by Pavolini and Guillén, 193–221. London: Palgrave Macmillan, 2013.

Quinn, Sandra Crouse, and Supriya Kumar. "Health Inequalities and Infectious Disease Epidemics: A Challenge for Global Health Security." *Biosecurity and Bioterrorism: Biodefense Strategy, Practice, and Science* 12, no. 5 (2014): 263–73. https://doi.org/10.1089/bsp.2014.0032.

Regidor, Enrique, David Martínez, Maria E. Calle, Paloma Astasio, Paloma Ortega, and Vicente Domínguez. "Socioeconomic Patterns in the Use of Public and Private Health Services and Equity in Health Care." *BMC Health Services Research* 8 (2008). https://doi.org/10.1186/1472-6963-8-183.

Ricciardi, Walter. *La battaglia per la salute*. Rome: Laterza, 2019.

Solar, Orielle, and Alec Irwin. "A Conceptual Framework for Action on the Social Determinants of Health." In *Social Determinants of Health Discussion Paper*, no. 2 (Policy and Practice). Geneva: WHO, 2010. https://apps.who.int/iris/bitstream/handle/10665/44489/9789241500852_eng.pdf.

Stefani, Silvia. "L'isolamento impossibile delle persone senza dimora." *Percorsi di secondo welfare*, April 8, 2020. www.secondowelfare.it/povert-e-inclusione/lisolamento-impossibile-delle-persone-senza-dimora/.

Terraneo, Marco. "Inequities in Health Care Utilization by People Aged 50+: Evidence from 12 European Countries." *Social Science & Medicine* 126 (February 2015): 154–63. http://dx.doi.org/10.1016/j.socscimed.2014.12.028.

______. "Studiare le disuguaglianze di salute in tempo di pandemia: Una cornice teorica." *Sociologia italiana* 16 (2020): 87–97. https://doi.org/10.1485/2281-2652-202016-6.

______, Linda Lombi, and Hannah Bradby. "Depressive Symptoms and Perception of Risk during the First Wave of the COVID-19 Pandemic: A Web-based Cross-Country Comparative Survey." *Sociology of Health & Illness* 43, no. 7 (2021): 1660–68. https://doi.org/10.1111/1467-9566.13350.

Vicarelli, Giovanna. "Regionalismo sanitario e Covid-19: Punti di forza e di debolezza." In *Libro bianco*, edited by Giarelli and Vicarelli, 23–30. Milan: FrancoAngeli.

Whitehead, Margaret. "The Concepts and Principles of Equity and Health." *Health Promotion International* 6, no. 3 (1991): 217–28.

World Health Organization (WHO). *The World Health Report, 2000: Health System; Improving Performance*. Geneva: World Health Organization, 2000. www.who.int/iris/handle/10665/42281.